ITI Treatment Guide
Volume 9

ITI Treatment Guide

Editors:
D. Wismeijer, S. Chen, D. Buser

ITI International Team
for Implantology

Authors:
F. Müller, S. Barter

Volume 9

Implant Therapy in the Geriatric Patient

Quintessence Publishing Co, Ltd
Berlin, Chicago, Tokyo, Barcelona, Istanbul,
London, Milan, Moscow, New Delhi, Paris,
Prague, São Paulo, Seoul, Singapore, Warsaw

German National Library CIP Data

The German National Library has listed this publication in the German National Bibliography. Detailed bibliographical data are available at http://dnb.ddb.de.

© 2016 Quintessence Publishing Co, Ltd
Ifenpfad 2 – 4, 12107 Berlin, Germany
www.quintessenz.de

Illustrations:	Ute Drewes, Basel (CH), www.drewes.ch
Copyediting:	Triacom Dental, Barendorf (DE), www.dental.triacom.com
Graphic concept:	Wirz Corporate AG, Zürich (CH)
Production:	Juliane Richter, Berlin (DE)
Printing:	Bosch-Druck GmbH, Landshut (DE), www.bosch-druck.de

Printed in Germany
ISBN: 978-3-86867-311-1

The materials offered in the ITI Treatment Guide are for educational purposes only and intended as a step-by-step guide to treatment of a particular case and patient situation. These recommendations are based on conclusions of the ITI Consensus Conferences and, as such, in line with the ITI treatment philosophy. These recommendations, nevertheless, represent the opinions of the authors. Neither the ITI nor the authors, editors, or publishers make any representation or warranty for the completeness or accuracy of the published materials and as a consequence do not accept any liability for damages (including, without limitation, direct, indirect, special, consequential, or incidental damages or loss of profits) caused by the use of the information contained in the ITI Treatment Guide. The information contained in the ITI Treatment Guide cannot replace an individual assessment by a clinician, and its use for the treatment of patients is therefore in the sole responsibility of the clinician.

The inclusion of or reference to a particular product, method, technique or material relating to such products, methods, or techniques in the ITI Treatment Guide does not represent a recommendation or an endorsement of the values, features, or claims made by its respective manufacturers.

Some of the manufacturer and product names referred to in this publication may be registered trademarks or proprietary names, even though specific reference to this fact is not made. Therefore, the appearance of a name without designation as proprietary is not to be construed as a representation by the publisher that it is in the public domain.

The tooth identification system used in this ITI Treatment Guide is that of the FDI World Dental Federation.

The ITI Mission is ...

"... to promote and disseminate knowledge on all aspects of implant dentistry and related tissue regeneration through education and research to the benefit of the patient."

Preface

With the previous eight volumes of this series, the ITI Treatment Guides have established their place as a valuable reference work for practitioners in the field of implant dentistry. Having dealt with all the classical aspects of implant therapy in those eight volumes, volume 9 closes the life-cycle loop by addressing the situation of the elderly and ailing patient.

It is a fact that the demographics of society today reflect a significant change: not only do we live much longer while still retaining high expectations in terms of health and quality of life, but the ratio of old to young people has also shifted, with the older generation significantly outnumbering the younger.

This has brought with it a new set of demands on implant dentistry and on its practitioners, who more routinely encounter elderly patients. The treatment of these patients is subject to certain limitations and requires compromises. And along with elderly patients who still lead an active life, there are also those who are more frail, whose health has been compromised, or who require special dental care. This changing situation requires well-considered and adequate solutions.

Volume 9 of the ITI Treatment Guide series addresses the situation and needs of the elderly patient, from systemic changes and physical and mental limitations to considerations of quality of life, and also illustrates these using well-chosen clinical cases.

D. Wismeijer   S. Chen   D. Buser

Acknowledgment

We would like to express our gratitude to Ms. Juliane Richter (Quintessence Publishing) for the typesetting and for the coordination of the production workflow, Mr. Per N. Döhler (Triacom Dental) for the editing support and Ms. Ute Drewes for the excellent illustrations. We also acknowledge Straumann AG, the corporate partner of the ITI, for their continuing support.

Editors and Authors

Editors:

Daniel Wismeijer
    DMD, Professor
    Head of the Department of Oral Implantology and
    Prosthetic Dentistry
    Section of Implantology and Prosthetic Dentistry
    Academic Center for Dentistry Amsterdam (ACTA)
    Free University
    Gustav Mahlerlaan 3004
    1081 LA Amsterdam
    Netherlands
    E-mail: d.wismeijer@acta.nl

Stephen Chen
    MDSc, PhD, FICD, FPFA, FRACDS
    Clinical Associate Professor
    School of Dental Science
    University of Melbourne
    720 Swanston Street
    Melbourne VIC 3010
    Australia
    E-mail: schen@balwynperio.com.au

Daniel Buser
    DDS, Dr med dent, Professor
    Chair, Department of Oral Surgery and Stomatology
    School of Dental Medicine
    University of Bern
    Freiburgstrasse 7
    3010 Bern
    Switzerland
    E-mail: daniel.buser@zmk.unibe.ch

Authors:

Frauke Müller
    Dr med dent, Professor
    Division of Gerodontology and Removable
    Prosthodontics
    University Clinics of Dental Medicine
    University of Geneva
    19, rue Barthélemy-Menn
    1205 Genève
    Switzerland
    E-mail: frauke.mueller@unige.ch

Stephen Barter
    BDS MSurgDent RCS
    Specialist in Oral Surgery
    Clinical Director, Perlan Specialist Dental Centre
    Hartfield Road
    Eastbourne
    East Sussex BN21 2AL
    United Kingdom
    E-mail: s.barter@gmx.com

Contributors

Daniel Buser
  DDS, Dr med dent, Professor
  Chair, Department of Oral Surgery and Stomatology
  School of Dental Medicine
  University of Bern
  Freiburgstrasse 7
  3010 Bern
  Switzerland
  E-mail: daniel.buser@zmk.unibe.ch

Anthony Dickinson OAM
  BDSC, MSD
  1564 Malvern Road
  Glen Iris VIC 3146
  Australia
  E-mail: ajd1@iprimus.com.au

Shahrokh Esfandiari
  BSc, DMD, MSc, PhD
  Associate Dean, Academic Affairs
  Associate Professor
  Faculty of Dentistry, McGill University
  Division of Oral Heath and Society
  2001 McGill College Avenue, Suite 500
  Montreal, Québec H3A 1G1
  Canada
  E-mail: shahrokh.esfandiari@mcgill.ca

Richard Leesungbok
  DMD, MSD, PhD
  Head Professor and Chair, Department of
  Biomaterials and Prosthodontics
  Kyung Hee University School of Dentistry
  892, Dongnam-Ro, Gangdong-Gu
  05278 Seoul
  Republic of Korea
  E-mail: lsb@khu.ac.kr

Gerry McKenna
  BDS, MFDS RCSEd, PhD, PgDipTLHE, FDS (Rest
  Dent) RCSEd, FHEA
  Senior Lecturer/Consultant in Restorative Dentistry
  Centre for Public Health
  Institute of Clinical Sciences
  Queens University Belfast
  Block B, Grosvenor Road
  Belfast BT12 6BJ
  Northern Ireland, United Kingdom
  E-mail: g.mckenna@qub.ac.uk

Robbert Jan Renting
  Tandarts, implantoloog i.o.
  Section of Implantology and Prosthetic Dentistry
  Academic Center for Dentistry Amsterdam (ACTA)
  Free University
  Gustav Mahlerlaan 3004
  1081 LA Amsterdam
  Netherlands
  E-mail: r.j.renting@gmail.com

Mario Roccuzzo
DMD, Dr med dent
Corso Tassoni 14
10143 Torino
Italy
E-mail: mroccuzzo@icloud.com

Martin Schimmel
Dr med dent, MAS Oral Biol, Professor
Department of Reconstructive Dentistry
and Gerodontology
Division of Gerodontology
School of Dental Medicine
University of Bern
Freiburgstrasse 7
3010 Bern
Switzerland
E-mail: martin.schimmel@zmk.unibe.ch

Shakeel Shahdad
Consultant and Hon. Clinical Senior Lecturer
Department of Restorative Dentistry
The Royal London Dental Hospital
Queen Mary University of London
Turner Street
London E1 1BB
England, United Kingdom
E-mail: shakeel.shahdad@bartshealth.nhs.uk

Murali Srinivasan
Dr med dent, BDS, MDS, MBA
Lecturer
Division of Gerodontology and Removable
Prosthodontics
University Clinics of Dental Medicine
University of Geneva
19, rue Barthélemy-Menn
1205 Genève
Switzerland
E-mail: murali.srinivasan@unige.ch

Ulrike Stephanie Webersberger
Priv Doz, Dr med dent, Dr sc hum, MSc
Restorative and Prosthetic Dentistry
Dental Clinic
Innsbruck Medical University
MZA, Anichstraße 35
6020 Innsbruck
Austria
E-mail: ulrike.beier@i-med.ac.at

Table of Contents

1 Introduction

F. Müller, S. Barter

Geriatric dentistry?

Some readers may wonder what has this to do with the ITI. Is not geriatric dentistry usually all about no treatment? Why would we need a Treatment Guide for this?

After a very successful series of eight previous Treatment Guides, it would seem logical to think about our patients' destiny as they become old, very old, and finally frail and dependent on care. This book is testament to the ITI's holistic approach to implant dentistry and the professional responsibility it takes—not only for those patients who have aged with implant restorations but also those who have reached an advanced age and may now benefit from the progress in materials and techniques that implant dentistry has to offer today, until late in their lives.

Implants have become an integral part of restorative dental care, and the number of implants placed increases steadily. Worldwide, an estimated 15 million implants are inserted per year to replace missing teeth, mostly in the adult and young elderly age groups. Economic growth and technological advances in almost all domains of our lives have led to a more exigent attitude of adult patients, who increasingly demand higher levels of functional and esthetic outcomes from restorative dentistry. Consequently, any treatise on implant therapy in the elderly population cannot be restricted to options for edentulous jaws.

A raised awareness for the biological and physiological value of natural teeth also increases the desirability of prostheses that protect the neighboring dental tissues and avoid the unfavorable side effects of removable appliances. Despite the cost involved and the physiological limitations of implant therapy, such treatment can fulfil the high demands of the elderly generation. Progress in terms of implant materials and design and also in surgical techniques, including regenerative procedures such as bone grafting, means that almost any partially or fully edentulous patient can be restored with a fixed implant-supported restoration, provided that he or she accepts the costs, time, and burden of treatment procedures involved.

But what is the future of these complex restorations when the patient ages? And what treatment concepts do we offer patients whose lives are already dominated by age, frailty, and multimorbidity? Treatment concepts for the elderly have to consider their physical and cognitive functions, their motivation, and their ability to manipulate and clean a sophisticated implant restoration.

For over 25 years, the ITI has produced numerous publications in its mission to promote and disseminate knowledge in all aspects of implant dentistry and related tissue regeneration through research, development, and education. ITI Consensus Conferences have produced systematic reviews of the latest research resulting in treatment guidelines, distilling the science into practical advice and recommendations for the busy clinician. The widespread use of the SAC Classification and the adoption (sometimes in modified form) of this tool by national implant and dental organizations bears witness to the value of the hard work done by the scientists and clinicians of the ITI for the benefit of both the patient and the practitioner. Books such as the Glossary of Oral and Maxillofacial Implants, an impressive reference volume with over 2,000 definitions of terms, further help establish common standards that facilitate more sharing of information and a better understanding of the fascinating field in which we work.

The ITI Treatment Guides have made a major contribution to further education. This ninth volume addresses an aspect of implant dentistry that has received far less attention than others: implant therapy in the elderly patient.

It has long been known that age alone is not a barrier to implant placement and that the process of osseointegration can be as successful in an older person as in a young adult. There is a growing awareness that in all fields of healthcare, chronological age alone does not govern the health status of an individual; rather, aging is a biological process that may progress at a variable rate, which can be affected by genetic and environmental factors and result in a considerable discrepancy between calendar age and biological age.

This is an increasingly relevant fact with a growing elderly global population. Advances in all fields of healthcare mean that people live longer, often with conditions that would previously have been life-limiting. Elderly patients frequently have multiple chronic conditions treated with a complex regime of multiple medications. This can bring them a longer period of healthy living in their communities. Quite reasonably, they want and need this to be accompanied by good oral health, function, and appearance, so that they may continue to enjoy life and preserve their self-esteem. It is possible to provide dental implants for the elderly and to replace missing teeth; a comfortable and effective tooth replacement is also an important aspect in the maintenance of good nutrition.

There is considerable evidence to support these statements. Many publications testify to the success and usefulness of dental implants in older persons. There is also an, albeit smaller, body of literature that examines the situation of elderly and geriatric patients who, having received dental implants at a younger, healthier age, now require care for their prostheses in times of advancing age, frailty, and declining health.

Few dental treatments last forever. Biological and technical complications will inevitably occur with all dental prostheses—whether implant- or tooth-supported. The treatment can be more challenging in the case of implant complications—even when the patient can be seen in an ideal facility. The management of complications in cases where there are issues of physical or mental health, access to healthcare, and other social or economic considerations may be quite different.

Implant therapy has been a common, successful, and accepted treatment modality for over 30 years. It is time to consider the aspects highlighted above. The aim of this Treatment Guide is to raise awareness of the inevitability of increasing demands on the profession to provide care and treatment for a growing population of patients who, having benefitted from our successes in implant treatment over the past decades, are now growing older with different care needs.

We hope you enjoy reading about the real future of implant dentistry!

2 <u>Implant Treatment in Old Age: Literature Review</u>

S. Barter, F. Müller

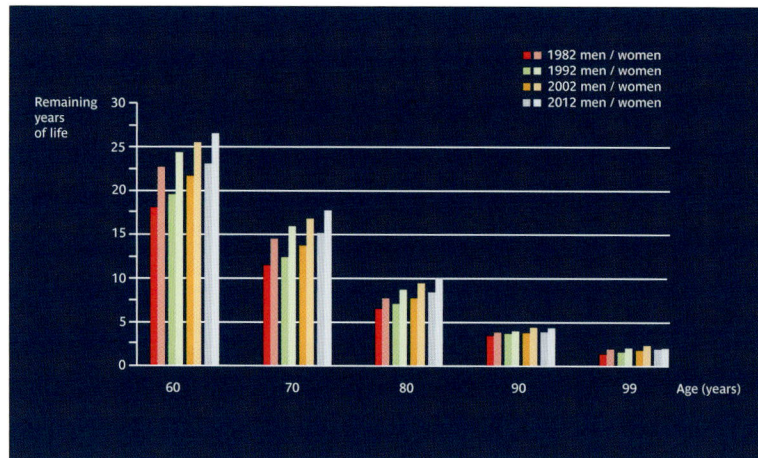

Fig 1 Life expectancy in Switzerland since 1982. (Data: Swiss Federal Statistical Office.)

Implants are used to replace missing teeth. It seems intuitive that their prevalence should be highest in the group of patients with the highest number of missing teeth. However, the prevalence of implants in old and geriatric patients is still negligible compared to tooth replacement using conventional fixed or removable dental prostheses. This is even more surprising in that almost 9 out of 10 persons aged 85 years or over are wearing removable prostheses in Switzerland, with well-documented functional and esthetic shortcomings (Zitzmann and coworkers 2007). Limited financial resources, a negative attitude towards both tooth replacement and implants themselves, a lack of knowledge, and reluctance to undergo invasive surgery may be amongst the factors that could explain this situation.

In the institutionalized elderly, a loss of autonomy and the consequently complex logistics for access to health care may further limit access to more complex dental treatment. There is considerable published literature suggesting that chronological age in itself is not a barrier to successful implant osseointegration in healthy individuals or in older people with controlled medical conditions (de Baat 2000; Ikebe and coworkers 2009). However, to focus only on the success of osseointegration and the ongoing survival of individual implants, which is often the level of evidence used, fails to consider the wider implications of such treatment. Other important considerations include patients' experience and their subjective opinion of the treatment and its benefits, how technical and biological maintenance and complications are managed in aging patients who are becoming progressively infirm, and the objective oral and general health implications, both favorable and unfavorable, of implant-supported prostheses.

Of at least equal importance are the holistic care of old patients and the need for a proper understanding of the physiology of aging and its effect on general health and well-being. Today's progress in health care enables elderly patients to survive with conditions that only relatively recently would have caused death at an earlier age (Fig 1). This in turn leads to an increasingly aged population that acquires more conditions, in turn leading to a higher prevalence of disability as well as to multiple chronic conditions, known as multimorbidity (Barnett and coworkers 2012). Consequently, these patients are placed on longer and more complex medication regimes, known as polypharmacy (Hajjar and coworkers 2007; Mannucci and coworkers 2014).

Besides the classic "geriatric giants" (immobility, instability, incontinence, and impaired intellect/memory), many other age-related features have been described, such as neurodegenerative diseases, sensory decline, adverse drug events or medication non-compliance, frailty, and the multiple organ or systemic diseases mentioned above. We have a role to play not only in the essential consideration of how these conditions may affect our treatment but also vice versa. We must also be aware and vigilant in order for us, as healthcare providers, to contribute to the general care of our population in its later years.

This chapter gives a brief overview of the current state of the literature at the time of writing. Readers should be aware that limited high-level evidence is available; only recently has there been a growing awareness of the need for further well-designed studies into many of these aspects.

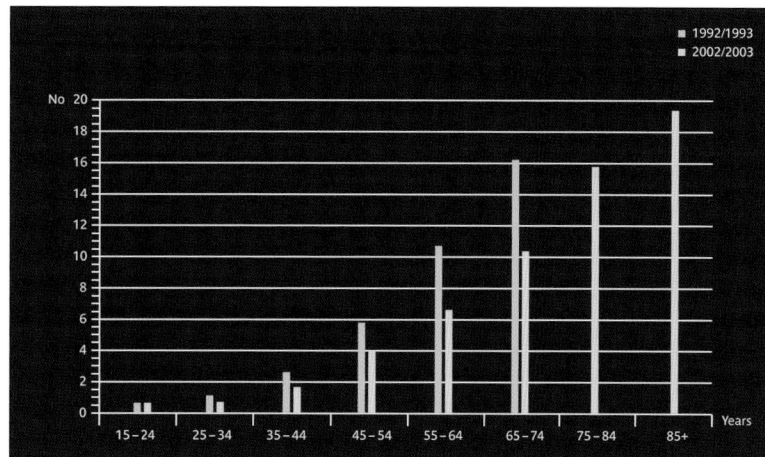

Fig 2   Number of missing teeth in different age cohorts. (Data from the Swiss National Health Surveys 1992/93 and 2002/03, cited after Zitzmann and Berglundh 2008b.)

Awareness and acceptance of implant therapy

Thanks to improved oral-health education, better preventive intervention, minimally invasive dentistry, and the increased quality of medical and dental care available to the populations of many developed countries, as well as increasing financial resources and social security, more and more people reach an advanced and very advanced age with their natural teeth. They often have fixed tooth-supported prostheses or, increasingly, fixed and removable implant-assisted prostheses (Joshi and coworkers 1996; Petersen 2003). The shift in oral health is reflected in the Swiss health survey: while in the 1992/1993 survey, the 65- to 74-year-old age group was missing on average 15.4 teeth, the same age group was missing only 10.4 teeth 10 years later (Zitzmann and coworkers 2008b; Fig 2). Thanks to the newly introduced age group of 85 years and over in this health survey, we know that 97.4% of this population group are wearing dentures, of which 11.5% are fixed and 85.9% are removable (Table 1). The percentage of complete-denture wearers in this age group is still 37.2%. A similar situation has been reported for most developed countries, where tooth loss also occurs later in life (Mojon 2003; Müller and coworkers 2007).

Age group (in yr)	Yes	Fixed	Removable	CD upper and lower jaw
15 – 24	10.9	8.2	1.5	0.2
25 – 34	24.4	20.5	1.8	0.1
35 – 44	42.0	36.3	3.6	0.4
45 – 54	67.8	52.2	14.5	1.9
55 – 64	82.6	52.2	29.0	5.1
65 – 74	89.5	38.7	49.4	13.1
75 – 84	93.6	23.3	69.7	25.7
85+	97.4	11.5	85.9	37.2
Total	54.4	34.0	18.9	4.7

Table 1   Prevalence of fixed and removable prostheses in different age cohorts. (Data from the Swiss National Health Survey, cited after Zitzmann and Berglundh 2008b.)

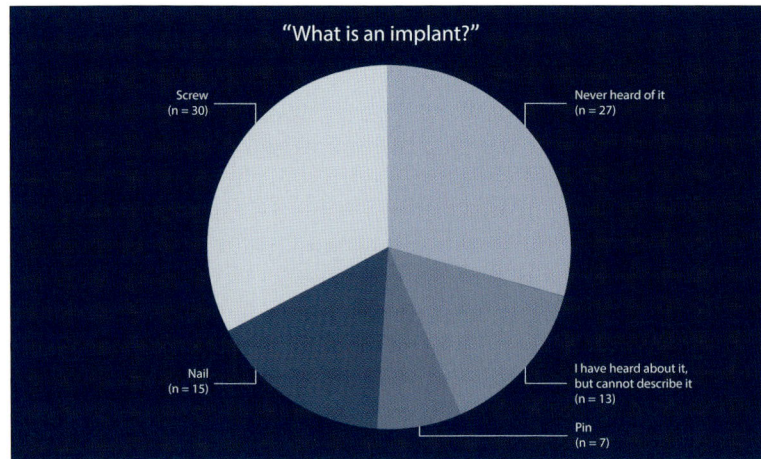

Fig 3   Out of 92 persons interviewed with an average age of 81.2 years, almost half had not heard of implants or could not describe them. (Cited after Müller and coworkers 2012a.)

Despite the progress in oral health promotion and restorative techniques, tooth loss is still a reality in old age; there is a widespread need for tooth replacement in the elderly population (Müller and coworkers 2007). Nevertheless, implants in elderly adults are disproportionately rare, especially in the very old and institutionalized population (Visser and coworkers 2011; Zitzmann and coworkers 2007). The prevalence of implants in a representative Swiss population sample was 4.4% (Zitzmann and coworkers 2008a); in Germany, it was 2.6% in the 65- to 74-year-old adult population (Micheelis and Schiffner 2006). In Europe, the highest frequency of implants in the edentulous population was found in Sweden, but despite substantial financial support from the public health system, it did not exceed 8% (Osterberg and coworkers 2000).

Evaluation of the awareness of implants in elderly persons is difficult, as there may be many factors involved in the dissemination of patient information, including the benefits of implant treatment. In a marketing-related study of the Austrian population, 42% of the cohort investigated was poorly informed and only 4% felt well informed. Approximately one-third of the study participants indicated a desire to receive more information and would prefer it to be provided by their dentist (Tepper and coworkers 2003).

Awareness of dental implants is not necessarily correlated with a correct understanding of the nature and benefits of treatment. Various studies indicate that approximately 70% of elderly patients questioned are aware of the existence of dental implants as a treatment option. The number of interviewees who had received information direct from a dentist appears to vary for reasons not fully understood. In the Tepper study, 68% had received an explanation from a dentist, whereas in a US-based study the level was 17% (Tepper and coworkers 2003; Zimmer and coworkers 1992). Similar results were found in a survey of Swiss adults in both in geriatric-care facilities and living at home (Müller and coworkers 2012a). The authors confirmed that in the elderly population, knowledge of dental implants is limited: almost half of the study participants had never heard of implants or could not describe them (Fig 3). Only one out of the 92 participants knew that implants were made of titanium (Fig 4). The rate of objection to implant treatment was high, mostly based on cost, the surgical nature of the therapy, and other psychological factors. A limited knowledge of implants as well as a poor state of general health—but not old age in itself—were not associated with a negative attitude toward implant treatment. Identifying further barriers and understanding patients' reluctance towards implant treatment could improve the acceptance of implant therapy in the elderly population. Providing further information in appropriate formats, with clearly worded and printed text complemented by simple illustrations, would help elderly patients to reflect on the novel information provided and give informed consent to implant treatment. Furthermore, the development of less invasive surgical techniques is another possible measure that could contribute to a greater uptake of an implant treatment.

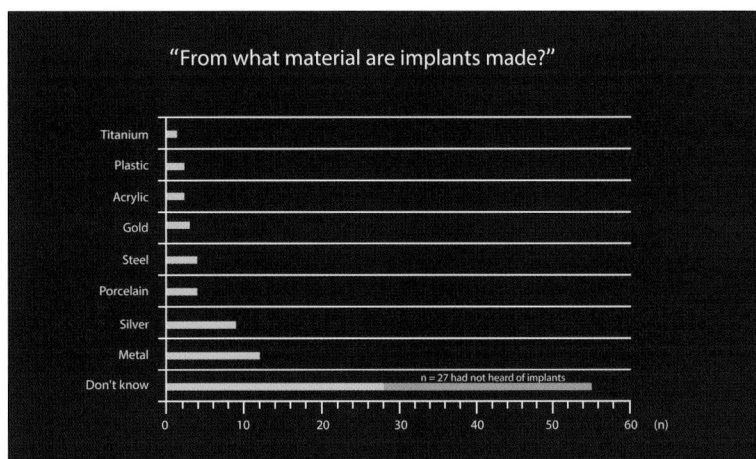

"From what material are implants made?"

Fig 4   Only 1 out of 92 persons interviewed with an average age of 81.2 years knew that implants were made from titanium. (Cited after Müller and coworkers 2012a.)

Of potentially greater concern is the awareness and understanding of implants and related prostheses by the caregivers of patients unable to access regular dental care or to manage adequate self-performed oral hygiene (Holtzman and Akiyama 1985). It has been suggested that in many elderly-care institutions, few staff members recognize an implant-supported prosthesis, let alone know how to handle and clean it. Even with a seemingly simple and straightforward overdenture supported by two implants, if the patient can no longer remove the denture, it is likely that nursing staff will not know how to help, and the denture may end up falling into disuse (Visser and coworkers 2011).

Considering the acceptance of proposed implant treatment, many elderly patients do not consider implants a preferred treatment option for reasons of cost. However, cost may not be the only issue, as demonstrated in a study showing that over one-third of patients with edentulous mandibles declined free treatment with an implant-supported overdenture. Elderly patients often object to surgical intervention, but may also consider any denture "improvement" unnecessary (Walton and MacEntee 2005). When presented with different treatment options for the replacement of missing teeth, they are frequently more conservative in their preferences and may be more tolerant of simpler solutions that the clinician may consider a compromise (Ikebe and coworkers 2011).

Implant success in the elderly patient—initial provision of therapy

The infinite variability of site- and patient-specific factors, implant and prosthetic designs, study methodologies and confounding factors, and many other interrelated considerations imply that considerations of age alone as a success factor in implant therapy are difficult to determine (Wood and coworkers 2004). A large part of the currently available literature is based on the treatment of the edentulous jaw, often with overdentures, and this does not fully reflect the emerging situation of a partially edentulous population with an increasing demand for implant treatment, historically restricted to younger age groups (Dudley 2015). There are also only few studies available that address the rate of biological and technical complications in geriatric patients who have previously had implants and prostheses for decades and who are now more infirm; perhaps more importantly, neither is there a body of literature outlining the issues of providing remedial treatment in such situations.

As previously mentioned, age alone appears to be unrelated to the success or failure of initial implant integration, with success rates similar to younger age groups but with a seemingly greater incidence of problems in adapting to a new prosthesis (Andreiotelli and coworkers 2010; Engfors and coworkers 2004). Osseointegration at an advanced age was well documented in an 83-year-old patient, who received four implants in the edentulous mandible. After passing away 12 years later, Lederman, Schenk and Buser had the opportunity to investigate the osseointegration histologically (Ledermann and coworkers 1998; Figs 5a-e). A close-up view confirms the intimate contact of the bone with the titanium implant surface.

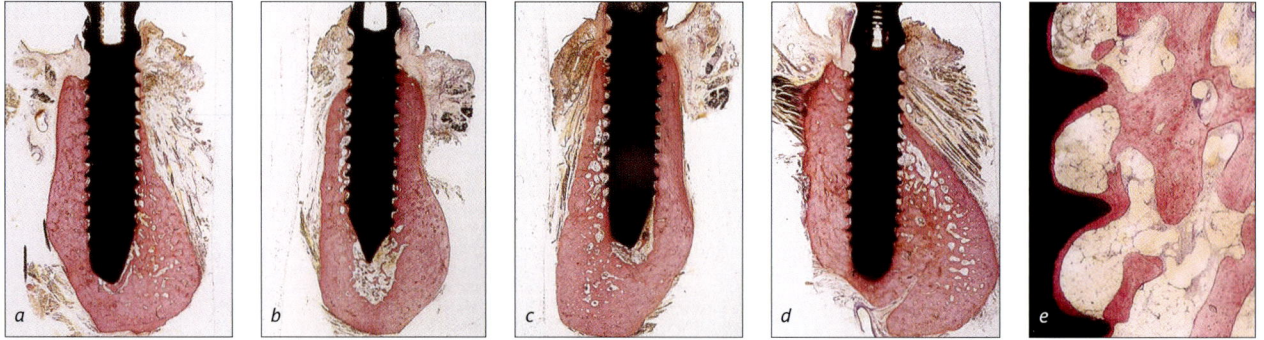

Figs 5a-e   This edentulous patient received his interforaminal implants at 83 years; 12 years later, at age 95, he passed away and donated his mandible to the University of Bern for histological analysis (Ledermann and coworkers 1998).

Very few studies have directly compared implant survival in young and old patients. Bryant and Zarb compared peri-implant marginal bone loss in 26- to 49-year-old patients with a cohort of 60- to 74-year-olds with fixed or removable restorations and found no difference over 17 years (Bryant and Zarb 2003; Fig 6). Hoeksema and co-workers, in a 10-year prospective study, followed a group of 52 young patients (age 35 to 50 years) and compared implant survival rates with those of 53 elderly edentulous wearers of overdentures (age 60 to 80 years). Despite the obvious larger dropout in the older cohort, due in part to death and health reasons, they found no statistical difference in implant survival and marginal bone loss between the two groups (Hoeksema and coworkers 2015). Even very old age—80 years and older—resulted in survival rates for fixed implant-supported prostheses that were similar to those of patients below 80 years over a 5-year observation period (Engfors and coworkers 2004).

While medical conditions exist that are considered relative contraindications that may affect successful osseointegration, the relative levels of associated risk may vary in different patients. There is a greater incidence of multimorbidity and polypharmacy in the older age group, and combinations of risk factors may increase the risk of an adverse outcome.

The most relevant factor of implant success may actually be the quantity and quality of the bone at the surgical site—and these may in part be age-related, reflecting changes in bone structure and quite simply the length of time that teeth had been diseased or missing (Bryant 1998).

A significant confounding factor in attempts to evaluate implant success is the lack of consistency amongst studies regarding what constitutes success. Indeed, many studies actually report implant survival, which is of course based only on the singular fact that the implant remains in situ. Different criteria exist for qualifying success, which generally include the following factors (Buser and coworkers 1990):

- Absence of persistent subjective complaints, such as pain, foreign body sensation and/or dysesthesia.
- Absence of recurrent peri-implant infection with suppuration.
- Absence of mobility.
- Absence of continuous radiolucency around the implant.
- Restorability.

However, success at the implant level is not a measure of treatment success, only of the biological achievement of osseointegration. Success has to be also measured at the prosthesis level and, perhaps most importantly, at the patient level—the patient should remain our prime concern. The possibility of autonomous management of the implant-supported denture, including proper oral hygiene, should therefore be added to the outcome measures.

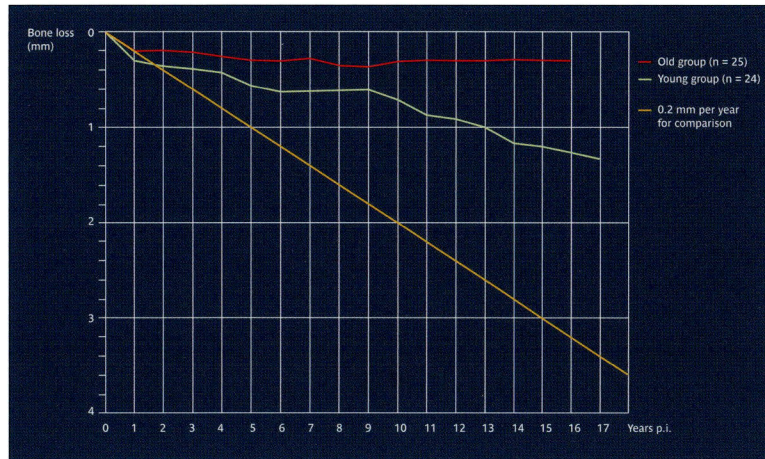

Fig 6   Cumulative peri-implant bone loss in mandibular implant-supported prostheses in a young and an old cohort. (Redrawn after Bryant and Zarb 2003.)

Nor can we be reassured by short-term success. Given the increasing life expectancy of the middle-aged and young-old patients who have received implant treatment, the rehabilitation will inevitably require both maintenance and repair or replacement. Furthermore, with the growing number of healthy and fit very old persons, implant treatment should not be withheld, even at a very high age, if close monitoring of the patient's denture management and oral hygiene are assured and the attachments can be removed easily if necessary.

Implant success in the elderly patient—maintenance and complications

There is ample evidence that the accumulation of bacterial plaque on the surfaces of implants and associated restorations can lead to inflammation of the soft tissues and, in susceptible sites and individuals, to peri-implant bone loss (Zitzmann and Berglund 2008b). Concerning the susceptibility of an individual to periodontal disease, Mombelli considered whether or not there are specific age-related changes in the oral microbiota that may affect the progression of periodontal disease. He concluded that other age-related general and oral health conditions might have a greater impact (Mombelli 1998). Declining manual dexterity and visual acuity may be associated with a reduced ability to maintain adequate plaque control. Several studies have observed that osseointegration can be maintained even under conditions of poor or moderately successful self-performed or caregiver-assisted oral hygiene procedures (Isaksson and coworkers 2009; Olerud and coworkers 2012). The impact of immunosenescence on the reaction of the peri-implant tissues to substantial bacterial load remains to be investigated. It is also recognized that the host response is as important a factor in peri-implant disease as it is

in periodontal disease (Heitz-Mayfield 2008), and that the risk of biological complications in periodontitis-susceptible patients is greater than in less susceptible individuals (Ong and coworkers 2008). Given the greater difficulty of treating such complications in patients with compromised oral hygiene and general health, it would be unwise to be complacent in situations of inadequate oral hygiene.

It is recognized that the role of staff and caregivers in maintaining oral health in such patients is important (Ettinger and Pinkham 1977; Mersel and coworkers 2000) and is an essential part of general healthcare, particularly in multimorbid and fragile elderly patients. An example of this is the prevention of complications such as aspiration pneumonia precipitated by oral pathogens (Quagliarello and coworkers 2005; Sjögren and coworkers 2008; van der Maarel-Wierink and coworkers 2011; Yoneyama and coworkers 1999).

As mentioned above, the awareness of care providers, relatives, and occasionally even patients of the presence and maintenance requirements of implants and related prostheses is low (Kimura and coworkers 2015; Sweeney and coworkers 2007). In the multimorbid and fragile elderly, adequate oral hygiene may not be the most important factor for the general well-being of the patient, especially when chronic disease and disability dominate daily life. However, the neglect of oral health can have serious implications, caused for example by the inability of some caregivers to as much as recognize the presence of implants. Examples are given of food refusal and weight loss in patients unable to inform the staff of oral discomfort from overdenture abutments where the overdenture is no longer worn (Visser and coworkers

2011). Adequate nutrition and weight are of vital importance for the morbidity and mortality of elders, and such incidents can have consequences of greater significance than oral health alone (Weiss and coworkers 2008).

All studies reporting on technical complications observe that while implant survival rates are high, there is a considerable rate of technical complications with all implant-retained prostheses that increases with the length of time in service (Albrektsson and coworkers 2012; Berglundh and coworkers 2002; Brägger and coworkers 2005; Zembic and coworkers 2014a). This has an impact on the health economics of implant treatment and requires considerable chairside time. This may be particularly relevant for a patient who is no longer able to access the dental office and/or who may no longer be able to afford the maintenance for an implant-supported denture to which they committed when in a more privileged financial situation.

Technical complications may in fact be more prevalent with overdentures than with fixed reconstructions, especially regarding the overdenture attachment system (Bryant and coworkers 2007). However, addressing such issues with an implant overdenture may be considerably more straightforward than with a complex fixed prosthesis in an elderly patient with general or mental health conditions that preclude care in a conventional clinical setting.

Implants in the fully edentulous elderly patient
As the population of elderly patients increases, the average age of that population also increases. Improved health care in developed countries reduces the proportion of edentulous patients, and this trend is expected to continue (Müller and coworkers 2007). However, there are indications that the growing elderly population will still result in many edentulous adults to treat and that these patients may benefit from implant therapy rather than being constrained to removable complete dentures (Turkyilmaz and coworkers 2010). We know that clinicians and patients often view the efficacy of treatment differently (Heydecke and coworkers 2003b) and that the acceptance of complete dentures by patients varies considerably, with some adapting better than others (Boerrigter and coworkers 1995a; Müller and Hasse-Sander 1993). Even among those patients who do not report high levels of chewing ability, there are many who do not consider such functional limitations any handicap (Allen and coworkers 2001).

It is frequently said that implant-retained overdentures are "better" than conventional complete dentures. However, it is important to distinguish between maxillary and mandibular prostheses, as much of the available literature relates to mandibular implant-retained overdentures. Indeed, many reviews of the literature do not explicitly differentiate these two distinct clinical situations.

It has been suggested that implant-supported maxillary complete overdentures have few advantages over conventional maxillary complete dentures (Watson and coworkers 1997). There is evidence that the simpler overdenture approach is favored by patients over a complex fixed bridge on implants, or even that there is no advantage of an implant-supported complete maxillary prosthesis over a conventional complete denture (de Albuquerque Júnior and coworkers 2000). Few studies include sufficient long-term follow-up to evaluate the differences between implant and prosthetic success, or between different types of restoration. It is inevitable that the design of a prosthesis will affect the ease of cleaning and the rate of technical complications, even though there appears to be no correlation between designs and implant survival/success over relatively short observation periods (Bryant and coworkers 2007).

Nor is there any reliable evidence for an optimal number of implants to support an overdenture (Roccuzzo and coworkers 2012). However, there is evidence that implant-supported mandibular prostheses are associated with improved clinical and patient-related outcomes compared to mandibular complete dentures. While well-made replacement conventional complete dentures can provide improvements in speech, appearance, and comfort, there is frequently little or no improvement in function (Awad and coworkers 2003), and this is especially so in elderly patients (Allen and McMillan 2003).

The use of two implants in the interforaminal region of the mandible to support an overdenture is well documented. There is reliable evidence for the benefits of this treatment modality and its cost-effectiveness (Heydecke and coworkers 2005). Indeed, the two-implant mandibular overdenture is now regarded the first-choice standard of care (Feine and coworkers 2002; Thomason and coworkers 2009) and that a conventional mandibular complete denture may be inadequate in terms of comfort and function, with masticatory performance being less than 20% of that achieved with a natural dentition (Heath 1982; Kapur 1964).

A recent review from Andreotelli and coworkers confirmed excellent survival rates for implant-supported overdentures (Andreiotelli and coworkers 2010). The majority of studies in this review concerned mandibular implants placed in the interforaminal region to retain removable overdentures. Observation periods in four of the studies analyzed reached the critical 10-year mark, indicating implant survival rates between 93% and

100%. Although the quality of the available evidence often precludes combining the individual study outcomes within a meta-analysis, it seems that neither the number of implants used nor the attachment system chosen, or splinting the implants, has a significant impact on the treatment success (Meijer and coworkers 2004; Naert and coworkers 2004).

Treatment concepts for the maxilla, single implant mandibular overdentures (Bryant and coworkers 2015; Kronstrom and coworkers 2014; Srinivasan and coworkers 2016), and short or reduced-diameter implants have been less well documented (Müller and coworkers 2015; Srinivasan and coworkers 2014a). Although immediate, early, and conventional loading protocols of mandibular implant dentures are predictable treatment modalities, early and conventional loading tended to reduce failures of osseointegration within the first year (Schimmel and coworkers 2014). From a patient perspective, early loading seems particularly attractive, as the time of discomfort due to provisionalization is limited. There is still sufficient time for wound healing, hence the likelihood of a reline being needed shortly after denture insertion is lower than with immediate-loading concepts. It can be concluded that mandibular implant overdentures are a safe and successful treatment modality and present multiple functional, structural, and psychosocial benefits.

Implants in the partially edentulous elderly patient

As stated, an increasing number of patients in a growing elderly population retain natural or treated natural teeth well into old age. Failing older dental restorations can of course lead to a partially edentulous situation; it may be desirable to preserve natural teeth as much as possible and to avoid the preparation of teeth adjacent to gaps for tooth-supported fixed prostheses. The greater expectations patients have of dental treatment and their desire to avoid dentures, even partial ones, mean that implants in partially edentulous patients are a practical and beneficial treatment option for many. Especially in severely depleted dentitions, where abutment teeth may be positioned unfavorably, additional abutments in the form of implants may greatly enhance denture kinetics. The literature is replete with evidence that the same patient- and site-specific factors are the main considerations affecting future implant survival and that age alone is not a factor (Kowar and coworkers 2013).

Patient-centered outcomes in elderly patients

Patient-centered outcomes are an important measure of the "success" of a treatment, both subjectively and objectively, particularly in regard to health economics (Rohlin and Mileman 2000). Clinicians and patients often perceive and evaluate the outcome of treatment differently, and such variation can lead to problems in treatment planning. Involvement of the patient in clinical decision-making can lead to higher levels of satisfaction with treatment (Kay and Nuttall 1995). It is therefore important to consider patient preferences and attitudes to treatment when selecting treatment (Kay and coworkers 1992). It is equally important to accept that elderly patients will often place different values on the potential benefits of treatment than younger adults, based on medical, social, cultural, and economic considerations. It is necessary to respect their decisions when deciding on the use of implants and the type of prosthesis that will produce the most predictable and satisfactory outcome. Respecting the patient's decision becomes even more relevant in patients who have to be considered vulnerable, as ethical considerations strongly preclude "forcefully convincing" the patient towards accepting a given treatment plan.

Unfortunately, most of the current literature in patient-centered outcomes relates to the treatment of the edentulous older adult (Weyant and coworkers 2004). As older adults retain teeth for longer, perhaps losing teeth later in life and demanding implant-supported partial or complete prostheses, we may need modified assessment tools that are preferably standardized to eliminate heterogeneity in results in order to evaluate the true benefit of treatment at the patient level.

Assessing oral health-related quality of life (OHRQoL) essentially measures the degree to which oral health interrupts the well-being and social functioning of an individual. There are a large variety of instruments that have been used to assess the social impact of dental disease (Hebling and Pereira 2007; Slade 2002).

From the literature, there appear to be two most commonly used indices for evaluating the impact of oral and dental problems on an elderly patient's quality of life:

- *OHIP—Oral Health Impact Profile.* Used to evaluate the patient's perception of the social impact of poor oral health (Slade and Spencer 1994). Within this tool, there are refined questionnaires to assess different specific treatment modalities such as OHIP-EDENT, for edentulous adults.
- *GOHAI—Geriatric Oral Health Assessment Index.* Used to evaluate the impact of oral health problems in the older population (Atchison and Dolan 1990).

There is evidence to show that after treatment, patient satisfaction with implants is good, even when there is a substantial need for support in daily living that includes assisted oral hygiene (Isaksson and coworkers 2009; Olerud and coworkers 2012; Osterberg and coworkers 2007). Mandibular implant-supported overdentures seem to provide improved patient-centered outcomes from both the patients' and the clinicians' perspectives (Boerrigter and coworkers 1995a; Boerrigter and coworkers 1995b; Emami and coworkers 2009; Meijer and coworkers 1999).

OHRQoL outcomes can be similarly improved by providing elderly patients with partial fixed and removable implant supported prostheses, depending on the age of the patient and the particular clinical situation (Swelem and coworkers 2014). In a wide ranging "real-world" practice-based study evaluating GOHAI indices, marked benefits were perceived by patients receiving either single-tooth replacement, fixed partial dentures, or complete fixed or removable full prostheses (Fillion and coworkers 2013). However, in common with many clinical studies, the follow-up period was less than 5 years, so only limited conclusions can be drawn; maintenance is inevitably required and complications may develop, so the level of satisfaction will possibly decline over time.

Patients with medical conditions that can have a further adverse impact on oral health or function may also benefit from implant therapy in terms of chewing efficiency and OHRQoL. There are a few case reports and series reporting on patients with neurodegenerative diseases such as Parkinson's and Huntington's disease, or dementia (Faggion 2013; Packer and coworkers 2009), diabetes (Kapur and coworkers 1999), xerostomia, or oral mucosal conditions. However, the reported case numbers are so low that they may be considered anecdotal, and no observation beyond 12 months follow-up exists. The supportive maintenance of implants and related prostheses may well be important and very difficult in patients with such conditions. Indications for implant placement must be balanced individually and carefully between the estimated benefit for the patient and the potential risks from peri-implant infection and failure to manage the prosthesis while the underlying medical condition progresses. Where the slightest concern of dropout from the recall and maintenance scheme exists, it seems advisable to opt for a conventional tooth replacement.

Functional benefits of implants in edentulous elderly patients

Improvements in orofacial function with implant-supported dental restorations are well documented, especially for edentulous subjects with upper complete dentures and lower implant-supported overdentures (Müller 2014). Besides the protection of the peri-implant bone through reduced atrophy (Bryant and Zarb 2003; Jemt and coworkers 1996a; Lindquist and coworkers 1988; Naert and coworkers 1991), such improvements comprise increased biting force (Muller and coworkers 2013) and improved masticatory efficiency and ability (van der Bilt and coworkers 2006; van Kampen and coworkers 2004). Furthermore, the positive impact on oral health-related quality of life (OHRQoL) from supporting complete dentures with implants has been demonstrated (Awad and coworkers 2014). The benefits of implants in overdentures will be discussed in more detail in Chapter 3.

3 Aging: a Biological, Social, and Economic Challenge

F. Müller

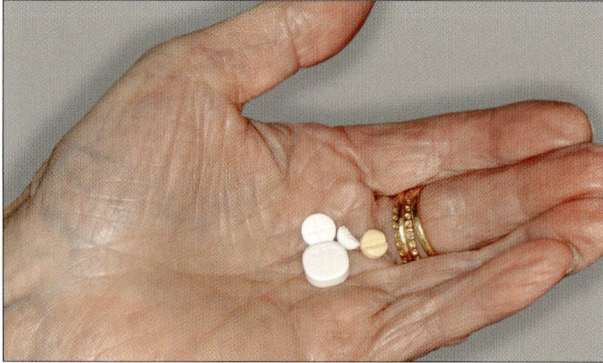

Fig 1 *Drug intake increases dramatically with age; in most elderly patients, the drugs are relevant for the dental treatment.*

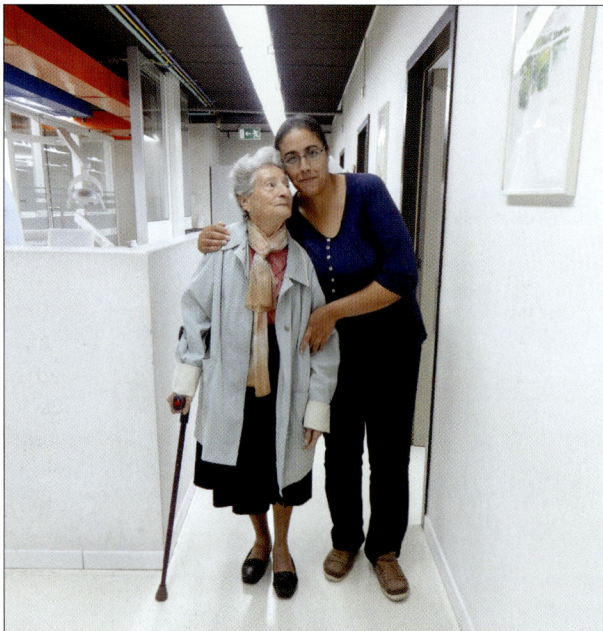

Fig 2 *Most elderly persons need help or special transportation to reach the dental office, so dental appointments require special logistics.*

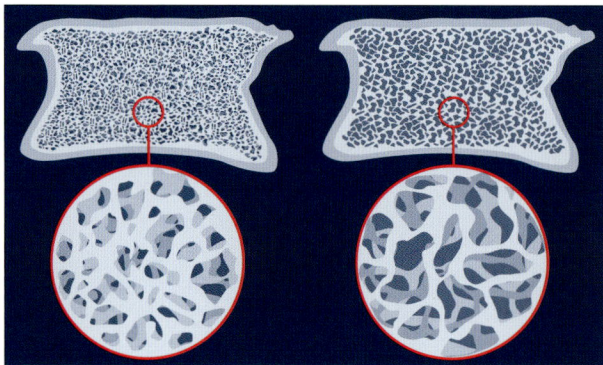

Fig 3 *Macroscopic changes in the bone structures occur with age that are similar to those described in osteoporotic patients (displayed here for the vertebral bone).*

Treating the elderly patient inevitably requires some adjustments compared to the treatment of younger adults.

First of all, physiological aging taxes the physiological reserve, and age-related changes become evident, in terms of both physiognomy and function. Secondly, the prevalence of chronic disease and functional handicaps increases with age, requiring adjustments to treatment planning.

Patients with three or more chronic diseases requiring drug intervention are considered multimorbid (Fig 1). In addition to the impact of the diseases themselves, the side effects of their treatment have to be taken into consideration. Given the large number of drugs that induce dry mouth as a side effect, xerostomia is one of the most prevalent symptoms in geriatric dentistry. In addition, the limited mobility of some patients requires special logistics to take them to the dental practice or, more rarely, to treat them at home (Fig 2).

Age-related functional and structural changes in the orofacial system

Bone and alveolar ridge. Aging results in a reduction in both cortical and trabecular bone mass in both men and women (Fig 3). Functional changes related to age imply increased brittleness, leading to a higher incidence of microfractures and fractures. The reduced activity of osteoblasts slows down the healing process, and bone remodeling takes longer. The age-related discrepancy between the activity of osteoblasts and osteoclasts is accelerated in women during menopause due to a decrease in estrogen levels.

The aging alveolar bone is subject to the same changes, but periodontal disease and tooth loss may result in atrophy beyond the physiological aging process. The bone mass responds positively to physiological stimulation such as the occlusal loading of natural teeth, which are suspended in the sockets via Sharpey fibers. In contrast, pressure is not considered a physiological stimulus, so occlusal loads from dentures are not an appropriate stimulus to prevent atrophy. The maxillary edentulous ridge has been reported to lose substantially less vertical height following an extraction than the mandibular ridge. Three to seven years following tooth loss, the annuals rate of vertical atrophy of the alveolar ridge are estimated at 0.2 mm in the maxilla and 0.7 mm in the mandible. In subsequent years, annual rates of atrophy slow down to 0.1 mm for the maxillary and 0.4 mm for the mandibular ridge (Tallgren 1972).

Bone atrophy never really comes to a standstill. This is of particular relevance in prosthetic dentistry, as the maxillary edentulous ridge tends to become smaller, whereas the mandibular alveolar ridge tends to widen, which may present a considerable challenge in setting up teeth for a complete denture (Fig 4).

Although implants are osseointegrated and not surrounded by periodontal tissues such as Sharpey fibers, they still exert some sort of stimulus to the bone when an occlusal load is transferred to the bone-implant interface, leading to a micro-deformation of the bony tissues under occlusal load or to deformation of the mandible. In the literature, peri-implant bone loss has been reported to be significantly lower than the equivalent loss in vertical height of an edentulous alveolar ridge. However, if denture kinetics implies a fulcrum line, bone loss may even be accelerated in non-supported (mostly posterior) regions of the alveolar ridge (de Jong and coworkers 2010).

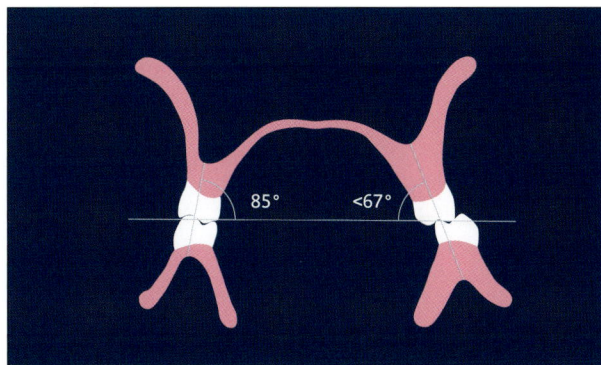

Fig 4 Atrophy of the alveolar ridges progresses with age, which finally leads to an unfavorable inclination of the intercrestal line. The posterior teeth may have to be set up in crossbite occlusion.

Temporomandibular joint. The temporomandibular joint has a higher prevalence of degenerative signs and symptoms with age, but mostly without a corresponding clinical treatment need (Tzakis and coworkers 1994). Atrophy of the skull includes the articular tuberculum, such that the inclination of the condylar path becomes more closely parallel to the Camper plane. The ligaments of the joint, which guide the mandibular border movements, lose elasticity in old age, resulting in greater joint mobility. In the prosthodontic treatment of elderly patients, these changes translate in a lower inclination of the molars' occlusal cuspids as well as a "freedom in centric" occlusal concept.

Muscles. One of the most obvious consequences of physiological aging is the loss of muscle bulk (sarcopenia); this is also true of the masticatory musculature. When studying the cross-sectional area (CSA) of the masseter and lateral pterygoid muscles, a 40% loss in CSA has been reported between 25 and 85 years of age, and even more pronounced in individuals who have lost their teeth (Newton and coworkers 1993).

According to the physiological principle of "use it or lose it," muscles need frequent and regular training to maintain their function. The speed of atrophy is well demonstrated when a leg is plastered after a fracture, where a significant loss in muscle strength is seen after only a few weeks of inactivity, thus requiring physiotherapy to regain normal function. For the closing muscles of the mandible, accelerated atrophy may also be related to reduced physical exercise, caused for example by poor chewing performance associated with conventional complete dentures. Fear of denture displacement limits mandibular excursions, and pain from the denture-bearing tissues restrict the force exerted on the replacement teeth. Occlusal support via dental implants limit the immediate load on the denture-bearing tissues and encourage muscle training while chewing.

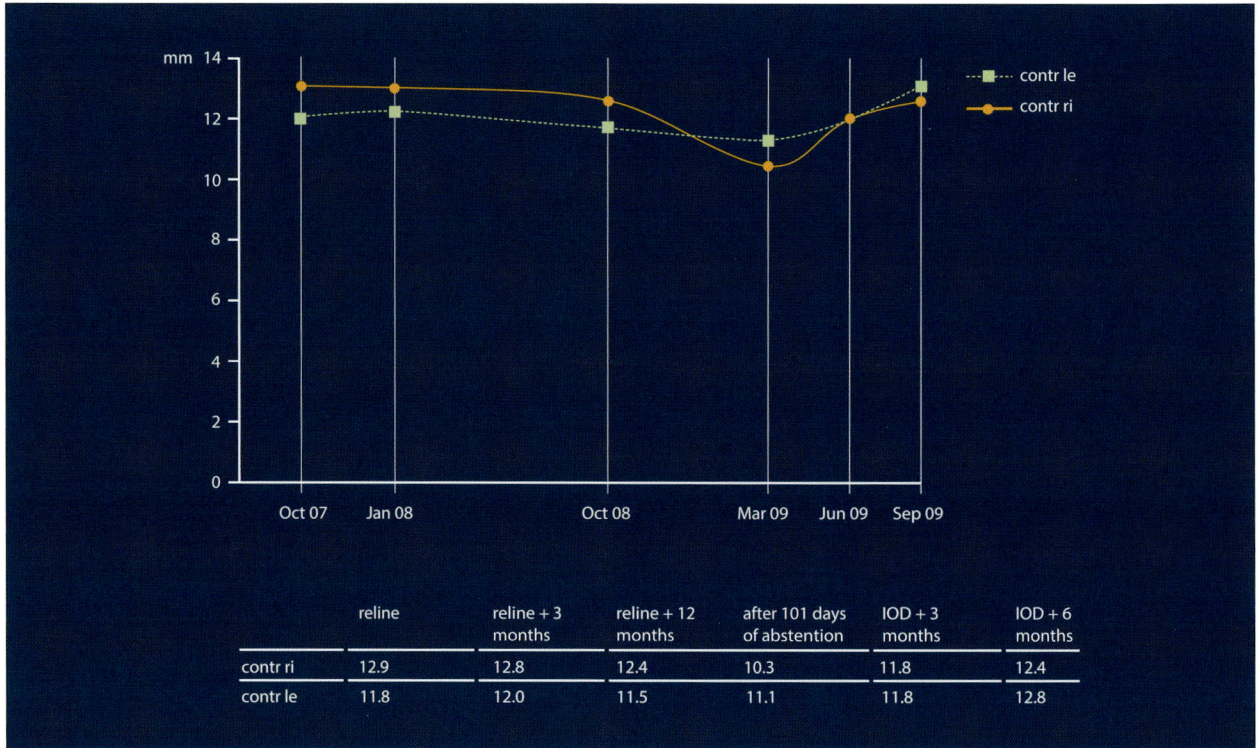

	reline	reline + 3 months	reline + 12 months	after 101 days of abstention	IOD + 3 months	IOD + 6 months
contr ri	12.9	12.8	12.4	10.3	11.8	12.4
contr le	11.8	12.0	11.5	11.1	11.8	12.8

Fig 5   97-year-old patient with significant muscle atrophy after (voluntary) denture abstention during implant osseointegration. Once provided with his mandibular overdenture, he regained muscle bulk along with the exercise through efficient chewing (Schimmel and coworkers 2010).

A training and detraining effect on thigh muscle bulk was reported for older adults (Tokmakidis and coworkers 2009). Little is known about whether masticatory muscle thickness can be regained once lost, especially in elderly and frail individuals. A recent case report from our group showed that 3 months of mandibular denture abstention in a 97-year-old patient induced a loss of up to 17% of his masseter muscle thickness, but was regained during 6 months after chewing function was restored with a mandibular implant-supported overdenture (Schimmel and coworkers 2010; Fig 5).

Aging processes in the muscles also include the motor units, which become larger as individual motor fibers disappear and some muscle fibers are adopted by neighboring motor units. With larger motor units, movements become less precise and controlled. Very obvious examples are the handwriting of elderly persons, which graphically depicts the physiological decline in motor control (Fig 6); controlling shoes, handbags, or other objects also becomes difficult (Fig 7). The mandibular closing trajectory can be more erratic, and a carefully adjusted balanced occlusion not only helps with denture reten-

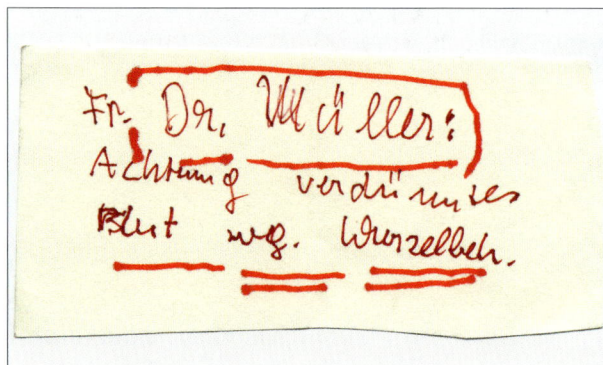

Fig 6   The deterioration of muscle skill is most obvious in the handwriting of an elderly person. Similar changes occur in the motor coordination of mandibular movements.

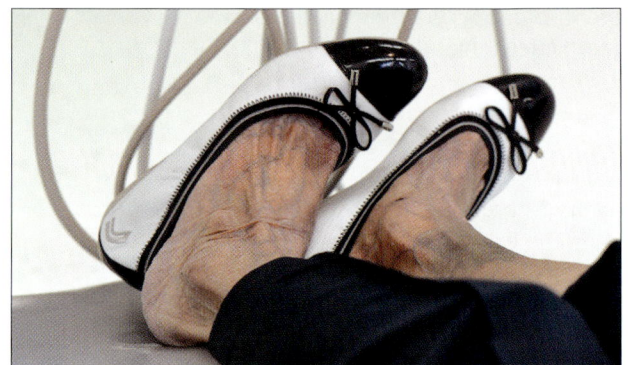

Fig 7   Motor control deteriorates with age, rendering motor tasks such as denture wearing difficult. This patient even had difficulties to control her shoes.

tion, but also gently guides the mandible to centric occlusion. A freedom-in-centric occlusal concept therefore seems most appropriate for elderly patients. Impaired muscle skill also affects denture control, especially in patients with neurodegenerative diseases such as Parkinson's disease, dementia, or mandibular dyskinesia.

Salivary glands. Although physiological aging reduces the total amount of saliva that can be produced by the glands, the quantity produced in healthy elders should be sufficient to keep the mouth in good shape. Saliva is also important for the taste; it can be noted that elderly persons tend to add more spices and more salt to their dishes. With age, parts of the acinar cells are replaced by connective tissue, and the ratio between active cells and ducts is shifted. The high percentage of elderly persons with dry mouth is more related to underlying pathology or to side effects of their treatment.

Oral mucosa. With age, the appearance of the oral mucosa becomes pale and thin or delicate, with a silky shine. Histologically, the oral mucosa becomes thinner and less elastic, and more fibrous fibres are present with age, with less interstitial fluid, rendering the tissues more vulnerable to mechanical injury. A reduced number of cell bodies and increasing surface keratinization can also be noted (Scott and coworkers 1983). The papillae of the tongue atrophy, and deep macroscopic fissures may appear in the dorsum.

Periodontium. Old age alone does not cause gingival recession or the loss of periodontal tissues. However, age is often associated with less meticulous oral hygiene; the cumulative effect of exposure to biofilm may account for the high prevalence of periodontal breakdowns and ultimately tooth loss in old age. In contrast, a true sign of physiological aging of the periodontium is the apposition of cementum—which is even used to determine age forensically.

Teeth. Of all structures of the orofacial system, the teeth present the most evident signs of aging. Functionally, teeth become less sensitive to external stimuli, and pulpal tissue becomes less resistant to trauma such as cutting with a dental turbine. Attrition, abrasion, and wear lead to a loss of hard tissue on the incisal and occlusal aspects, often exposing the underlying dentin. Nutritional habits, bruxism, and the hardness of the enamel modulate the extent of these changes.

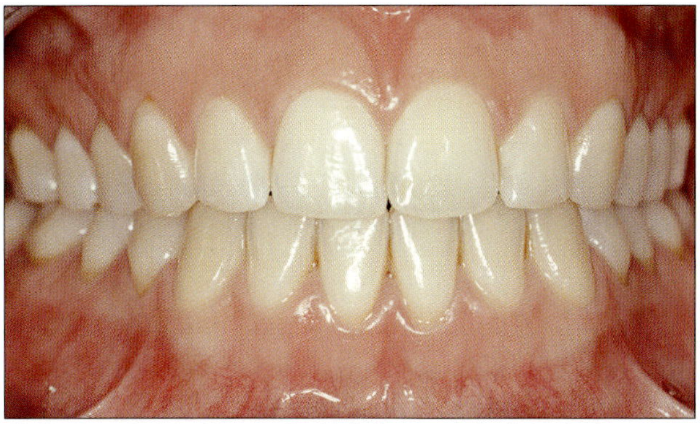

Fig 8 Young adults have teeth with little wear and a light shade.

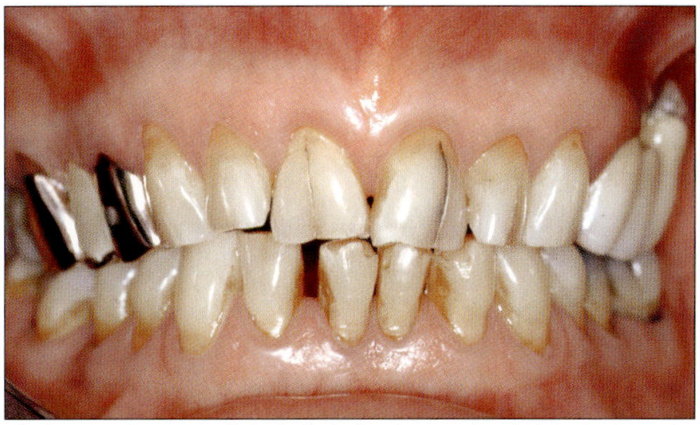

Fig 9 Age shows mostly in incisal abrasions and a darker shade; stains and cracks also become more frequent.

The tooth surface appears smoother and is less transparent and duller. Abrasive toothpastes and certain brushing techniques may accelerate these age-related changes. Hartmann and Müller (2004) showed in their studies on the age-related changes in appearance that the unrestored tooth of a 21- to 33-year old person is one to two shades lighter than that of 67-year-old volunteers. They also confirmed that aged teeth are more likely to exhibit cracks, discolorations, abrasions, and crowding of the incisors (Figs 8 and 9; Table 1). A knowledge of these age-related changes allows the restorative dentist to suggest an age-appropriate appearance to a patient when tooth replacement becomes necessary.

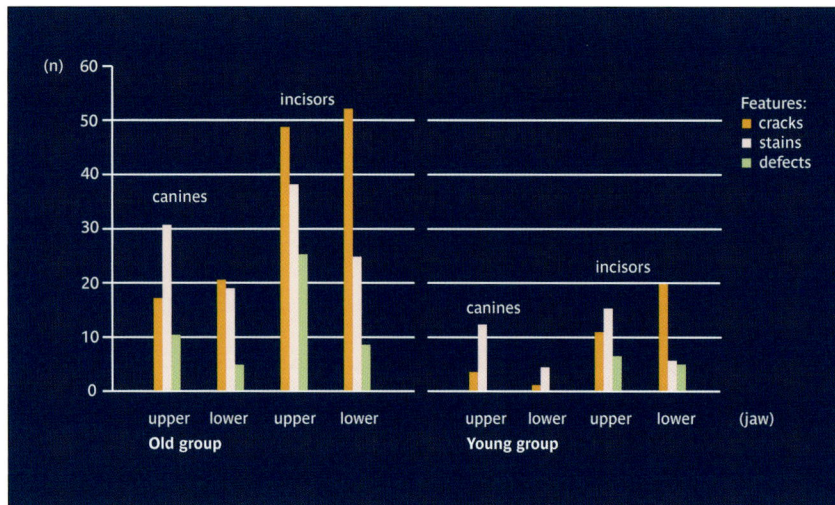

Table 1   Features like cracks, stains, and defects in a group of young volunteers with unrestored dentitions (n = 64; mean age 25.8 years) and a group of older persons (n = 64; mean age 67.3 years) with an unrestored anterior dentition (after Hartmann and Müller 2004).

Nerves. The peripheral and central nervous systems also undergo changes along with physiological aging. The conduction speed of the peripheral nerves decreases and the sensitivity of mechanoreceptors diminishes. Large particles of food debris can often be found in the vestibulum of elderly patients, as they cannot feel the foreign body. However, in prosthodontics the most important age-related neurological change is reduced neuroplasticity. The insertion of a new prosthesis implies the stimulation of different mechanoreceptors in the oral mucosa and requires the modification of existing movement patterns and reflexes. Elderly persons with a reduced capacity for adaptation should therefore be provided with replacement dentures similar in form and function to the previous well-adapted set. Duplication techniques may be employed to transfer the maximum number of a denture's successful features to the new prosthesis. Mechanical retention may also be helpful, as neuroplasticity is less challenged when denture function does not rely on motor control (Müller and coworkers 1995).

Multimorbidity and frailty
The transition of the stable stage of life (third age) to the stage of dependency for the activities of daily living, also called the fourth age or old age, is generally not linear. Signs of frailty include rapid weight loss, weakness, fatigue, anorexia, and physical inactivity. Clinically frail patients may present with undernutrition, sarcopenia, osteopenia, slow walking, balance problems, and poor physical fitness (Fried and Walston 1998).

Whereas medical events often initiate the transition from the third to the fourth age, we also note that psychological stress or life events like the loss of a partner or shifting to a new residence trigger a rapid and steep functional decline. Patients may suddenly appear less well dressed, poorly shaved, and sometimes a little "smelly." Their oral hygiene often seems unusually neglected, and a severe and comprehensive periodontal breakdown is often the consequence. Whereas healthy adults can regain their pre-event level of functioning, frail persons will remain permanently impaired. As frailty progresses, they become dependent on help for normal activities of daily living (ADL). Their functional decline can be evaluated and monitored by a geriatric assessment comprising a comprehensive battery of instruments. Only a few very commonly used tests are listed here:

Base activities of daily living can be evaluated by means of

- Barthel Index for the Activities of Daily Living (Mahoney and Barthel 1965)

Cognitive function and psychological health can be assessed by

- Geriatric Depression Scale (GDS) (Sheikh and Yesavange 1986)
- Mini Mental State Examination (MMSE) (Folstein MF 1975)
- Clock-drawing test (Shulman 2000)

The nutritional state may be evaluated by

- Mini-Nutritional Assessment (MNA) (Guigoz and coworkers 1994)

Although some of these tests may be not practical in daily dental practice, the well-established but less well-documented "denture-upside-down test" is easy to implement. When a patient is handed a denture upside down and places it in the mouth without first turning it over, this may be a first sign of cognitive impairment, and the patient may benefit from an in-depth examination at a specialized memory clinic (Figs 10a-c).

The most common chronic diseases in elderly adults on average 84 years of age who live in long-term care facilities are hypertension (men, 53%/women, 56%), dementia (45%/52%), depression (31%/37%), arthritis (26%/35%), diabetes (26%/23%), reflux (23%/23%), arteriosclerosis (24%/20%), cardiac insufficiency (18%/21%), cerebrovascular diseases (24%/19%), and anemia (17%/20%) (Moore and coworkers 2012). In Switzerland, about half of the population over 75 years indicated that they had a permanent health problem. This percentage increases steeply in the institutionalized population.

Physical limitations

Frail and multimorbid elderly persons often present with physical limitations when it comes to dental treatments. Appointments have to be adjusted to individual habits, not too early in the morning, as dressing takes longer, not during fixed mealtimes, and preferably during daylight (Fig 11). Winter months have to be avoided for non-urgent treatments, as falls on slippery and icy roads all too often result in hip fractures, an incident with a mortality of 20% in old age. Appointments should be made in writing with clear and large letters on a sheet with no distracting advertising. Financial agreements should also be clear and equally made available in writing, as children and family often advise their elderly relatives, even if they are not officially appointed as legal representative. Elderly persons should be discouraged from carrying large amounts in cash when they attend for treatment, as they may become easy victims for burglary and violence in the streets. Their physical frailty also precludes long and invasive treatment sessions, and often the necessary dental procedures have to be performed with high precision in a short time, which requires a significant degree of skill and experience on the part of the operator.

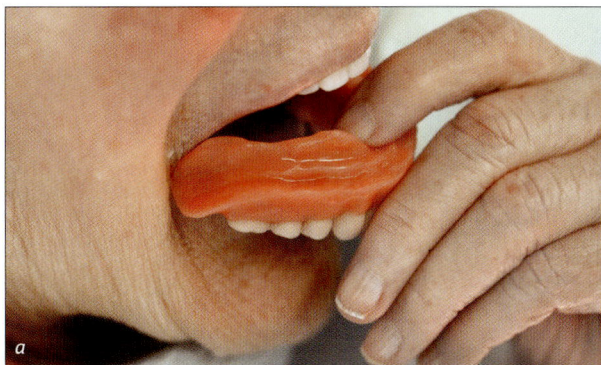

Figs 10a-c   Denture-upside-down test.

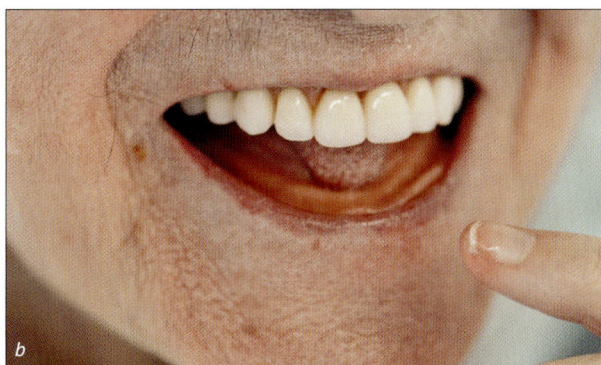

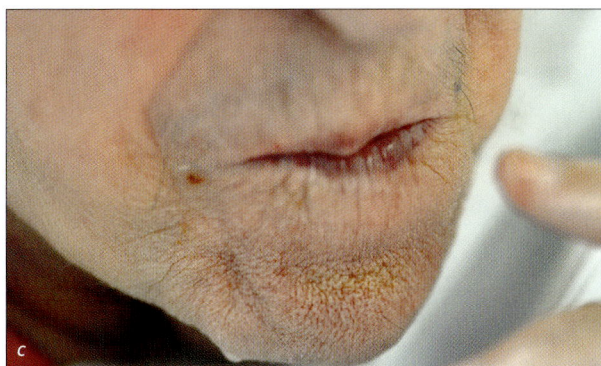

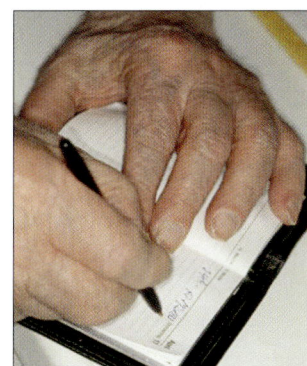

Fig 11 Even if older patients' calendars seem "empty" compared to ours, these patients are not always available for dental appointments.

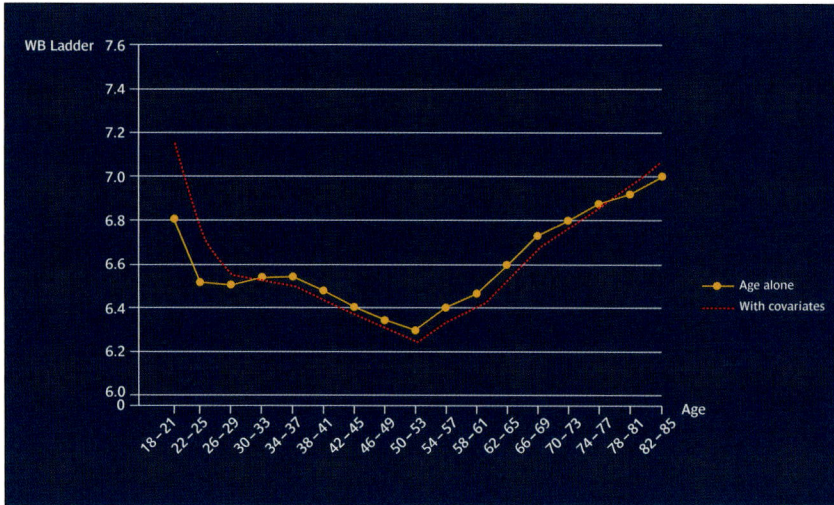

Fig 12 Psychological well-being increases with age beyond 50 years (after Stone and coworkers 2010).

Psychological and social aging

The U-shaped curve of psychological well-being in a cohort of 340,847 participants in the United States showed that aging is accompanied by a constant increase in psychological well-being (Stone and coworkers 2010; Fig 12). Little is known about psychological aging, although this may be a very relevant factor in medical treatment outcomes. While everything is not all that marvelous in old age, some suggest the elderly adopt a more accepting attitude and more realistic expectations, along with less stress, which renders them more content. On the other hand, there is an increasing prevalence of depression and social isolation in the elderly population, as their partners and friends pass away, or when relocation to a more age-adequate and "practical" abode reduces their usual social contacts and familiar environment. All this implies a certain risk that oral health is neglected, as oral pathologies and functional impairment are no longer correctly perceived. It is well documented that the subjective demand of elderly persons for improvements in their oral health or regarding prostheses is less; this is in extreme contrast to the objective judgement of their treatment need by dental health professionals (Locker and Jokovic 1996; Figs 13a-c).

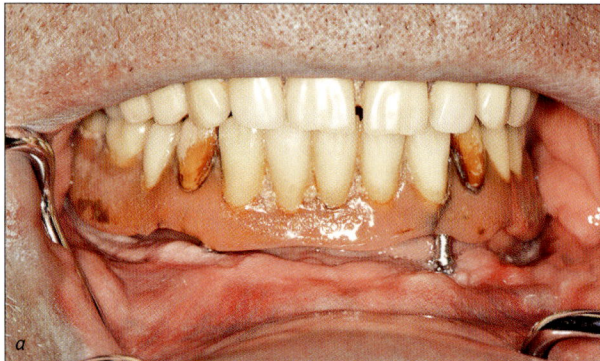

Figs 13a-c "Overadaptation" describes a situation where an elderly person accepts a traumatic and non-functional condition without demanding treatment. (a, b) This patient did not seek treatment to have the pins of his denture removed. (c) The gingiva showed chronic inflammation and keratinization where the pins were located.

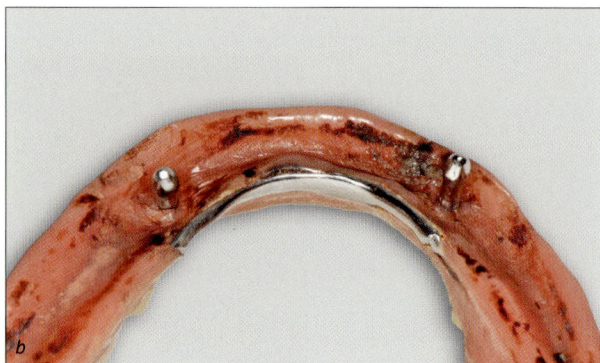

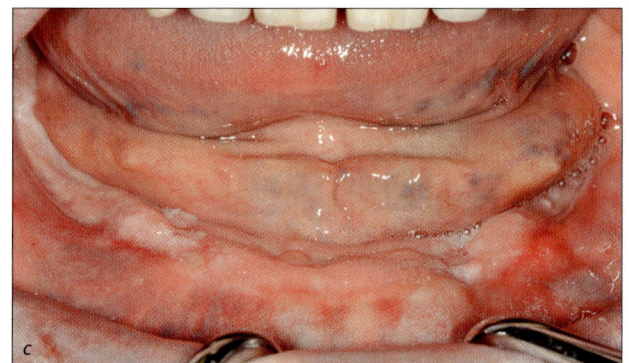

Old patients still have the right of self-determination of their medical treatment; patients may choose to decide against interventions that—from an objective and professional point of view—ought to be performed. It is easy to imagine that optional interventions, especially when they include a surgical procedure, are even less popular in elderly adults. The role of the health professional is to inform patients on their oral health and to propose, with professional knowledge and judgment, adequate treatment options, so that patients know everything necessary to give "informed consent." Written information sheets give patients the time necessary to thoroughly consider the proposed treatment options and discuss them with family and friends (Fig 14).

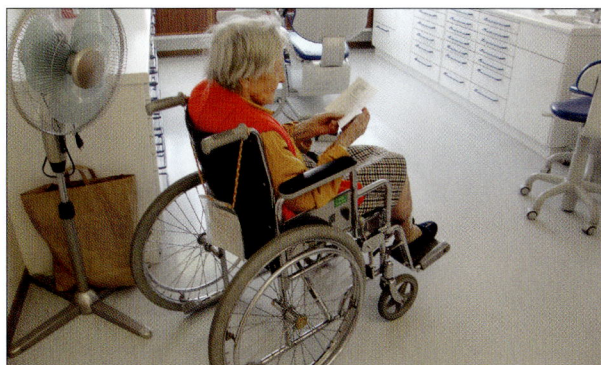

Fig 14 *Written information sheets allow the patient to spend as much time as needed to understand the proposed treatments and discuss them with family and friends before taking a final decision.*

Oral health in elderly persons

Despite all prevention and progress in restorative techniques, caries, periodontal disease, and tooth loss are still a reality in old age; 97.4% of the Swiss population have some sort of prostheses, and 85.9% wear removable dentures at 85 years or over (Zitzmann and coworkers 2008a). However, the prevalence varies between countries and studies, and comparisons are difficult as age groups and study contexts vary enormously (Müller and coworkers 2007).

As mentioned before, there is still a substantial proportion of edentulous persons in the higher age groups. In the USA, the total number of cases to treat is even expected to rise due to the growing percentage number of older persons (Douglass and coworkers 2002). When natural teeth are still present, they usually present with the above-mentioned signs of aging, but also show pathologies such as coronal and root caries, occlusal wear, and periodontal disease.

Oral health in elderly persons is further compromised by a high prevalence of xerostomia, with the accompanying painful infections of the oral mucosa (Locker 2003). The prevalence of oral squamous-cell carcinoma increases beyond the age of 60 years, so regular screening of the oral cavity is highly recommended (Dhanuthai and coworkers 2016). Another frequent pathology in old age is dysphagia, whose prevalence, 6%–9% in the adult population, rises to 15%–22% for those aged over 50 years and 40%–60% in institutionalized individuals (Aslam and Vaezi 2013). Dysphagia is the main risk factor for the development of aspiration pneumonia as food debris, biofilm, and saliva risk descending the bronchi (Quagliarello and coworkers 2005). In fragile and compromised patients, mortality rates of up to 48% were described for pneumonia (Welte and coworkers 2012).

Aspiration is not limited to small particles or objects. A case was reported where a four-unit bridge, failing due to rampant root caries in the abutment teeth, was aspirated by a patient who suffered from Alzheimer's disease (Oghalai 2002), and even several cases of aspirated "missing" dentures are known (Arora and coworkers 2005). Again, the mechanical retention of a removable denture may effectively prevent these incidents and protect patients with swallowing disorders from aspiration.

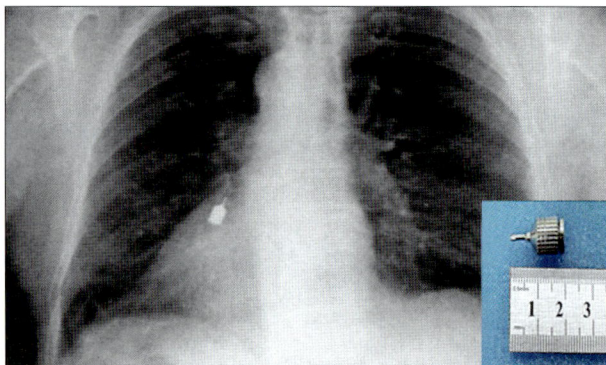

Fig 15   Particular risks such as swallowing disorders or mandibular dyskinesia have to be considered in treatment planning. This Parkinson's patient had accidentally aspirated an implant screwdriver (reprinted with permission from Deliberador and coworkers 2011).

>   Academic treatment plan (ideal)

        treatment demand
        oral examination
        complaints/pain
        medical reasons for a dental treatment

>   Clinical treatment plan (reasonable)

        general health and functional findings
        physical or mental handicap
        ratio cost/benefit
        autonomy

>   Practical treatment plan (possible)

        subjective treatment demand
        wishes of the family
        financial aspects
        dental preliminary treatment/invasive diagnostics

>   Modified treatment plan (up to date)

        changes in compliance
        changes in general and oral health

Fig 16   Treatment planning in gerodontology (after Riesen and coworkers 2002).

Treatment planning

As for younger patients, treatment planning for elderly patients starts with an ideal treatment plan where the patient's chief complaints and medical findings are the basis for a first suggestion to satisfy an ideal level of esthetics and function under healthy conditions. However, even in younger patients, such ideal conditions are rarely present, and a more reasonable approach for treatment planning has to be adopted, taking into consideration the cost-benefit ratio, patients' physical and mental condition, and their autonomy in denture handing and oral hygiene. Such a clinical treatment plan may vary considerably from the ideal one in terms of technical sophistication and invasiveness of a proposed prosthodontic rehabilitation. Whereas in younger patients, almost any agreed treatment goal can be achieved if the patient accepts the corresponding financial, logistic, physical, and psychological effort, this is no longer the case in elderly patients, or particular risks associated with the patient's condition may exist. In patients with swallowing disorders or dyskinesia, there may be an increased risk for aspiration—even of dental instruments (Deliberador and coworkers 2011; Fig 15).

Therefore, quite often the treatment plan will have to be reduced to a pragmatic level (Riesen and coworkers 2002; Fig 16). The treatment goal will have to be modified to what is achievable. The subjective treatment demands, the wishes of the family, or the socio-economic context may limit the available treatment options. The desires of the elderly patient may often be overshadowed by those of the family. Moreover, financial aspects may dominate the treatment options and reduce the reasonable treatment plan to a feasible level. In addition, the patient's physical condition and general health may not allow long and invasive treatment options, which further restricts the available treatment options. A preliminary treatment phase may be helpful to decide on these limits, as elderly persons may have days on which they are less resilient. A typical example would be a hot summer day, where elderly persons tend to dehydrate as the sensation of thirst diminishes with age. In the dental consultation, they may seem confused and disoriented, even though their only actual problem is that they did not drink sufficiently. This pre-treatment phase should be understood as a diagnostic tool to be reconsidered in later re-evaluations.

The elderly patient in the dental practice

Treating elderly patients in a dental practice may require some special arrangements. First of all, it seems important that the dental practice be equipped to meet the physical handicaps of elders, such as reduced mobility and vision. Absence of tripping hazards, good lighting, and chairs that are stable and not too deep are essential features of a dental practice. Wheelchair access may also be desirable (Fig 17). Forms should be prepared in a legible font size and the dental nurse should assist in filling the forms, if needed.

Once in the dental office, placing the patient on the dental chair may also be a challenge; tools are available to facilitate this task and prevent accidents. Simple interventions and oral examinations may even be performed with the patient still seated in a wheelchair (Fig 18). Radiographs are diagnostic essentials, but some elderly patients may not be able to have a panoramic radiograph taken due to their posture, reduced mobility, or fear (Fig 19). In these cases, intraoral radiographs may be an alternative.

Communication with elderly persons may not only be difficult because of hearing problems; it is also important to note that one is talking to a "different generation," who have many more years of experience and different values (Fig 20). Especially for dental students, it is difficult to imagine that their elderly patients may have experienced hunger and war, lived without the internet and mobile telephones. Technical progress, even when it concerns a dental prosthesis, may be regarded with a substantial degree of suspicion. Understanding suggested treatments and their implications is a key factor for treatment success and compliance. Finding the right words to explain the advantage of progress in the modern world (and in dentistry) is important in having elderly persons participating and benefiting in the recent developments of implant dentistry.

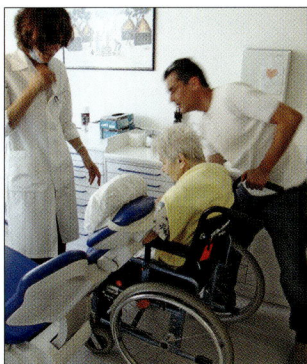

Fig 17 The dental office should have sufficient space for elderly patients with reduced mobility and—if possible—wheelchair access.

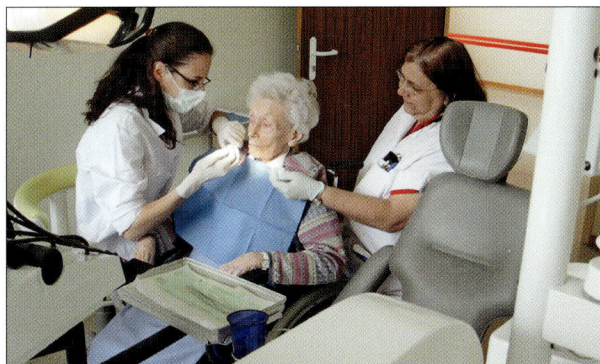

Fig 18 If the dental unit is sufficiently spacious, simple treatments may even be performed without transferring the immobile patient to the dental chair.

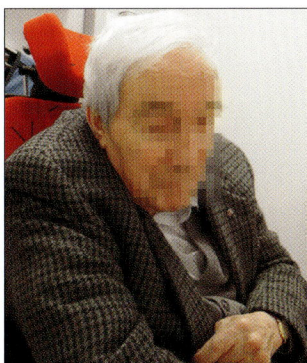

Fig 19 If the patient's posture or reduced mobility does not allow taking a panoramic radiograph, intraoral radiographs may be a good alternative for a radiological examination.

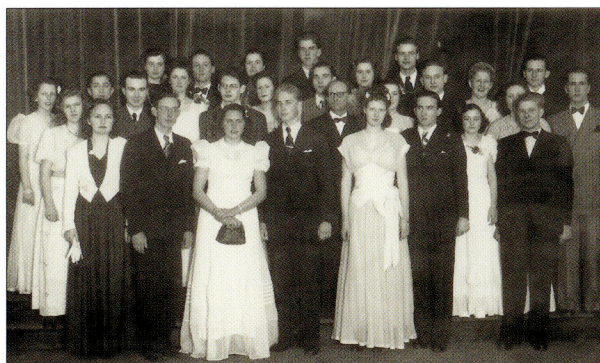

Fig 20 In the treatment of elderly patients it is important to take into consideration that they may have lived in different times (without internet!) and have had very different experiences (war) and values.

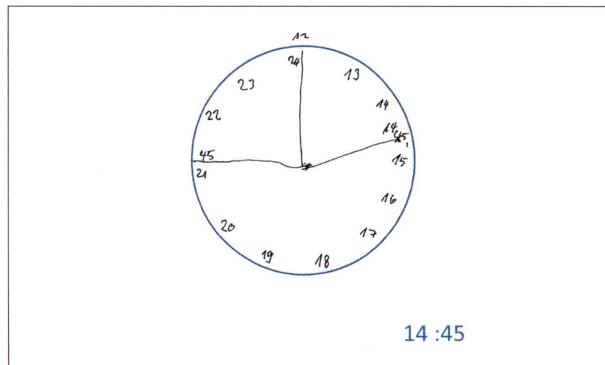

Fig 21   Clock-drawing test.

Legal context

Old age and dependency for the activities of daily living does not automatically imply the loss of the individual person's legal rights in terms of health decisions and financial agreements. As long as no official representative is allocated, old persons remain entitled to make their own business and health decisions. However, their family may increasingly wish to be involved and informed on any complex treatment decisions. Although this may be an agreeable arrangement, dentists need to be aware that reported elder abuse is frequent and the non-reported incidence rate is even higher. Unreasonable withholding of financial resources and psychological manipulation may constitute elder abuse and should be reported to the authorities where noted.

Dentists could also be the first person to suspect the onset of cognitive impairment. A first suspicion can be confirmed by the above-mentioned clock-drawing test (Fig 21). Depending on the results, a referral to a specialized memory clinic for a more comprehensive examination may be indicated. The drawing can be kept in the patient's file to document a responsible evaluation of their cognitive function.

Placing dental implants and fabricating a new prosthesis are never emergency treatments. It therefore seems important to give an elderly person sufficient time (at least one week) before agreeing to such interventions. Written proposals with a clear statement of the financial commitment can help to avoid allegations and conflicts. If a patient has a legal representative, it is important to know that some countries distinguish between "financial" and "other" decisions. So even if the patient's representative may have the right to take financial decisions, they may not be entitled to agree or disagree to a medical treatment. Elderly patients should also be invited to discuss the treatment options with their family and friends. Only after they are completely convinced of the proposed intervention and have signed the agreement should the treatment begin.

4 The Benefits of Implant-supported Prostheses in the Elderly Patient

F. Müller

The benefits of implant-supported prostheses in elderly patients are most evident in completely edentulous patients who have been wearing conventional complete dentures for years or decades. As mentioned before, the decision to extract or keep compromised natural teeth in elderly or very old patients is complex, as the possibilities of conventional or implant-supported tooth replacement may be limited by functional, medical, or economic factors. Hence, all efforts are made to retain an elderly patient's natural dentition and to apply, where possible, the "shortened dental arch" concept (Käyser and coworkers 1981), or manufacture overdentures on natural abutment teeth to avoid invasive procedures and overtreatment. Despite these efforts, there are still very many fully edentulous persons among the elderly population, particularly among the very old (Müller and coworkers 2007). Not only do these patients require dental prostheses, they also depend on continuous care to maintain oral function and hygiene and on the progressive adaptation of the denture to the aging oral environment.

Function of conventional dentures

Conventional complete dentures replace teeth and lost tissue, but fall short of restoring oral function. Mucosally supported dentures rely on three mechanisms. At insertion, they can exert physical suction, obtained by a precise impression with selective tissue compression or the creation of a posterior palatal seal. Physical suction requires the presence of a thin film of saliva, preferably of mucous consistency. Cohesive and adhesive forces are more easily achieved in maxillary complete dentures, as the ratio of denture-bearing surface to the length of the border seal is more favorable than with mandibular dentures. However, the physical retention decreases over time as the alveolar structures atrophy with age and protracted occlusal load (Tallgren 1972).

With the decrease of physical retention, denture function is increasingly assured by the second mechanism, "muscular" retention—a learned skill to keep the denture in place during function (Basker and Watson 1991; Müller and coworkers 2002; Fig 1). To perform this demanding task successfully, the brain processes afferent information from the oral cavity, which is then translated into a purpose-oriented motor activity pattern.

Oral perception is essential for denture control, but the sensitivity of the mechanoreceptors diminishes with age. The absence of this afferent information can be simulated by surface anesthesia of the denture-supporting mucosa; pertinent experiments clearly demonstrated the failure of denture control and the inability to speak or chew efficiently (Brill and coworkers 1959). Complete-denture wearers regularly "refresh" the central nervous system (CNS) with the afferent information on the denture position by unconscious denture-control movements.

In addition to physical retention and muscle control, conventional denture function relies on a third mechanism: occlusion. The positive effect of occlusal denture stabilization becomes most apparent when it is missing, such as when patients wear only their maxillary dentures, when surgical removal of the mandibular hard and soft tissues is required in the treatment of head and neck cancer, or simply when the mandibular denture is not worn because it causes discomfort. Denture kinetics during swallowing and the mentioned control movements also rely on occlusal contact. A bilaterally balanced occlusion helps guide the closing trajectory of the mandible to central occlusion without challenging the denture adhesion with unilateral occlusal loads.

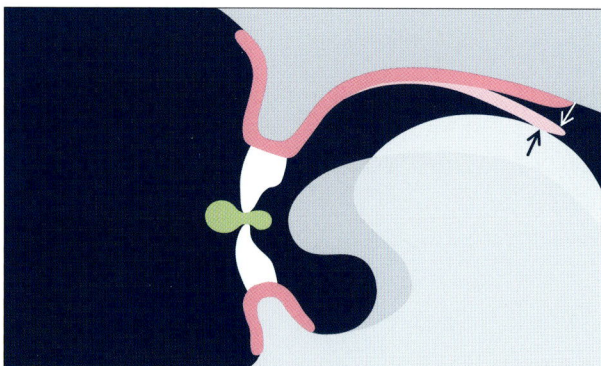

Fig 1   Motor control allows wearers of complete dentures to function with poorly fitting dentures, but the required motor skills diminish with increasing age and morbidity, and denture control becomes difficult. The image illustrates the reflex of stabilizing a dislodged maxillary denture in place (after Basker and Watson 1991).

Benefits of the implant-supported overdenture
Implant-supported overdenture retention and stability.
All three of the abovementioned mechanisms of denture function are assisted by the conversion of a conventional complete denture to an implant-supported overdenture. All implant-supported overdentures (IODs), regardless of implant number and positions, provide substantial improvement in terms of denture retention and stability. This is a particular advantage in compromised elders with xerostomia, as the available quantity of saliva may not be sufficient to assure denture retention. Despite the benefit of added retention from the insertion of implants, patients with xerostomia may still experience pain and discomfort when the denture base rubs on the dry mucosa during micro-movements.

IODs are further beneficial when oral motor control deteriorates due to age or disease, such as with Parkinson's disease or dementia. Also, drug-induced oral dyskinesia can often be observed in fragile and multimorbid elderly persons. This lack of motor control may render conventional dentures very difficult to wear, and dentures are worn much less by patients with these conditions. Although rare, reports confirm that complete dentures can even be aspirated in the absence of protective motor control, especially when the patient also presents with dysphagia (Arora and coworkers 2005). The additional retention and stability provided by implants replaces the need for muscular skill and prevents denture displacement during speech and chewing function.

Finally, implant-supported overdentures alleviate the need for a balanced occlusion. Although this occlusal concept is still adopted in IODs, denture stability is less at risk when the mandibular closing trajectory is not well controlled and the teeth contact the antagonistic arch in an eccentric position.

Denture adaptation. As mentioned earlier, the adaptation to replacement dentures comprises three components: psychological adaptation (not perceiving the prosthesis as foreign body), physiological adaptation (habituation, indicating a diminishing reflex response to a continuous or repeated stimulus), and muscle skills (indicating motor control of the prosthesis). Whereas psychological adaptation is complex and may be overshadowed by various aspects of tooth loss and denture wearing, the other two components may be greatly aided by implants.

Implants can ensure denture retention and facilitate continuous and consistent stimulation of the mechanoreceptors, which in turn enhances the habituation, as the reflex response to a continued stimulus generally weakens with time.

Implants also render muscular skills redundant when denture stability and retention are assured by way of mechanical attachment systems. Consequently, IODs present less of a challenge to the patient's neuroplasticity by lowering the amount of new muscular skills that the patient has to acquire.

Prevention of bone atrophy. Numerous scientific studies provide solid evidence on the beneficial effect of implants on the preservation of the peri-implant bone. Alveolar-ridge atrophy in edentulous persons has rarely been studied, yet long-term observations have reported an annual atrophy of 0.2 mm in the maxilla and 0.7 mm in the mandible (Tallgren 1972) 3 to 7 years after extraction. In the peri-implant area, atrophy is reduced by a factor of between 7 and 10 when implants are inserted (Jemt and coworkers 1996a; Lindquist and coworkers 1988; Naert and coworkers 1991; Table 1). However, IODs increase the chewing and biting forces and may accelerate bone resorption distant to the implant (de Jong and coworkers 2010; Jacobs and coworkers 1992). If the IODs are not regularly monitored and relined if needed, this might lead to an anterior occlusion and eventually even to "combination syndrome" (Kreisler and coworkers 2003; Tymstra and coworkers 2011). The beneficial effect of bone conservation through implants depends on the treatment concept in general and the occlusal load distribution in particular.

Table 1   Numerous studies have demonstrated that the annual peri-implant bone loss in overdenture wearers proceeds more slowly than the atrophy of the edentulous mandible in complete-denture wearers.

Authors	Year	Patients and implants	Mean age [a]	Observation	Bone loss [mm]	Indication	Survival rate [%]
Hoeksema and coworkers	2015	Young, n = 52 104 implants Old, n = 53 106 implants	45 (34–50) (60–80)	0–1 a 0–5 a 0–10 a	Y = 0.5 /O = 0.4 Y = 1.2 / O = 0.8 Y = 1.2 /O = 1.2 0.12 p.a.	Mandibular 2-IOD	Insertion IOD to 10 a: Young = 97.1 Old = 93.4
Heschl and coworkers	2013	39 patients 156 implants	61 (28–79)	5 a	1.4 0.3 p.a.	Mandibular 4-IOD	99.4%
Meijer and coworkers	2009	30 patients 60 implants	52.8–56.6 (35–79)	10 a	0–1 a = 0.2–0.8 0–5 a = 0.7–1.4 0–10 a = 0.7–1.4 0.07–0.01 p.a.	Mandibular 2-IOD	93%–100%
Vercruyssen and coworkers; Vercruyssen and Quirynen	2010a; 2010b	495 patients 1051 implants	60.8 (±10.2)	5–20 a	1–3 a = 0.08 p.a. 1–5 a = 0.07 p.a. 1–8 a = 0.06 p.a. 1–12 a = 0.04 p.a. 1–16 a = 0.05 p.a.	Mandibular 2-IOD	After 20 a 95.5%
Gotfredsen and Holm	2000	26 patients 52 implants	64 (52–78)	0–5 a	Ins – 0 = 0.5 0–1 a = –0.3 1–2 a = 0.2 2–3 a = 0.1 3–4 a = 0.2 4–5 a = 0 0–5 a = 0.2 Ins – 5 a = 0.1 p.a.	Edentate C/2-IOD	0–5 a 100%
Bilhan and coworkers	2011	51 patients 126 implants	59.4 (39–86)	3 a	0–1 a = 0.8 0–2 a = 0.9 0–3 a = 0.9 0–3 a = 0.32 p.a.	Mandibular 2/3/4-IOD	
Quirynen and coworkers	2015	89 patients 178 implants	65.8 (±8.4)	0–1 a 0–2 a 0–3 a 0–3 a	0.3/0.3 0.6–0.6 0.8/0.6 0.26 p.a./0.20 p.a.	Mandibular 2-IOD	97%–99%
Müller and coworkers	2015	47 patients 94 implants	72 (54–92)	5 a	0.60/0.61 0.12 p.a.	Mandibular 2-IOD	97.8%/98.9%
Tallgren	1972	9 patients 20 patients		0–1 a 3–7 a 10–25 a	C/– 0.7 –/C 2.4 C/– 0.2 –/C 0.7 p.a. C/– 0.05 –/C 0.2 p.a.	Edentate C/C	

Y = young; O = old; a = years; p.a. = per annum; C/C = complete maxillary/mandibular denture; IOD = implant-supported overdenture; 2/3/4 = on 2/3/4 implants

Chewing efficiency and bite force. Chewing efficiency and bite force with complete dentures is significantly impaired when compared to persons with a natural dentition. Analyses of mandibular movements revealed that complete-denture wearers present about one-third less vertical opening and about half of the frontal width of the chewing cycle compared to dentate volunteers (Hofmann and Pröschel 1982). The limiting factors are denture retention and stability, as the complete-denture wearer unconsciously limits mandibular excursions to avoid denture displacement. Furthermore, chewing forces may cause pain on the denture-bearing mucosa. Denture-related sore spots are alleviated when chewing forces are transferred to implants rather than fragile mucosal tissues. Supporting overdentures by implants significantly improves masticatory efficiency in independent complete-denture wearers (van der Bilt and coworkers 2010). Experiments with a test bolus consisting of a 5.6-mm silicone cube showed that only half the chewing cycles were necessary to obtain the same particle size, and this was independent of the attachment system (van Kampen and coworkers 2004; Fig 2). In fragile elderly patients, this effect is less pronounced, as the weak chewing muscles and occlusal wear may overshadow the positive effect of denture stability from implants (Müller and coworkers 2013). The bulk of the chewing muscle diminishes with age, and bite force is greatly reduced. Atrophy is even more pronounced after tooth loss, probably due to the lack of physiological stimulation (Newton and coworkers 1993). According to the physiological principle of "use it or lose it," it is possible, although unproven, that implant-supported overdentures slow down muscle atrophy by providing constant "training" via improved chewing activity (Müller and coworkers 2012b; Fig 3).

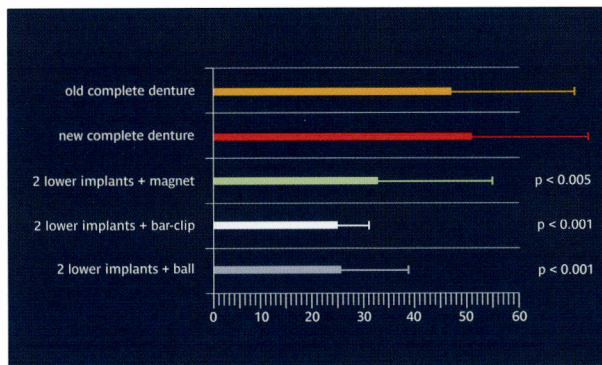

Fig 2   Number of chewing cycles needed to reduce to half the initial size of a 5.6-mm test bolus after stabilization of the mandibular denture with two implants. Significant improvements with all three attachment types (after van Kampen and coworkers 2004).

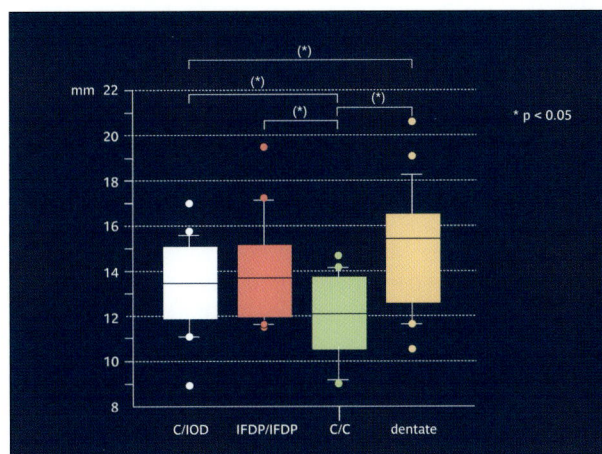

Fig 3   The well-documented decrease in muscle bulk after tooth loss seems to be partly compensated when implants are placed for fixed or removable restorations. This may be attributed to a training effect following the improved chewing function. Each group had 20 patients with an average age between 61.5 and 68.2 years (after Müller and coworkers 2012b).

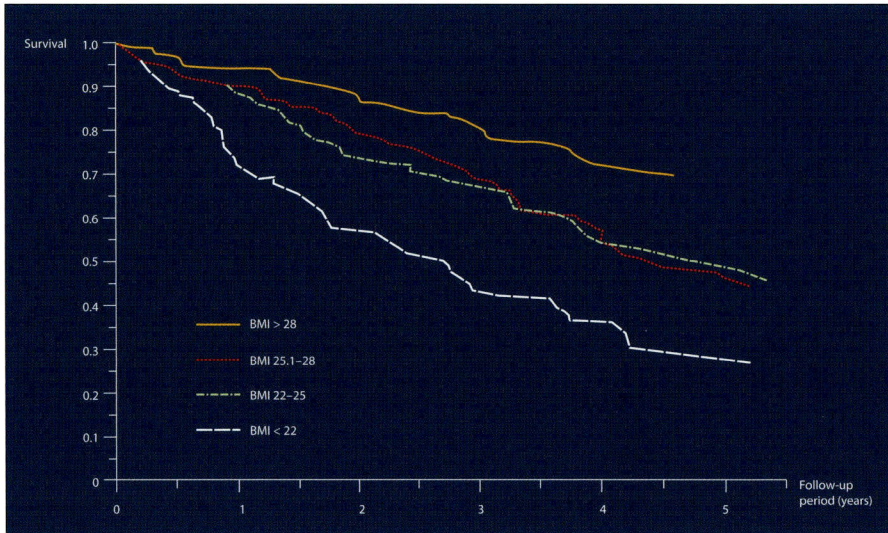

Fig 4   In a cohort of 470 hospitalized patients with an average age of 81.5 years over 4.2 years, the mortality was lowest in persons with a body mass index (kg/m²) of over 28 (after Weiss and coworkers 2008).

Nutritional state. Malnutrition is a widespread health problem in the elderly population with a prevalence of 5%–8% reported for community-dwelling elderly adults and 30%–60% in the institutionalized population (Guigoz and coworkers 1994), and may be in excess of 60% of long-term care home residents (Pauly and coworkers 2007). However, in elders a BMI of 28 or above is associated with reduced morbidity and mortality (Weiss and coworkers 2008; Fig 4). Food intake depends on multiple factors such as appetite, cognitive state, general health, knowledge, mobility, financial resources, culture, religious practice, and finally cooking skills. Chewing efficiency is only one factor affecting food intake. Still, there is an established correlation between the number of teeth and food intake (Sheiham and coworkers 2001). With the loss of teeth and the accompanying impairment of mastication, a silent change in diet occurs, often unnoticed by the denture wearer. This shows most clearly in the large discrepancy between the answers to the questions "is there any food that is difficult to eat?" and "What food do you not eat because it is too difficult to chew?" (Millwood and Heath 2000).

Denture wearers tend to shun hard food like nuts, raw carrots, or celery, as well as tough food such as meat or sticky food such as toffee and chewing gum, which tend to dislodge the prosthesis. Equally unpopular amongst denture wearers are foods with pips, like tomatoes, strawberry and raspberry jelly, or cakes and bread with small grains, as they could slip under the denture and cause severe discomfort during the rest of the meal. In public, this may lead to embarrassing situations, and it is known that denture wearers are self-conscious about these limitations, sometimes even preferring to eat alone. Although aged individuals have lower energy requirements and therefore need fewer calories, the amount of nutriments such as vitamins or micronutrients needed remains the same as in younger persons. This implies that the diet of elderly persons should be "nutrient-dense" (Moynihan 2007). The consumption of fruit and vegetables diminishes along with tooth loss, and the recommended five portions a day are rarely eaten by elderly denture wearers.

It can therefore be assumed that the stabilization of complete dentures by means of osseointegrated implants may improve the nutritional state of elderly complete-denture wearers (Morais and coworkers 2003). Implants avoid dislodging of the denture during chewing, provide support for the chewing forces and assure an intimate contact of the denture base to the denture bearing tissues, thus assisting in the prevention of food particles accumulating under the denture saddles. However, with surprising consistency, the literature proves that converting a complete denture to an implant-supported overdenture alone does not influence the patient's food choice, although most patients are aware of and are subjectively satisfied with the improved chewing efficiency. The group of Jocelyne Feine in Montréal recently completed a randomized controlled trial where 113 wearers of conventional dentures and 103 wearers of conventional maxillary and implant-supported mandibular overdenture were enrolled (Hamdan and coworkers 2013). One year after denture delivery, fiber intake, macro- and micronutrient composition, and consumed energy were assessed. They concluded that implant overdentures alone fail to improve the food intake and the nutritional state of edentulous persons.

Nutritional habits and food intake are largely determined by habits. To actively disrupt established nutritional habits, the patient should be encouraged to try out new recipes and food items after the delivery of the implant-supported denture in order to increase the consumption of fruit and vegetable and give more "exercise" to the masticatory muscles (Bradbury and coworkers 2006). Poor masticatory performance is also related to a higher intake of digestive drugs (Brodeur and coworkers 1993) and slower postprandial protein metabolism (Rémond and coworkers 2007). Hence, improvements in chewing efficiency might aid the patient's digestion and overall well-being. Professional counseling by a nutritionist may help increase the patient's nutritional benefit from an implant-supported overdenture (Bradbury and coworkers 2006).

Denture stability is not the only factor limiting the nutritional intake of elderly persons. Wear of the acrylic denture teeth may preclude cutting the thin leaves of salad. Food particles might still get under the denture base, even with implants. It has been shown that age-related atrophy of masticatory muscles results in lower mandibular chewing forces (Newton and coworkers 1987). Our chewing movements are already ingrained at the age of 4 to 5 years and remain stable throughout over our entire lifetime. However, for every 10 years of aging we add three to four chewing cycles to each sequence, leaving mandibular movements and chewing rhythms largely unchanged (Peyron and coworkers 2004). And finally, mastication relies on motor coordination and oral perception, both of which deteriorate with age.

Esthetic aspects. Can implants improve esthetics? This question seems intriguing, as implants are not visible per se. Again, we need to look into the function of the conventional complete denture to highlight the benefit of implants supporting overdentures. In conventional dentures, the maxillary anteriors are set up according to esthetic needs, providing a natural profile and lip support, as well as morphological needs, facilitating speech. In contrast, the mandibular incisors of a complete denture have to be placed according to functional and static needs, to accommodate the orbicularis oris muscle and preclude denture displacement during mouth opening. In complete-denture wearers, this may result in a substantial overjet that may even become evident in patient's profile.

Although the teeth of an overdenture should generally be set up as in a complete denture, the stability afforded by the implants allows for a wider range of possible tooth positions, helping reconstruct the patient's very personal profile and look. However, care must be taken to assess the patient's expectations before inserting the implants, as unrealistic expectations may lead to profound disappointment and may cause the patient to lose confidence in the dentist. Implants cannot restore the patient to the young look he or she had on old photos taken with natural teeth—very often the wedding picture. Vertical wrinkles in the lips, reduced mandibular lip tone with more mandibular and fewer maxillary front teeth being visible, as well as thinner lips with less vermilion border are signs of physiological aging and cannot be corrected by prosthodontic means.

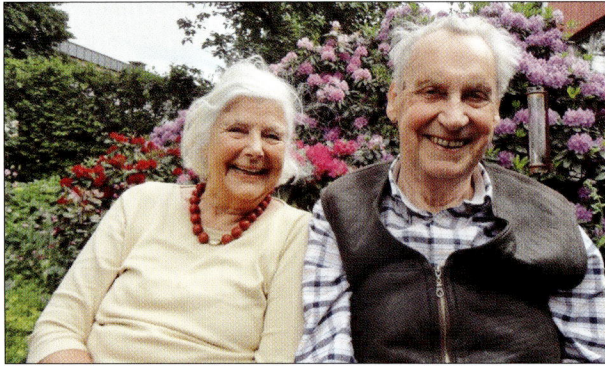

Fig 5   In complete-denture wearers, good retention seems to promote self-confidence in a social context. Being able to enjoy a meal in good company may help preventing social withdrawal.

Psychosocial aspects. Tooth loss and the wearing of a removable prosthesis can have a negative impact on self-esteem and psychosocial well-being. Just imagining the denture to come loose in a social context frightens most denture wearers. The inability to finish a meal within an acceptable time is feared and may lead to social isolation, even within an institutionalized environment (Fig 5). Wismeijer and his group achieved the convincing psychosocial rehabilitation of 104 complete-denture wearers by stabilizing their mandibular prostheses with Straumann implants (Wismeijer and coworkers 1997; Fig 6). Sixteen months after insertion, the patients were significantly more outgoing and sociable, visited their friends and family more often, and enjoyed going out to restaurants.

Oral health-related quality of life (OHRQoL) can also be measured with validated instruments that provide consistent information and allow comparing the situation before and after the treatment (Slade 2002). To assess the effectiveness of a treatment on the OHRQoL, a control intervention is necessary; it seems intuitive to compare patients with conventional complete dentures and patients with conventional maxillary and implant-supported mandibular overdentures. When randomized into one of these two treatment arms, both groups perceived an improvement in OHRQoL; however, only in the IOD group was the effect statistically significant. At the end of the 6-month observation period, the IOD patients indicated a significantly better OHRQoL (Heydecke and coworkers 2003b). This effect was confirmed in a context where patients were not randomized but received their treatment of choice (Rashid and coworkers 2011).

It seems intuitive to assume that satisfaction with IODs has to do with the cost involved, as humans tend to justify their expenses by expressing a high satisfaction with their purchase. However, within the context of a study, treatment is provided free of charge to the patient, so no financial bias is involved. Also, the higher satisfaction with complete IODs seems to last throughout the wearing period, even until 10 years after denture insertion (Meijer and coworkers 2003).

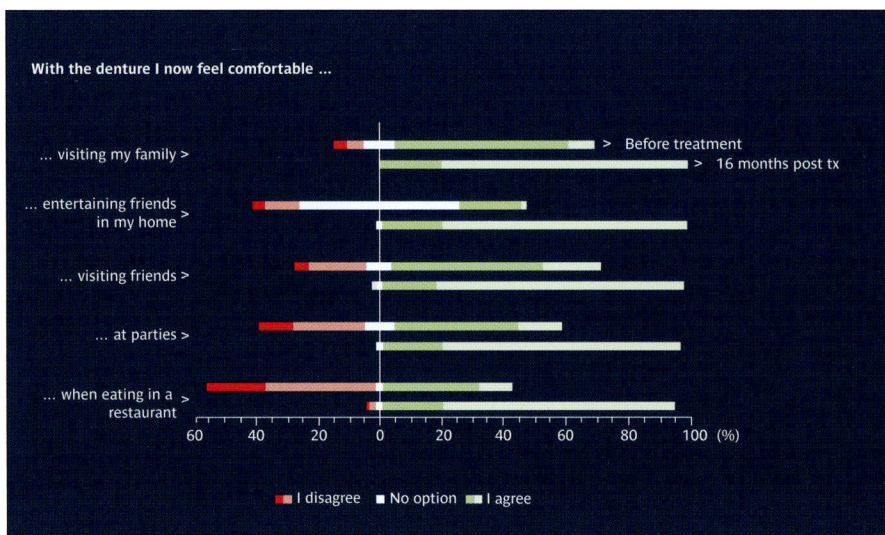

With the denture I now feel comfortable ...

... visiting my family >
... entertaining friends in my home >
... visiting friends >
... at parties >
... when eating in a restaurant >

> Before treatment
> 16 months post tx

60   40   20   0   20   40   60   80   100 (%)

I disagree   No option   I agree

Fig 6   Edentulous patients who had their mandibular dentures stabilized by two interforaminal implants participated much more in social activities 16 months after insertion of the overdenture (after Wismeijer and coworkers 1997).

Apprehensions and treatment acceptance

Besides the known and widespread barriers to oral health care for elderly adults, such as access to care and the lack of financial resources, implant treatment might be limited by poor general health. In addition to "objective" barriers, subjective apprehension influences the acceptance of implant treatment. Even with the treatment offered at no charge, 36% of elderly edentulous subjects refused implants within the context of a clinical study (MacEntee and coworkers 2005). Mostly, the fear of the surgical intervention accounted for the refusal, but there was also a lack of perceived need for improvement. In a survey conducted at the University of Geneva, the attitude towards and knowledge of implants and the hypothetical acceptance of implant treatment was investigated in 92 volunteers by means of a semi-structured interview. A stepwise backward multiple linear regression analysis revealed that not age as such but rather limited knowledge of implants, wearing (poor) dentures, and being a woman, as well as low autonomy in daily life are the predominant factors that give rise to apprehension in regard to implant treatment (Müller and coworkers 2012a).

Patient acceptance could therefore be increased by:

- Raising awareness for oral health and its impact on health and the quality of life.
- Providing professional information (in writing and pictures—neutral, legible).
- Suggesting treatment when the patient is still "fit" enough for the intervention and the surgical intervention is not perceived as an insurmountable burden.
- Proposing minimally invasive procedures.
- Proposing prosthodontic solutions which are easy to handle and straightforward to clean.

5 Medical Considerations for Dental Implant Therapy in the Elderly Patient

S. Barter

5.1 Introduction

The global population is aging due to decreasing mortality and declining fertility. Globally, the proportion of the over-60 population increased from 9.2% in 1990 to 11.7% in 2013 and is predicted to reach 21.1% by 2050—more than 2 billion people, of whom 20% will live in developed regions (United Nations 2013).

Improvements in health care and advances in medicine mean that people are living longer, even with chronic diseases; this in turn results in a greater incidence of elderly patients with multiple organ disease and as a consequence, more extensive and complex drug regimes.

Clinicians therefore more frequently see elderly patients with complex medical histories and long medication lists. While this chapter will examine the special considerations in the elderly patient for specific organ-system diseases, it must also highlight the need for an awareness of the effects of combinations of disease processes, the potential issues associated with multiple medications, and the impact not only of these issues on the treatment dental practitioners may provide, but also the impact our treatment may have on the general health and well-being of the patient.

Quality of life is in itself important in preserving health, and this can be in part reliant on the provision of good dental prostheses. Our patients frequently refuse to accept the esthetic, phonetic, and functional problems caused by the discomfort and limitations of loose complete dentures or a failing dentition—and why should they? Esthetics and self-esteem are no longer the privilege of the young. However, the more complex treatment we can now provide using dental implants is governed by the need for such treatment to be properly planned, executed with care and precision, and appropriately maintained, even if the aging patients become unable to do so themselves.

The treatment plan must address the general health and well-being of the patient, and there will have to be special considerations for elderly patients relating to:

- The elderly patient with a failing dentition and the selection of appropriate treatment options.
- Surgical considerations for elderly patients with medical problems, both intra- and postoperative.
- The management of medically compromised patients who already have dental implants, either for a replacement or modified prosthesis or as a result of biological/technical complications.
- Our responsibility as health-care providers to recognize possible changes in the overall health of a patient and notify other health-care providers accordingly.

A holistic approach to treatment is arguably even more important in elderly patients, where age-related vulnerability can mean a significant impact from treatment that in younger patients would be relatively innocuous; for dental implantology, this will include important considerations in the planning of surgical procedures. However, the prosthetic aspects of treatment will require equally careful planning to ensure that patients are able to cope with the associated procedures and to ensure that the prosthesis itself provides adequate comfort, function, ease of plaque control, and continuing mucosal health. We have a duty to ensure that in our efforts to "help" patients, we do not cause problems that become more significant as patients become increasingly frail.

Success (or more commonly, survival) rates for implants in healthy individuals have been reported as being as high as 99% over 15 years when implants are placed under ideal anatomical conditions (Lindquist and coworkers 1996). However, there is a lack of scientific literature regarding the use of dental implants in medically compromised patients, where outcomes can be significantly less favorable, and even less evidence relating to the elderly complex medical patient.

It is well documented that advanced age in itself is not a contraindication to successful implant treatment (Zarb and Schmitt 1993, de Baat 2000). However, one of the most important considerations related to the success of implant treatment is the matter of patient-related factors, of which the individual's medical health and the associated pharmacological considerations are paramount. This is especially so in elderly patients, when the increasing burden of age, multiple health issues, and increasing frailty result in a more complex series of interactions that may complicate the safe and successful provision of implant treatment and that can make a decision to provide implant-based treatment questionable. We have also to consider potential later problems in the maintenance of dental implants or the future treatment required for implants and related prostheses provided at an earlier age.

While most patients presenting for treatment with dental implants will be categorized according to the classification system of the American Society of Anesthesiology (ASA 2014) as P1 (normal healthy) or P2 (mild systemic disease), elderly patients with polymorbidities and polypharmaceutical therapies may increasingly move into P3 status (severe systemic disease). There is little evidence yet for the short and long-term performance of dental implants in these patients and even less for the practicality of such therapy. While we may reasonably decide that the initial provision of dental implants in more severely medically compromised patients should be delayed or abandoned, we can undoubtedly expect to see an increasing number of people who have received implant therapy in the past, are aging and becoming more medically compromised, but may require treatment for peri-implant diseases. Such treatment may be surgical, relating to the development of peri-implant disease, and could have important considerations regarding the patient's medical health. It has been observed that the elective dental treatment of patients classified as P4 (severe systemic disease that is a threat to life) or higher should ideally be postponed until the patient's medical condition has stabilized and improved to at least P3 (Maloney and Weinberg 2008).

Often, the goal of dental implant studies in medically compromised patients is to assess the success or survival of the implant itself. To ignore the possibility of wider health implications in providing surgical treatment with potential long-term care issues would be quite inappropriate. It is recognized that older adults require a different approach to oral health and dental treatment and that the dentist requires a more comprehensive knowledge of the effects of medical conditions and their treatment on oral health (Koller 1994). The progressive change in the health status of an increasing number of patients with dental implants presents a new challenge. Studies have shown that in the institutional setting there is little awareness of what dental implants are or how they should be cared for, although it was recognized that there were difficulties in caring for implants as compared to natural teeth (Kimura and coworkers 2015). It is therefore hoped that the present chapter will be helpful in highlighting the many interacting considerations governing the provision of care for the elderly patient who is considering, or has already received, implant therapy.

5.1.1 Aging and Multimorbidity

There is a greater prevalence of chronic, non-communicable disease and of disability in elderly people, and most developed countries already have significant aged populations that, moreover, are aging further. The global proportion of "oldest old" (persons 80 years or over) was 14% in 2013 and is predicted to rise to 19% by 2050—392 million people (United Nations 2013). As we age, our bodies undergo progressive changes in biology and physiology that will be influenced in different ways by psychosocial and genetic factors, functional and nutritional considerations, the side effects of drugs used to treat medical conditions, and both physical and mental disabilities. There are endless permutations of these factors, which makes it difficult to construct algorithms to deal with what has been described as comorbidity. Most guidelines are based on the diagnosis and treatment of single diseases and are often inapplicable to the polymorbid patient (Lugtenberg and coworkers 2011). The term "comorbidity" implies that a patient may have one major disease and one or more additional conditions or diseases that may or may not be interrelated. However, the real situation is of multiple chronic disorders in one patient—"polymorbidity" (or "multimorbidity")—all of which may interact on a constant, dynamic basis.

Population aging will have a significant effect on the prevalence of polymorbidity. One estimate based on the US population estimates between 2000 and 2030, the number of Americans with one or more chronic conditions will increase from 125 million to 171 million, an increase of 37% (46 million people) (Robert Wood Johnson Foundation 2010).

In a cross-sectional study of more than 175,000 patients, examining data on 40 conditions, it was reported that 65% of 65- to 84-year-olds have two or more diseases and that 82% of persons over 85 years have three or more diseases (Fig 1). However, the current total number of people with polymorbidity is highest in those younger than 65 years (Barnett and coworkers 2012; Table 1).

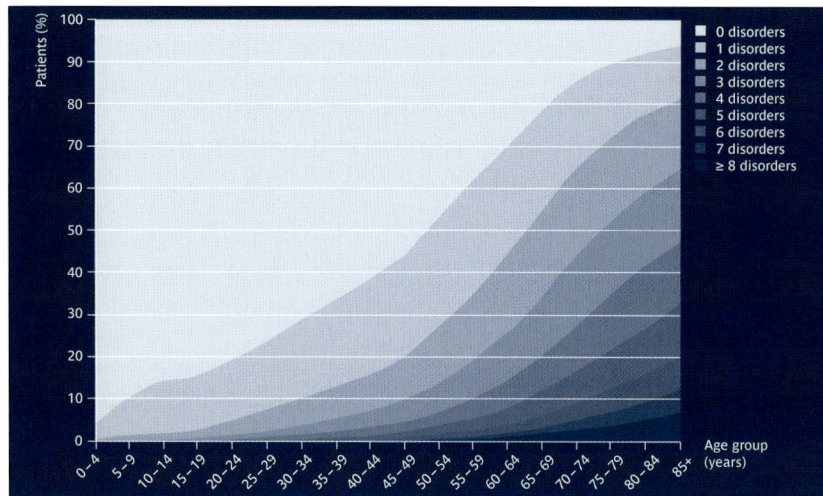

Fig 1   Number of chronic disorders by age group (Barnett and coworkers 2012).

This is an important consideration, as it brings the possibility that as these patients age, the number of elderly polymorbid patients will increase further. Polymorbidity is most prevalent in women, the very elderly, and in patients from lower socioeconomic classes (Marengoni and coworkers 2011), where polymorbidity is increasingly found in young and middle-age groups (Barnett and coworkers 2012). The prevalence of mental health disorders, including depression, is also greater in polymorbid individuals (Moussavi and coworkers 2007).

Scientific understanding of the combinations of diseases is poor due to innumerable permutations of the factors discussed above (van den Akker and coworkers 2001). Medical specialization can lead to the diseases rarely being investigated for their combined effect (Nobili and coworkers 2011). The interaction of two or more disease processes can be greater than the effect of each individual disease or it can be inhibitory, such as the effect of neurodegenerative disease on some neoplastic diseases (Plun-Favreau and coworkers 2010). The polymorbid elderly individual requires a more patient-centered approach in medicine, rather than the disease-centered approach engendered by the development of medical subspecialties.

It could perhaps be considered that there are not "seven ages of man" (Shakespeare) but three: biological, chronological and dental. There is evidence to suggest that polymorbidity will have a greater impact on immune function than age alone (Castle and coworkers 2005). Results of studies assessing surgery outcomes among the elderly do not support making decisions based only on patient age. In general, for surgical patients it appears that preoperative medical fitness is of greater importance than chronological age (Seymour and Vaz 1989).

Multimorbidity is certainly correlated with increasing mortality. It also seems clear that polymorbidity in the elderly is associated with an increased rate of functional decline, and this may be taken into consideration when planning implant treatment.

The most prevalent polymorbidity is that of cardiovascular disease (including hypertension), type 2 diabetes, and depression, and this cluster is associated with poor physical and mental health outcomes, significant morbidity, and mortality (Katon and coworkers 2010; Gallo and coworkers 2005). Indeed, depressive illness can have a greater detrimental impact on health than chronic angina, arthritis, asthma, or diabetes. Depression combined with other comorbidities will worsen health more than the same comorbidities without depression (Moussavi and coworkers 2007).

Such patients can be challenging to treat when considering complex dental rehabilitation, and expectation management with clear communication of the outcome that can realistically be achieved, is of paramount importance.

In addition, polymorbid patients have higher rates of disability and adverse drug events (ADEs) or lower health-related quality of life (Vogeli and coworkers 2007). Comorbidities such as coronary artery disease, diabetes mellitus, or anticoagulation may compromise wound healing. The main causes of deep neck infections are odontogenic (Boscolo-Rizzo and coworkers 2012); elderly polymorbid patients with dentoalveolar abscesses or deep peri-implant infections may present the surgeon with difficulty in the management of severe infections, which can develop and worsen rapidly.

Table 1   Odds ratios (OR) for any mental health disorder by age, sex, socioeconomic status, and number of physical disorders (Barnett and coworkers 2012)

	n (%)	Mean number of morbidities (SD)*	Percentage (95% CI) with multimorbidity[†]	Percentage (95% CI) with physical-mental health comorbidity[†]
All patients	1,751,841 (100%)	0.96 (1.56)	23.2% (23.1 – 23.2)	8.34% (8.3 – 8.4)
Sex				
Female	884,420 (50.5%)	1.09 (1.65)	26.2% (26.1 – 26.3)	10.2% (10.2 – 10.3)
Male	867,421 (49.5%)	0.84 (1.46)	20.1% (20.0 – 20.1)	6.4% (6.4 – 6.5)
Age, years				
0 – 24	479,156 (27.4%)	0.16 (0.44)	1.9% (1.9 – 2.0)	0.5% (0.5 – 0.6)
25 – 4	508,389 (29.0%)	0.50 (0.92)	11.3% (11.2 – 11.4)	5.7% (5.6 – 5.7)
45 – 64	473,127 (27.0%)	1.18 (1.50)	30.4% (30.2 – 30.5)	12.4% (12.3 – 12.5)
65 – 84	254,600 (14.5%)	2.60 (2.09)	64.9% (64.7 – 65.1)	17.5% (17.4 – 17.7)
≥ 85	36,569 (2.1%)	3.62 (2.30)	81.5% (81.1 – 81.9)	30.8% (30.3 – 31.3)
Deprivation decile				
1 (affluent)	163,283 (9.3%)	0.82 (1.42)	19.5% (19.3 – 19.6)	5.9% (5.8 – 6.0)
2	171,296 (9.8%)	0.83 (1.44)	19.9% (19.7 – 20.1)	6.2% (6.1 – 6.3)
3	165,199 (9.4%)	0.92 (1.50)	22.2% (22.0 – 22.4)	7.0% (6.9 – 7.1)
4	207,129 (11.8%)	0.95 (1.54)	23.0% (22.9 – 23.2)	7.5% (7.4 – 7.7)
5	198,419 (11.3%)	1.02 (1.60)	24.5% (24.3 – 24.7)	8.6% (8.5 – 8.7)
6	198,526 (11.3%)	0.97 (1.57)	23.4% (23.2 – 23.5)	8.4% (8.3 – 8.5)
7	186,083 (10.6%)	1.00 (1.59)	24.4% (24.2 – 24.6)	9.1% (9.0 – 9.2)
8	147,836 (8.4%)	1.00 (1.59)	24.2% (24.0 – 24.4)	9.3% (9.2 – 9.5)
9	164,386 (9.4%)	1.09 (1.70)	26.3% (26.1 – 26.5)	10.7% (10.6 – 10.9)
10 (deprived)	149,684 (8.5%)	1.01 (1.65)	24.1% (23.9 – 24.4)	11.0% (10.9 – 11.2)
Number of disorders				
0	1,012,980 (57.8%)	–	–	–
1	333,365 (19.0%)	–	–	–
2	167,518 (9.6%)	–	–	22.2% (22.0 – 22.4)
3	99,487 (5.7%)	–	–	36.1% (35.8 – 36.4)
4	60,417 (3.4%)	–	–	44.8% (44.4 – 45.2)
5	35,641 (2.0%)	–	–	52.1% (51.6 – 52.6)
6	20,507 (1.2%)	–	–	59.0% (58.3 – 59.7)
7	11,080 (0.6%)	–	–	65.7% (64.8 – 66.6)
≥ 8	10,846 (0.6%)	–	–	73.9% (73.1 – 74.7)

* Differences between means within each variable differed significantly $p < 0.0001$ (t-test for independent samples for sex; one-way ANOVA for age group and deprivation)
† Differences between categories within each variable differed significantly $p < 0.0001$ (χ^2 test for 2xn tables)

There is little evidence to provide a scientific basis for the evidence-based care of patients affected by polymorbidity. Reports in the surgical field tend to be condition- or procedure-based, with no data being available that could be used to provide collaborative guidelines. Clinicians continue to find it difficult to apply disease-specific guidelines to elderly patients with multiple conditions and to reconcile perceived clinical needs with patients' treatment priorities (Fried and coworkers 2011a).

The most commonly used prognostic tool in clinical research for assessing risks from polymorbidity is the Charlson index. Although first published over 25 years ago (Charlson and coworkers 1987), it is increasingly viewed as the gold standard in assessing and highlighting the clinical risk of the burden of multiple illness (de Groot and coworkers 2003).

Models for the successful treatment of elderly patients with polymorbidities have been demonstrated as successful, designed as they are around multidisciplinary teams working in very close collaboration. However, the uptake of such programs will likely be restricted by operational and financial barriers, as well as by the low availability of experts in chronic care (Boult and coworkers 2009).

In the dental field, in particular where systemic risk factors for implant therapy are concerned, there is little information on the use of oral implants with individual systemic diseases, nor in situations of polymorbidity (Cochran and coworkers 2009). Risks of implant complications are frequently reported, but there is little associated reporting of general medical complications, with the possible exception of conditions such as osteoradionecrosis or bisphosphonate-related osteonecrosis. There is a need for the reporting of complications; calls for well-designed prospective trials may be unrealistic, given the cohort-based problems of studying this subject. However, clinicians must be encouraged to submit case reports in a structured manner that may allow the gathering of useful data.

We need to be aware of the wide-ranging possible issues that may affect our patients, and we must be vigilant. In assessing the multiple factors of implant treatment for the geriatric patient, dentists must understand the prevailing medical conditions, their pharmacologic management, and possible functional limitations in terms of patients' ability to cope with and contribute to different aspects of care, as well as pitfalls that may arise (Shay 1994). Examples of such considerations are listed in the following sections of this chapter.

In conclusion, polymorbidity affects more than half of the elderly population, with increasing prevalence in the oldest old, women, and people from lower social classes. Very little is known about risk factors for polymorbidity; however, it is recognized that polymorbidity can have a major impact on functional impairment, poor quality of life, and increased usage of health-care services, with a detrimental impact on health economics.

5.1.2 Polypharmacy

Older patients are more likely to be taking medications, and inevitably greater numbers of drugs, for multiple chronic conditions, with prevalence increasing for each decade of aging after the age of 60. The incidence of adverse drug effects (ADEs) associated with unexpectedly high plasma concentrations is increased in the elderly, as is the rate of reactions to normal therapeutic blood levels, although drug allergies are no more prevalent than in younger age groups (Iber and coworkers 1994). This requires an understanding of the effects of the drugs and the possibility of interactions with drugs prescribed by the dentist.

The effects of drugs are different in elderly patients when compared to younger adults, with significant variation in sensitivity to certain drugs. Absorption rates may be similar in the two age groups, but changes in body fat and water composition may affect therapeutic drug levels. As fat stores increase, the half-life of lipid-soluble drugs also increases. Similarly, as total body water content decreases with age, the concentration of water-soluble drugs may increase. The metabolism and excretion of drugs will also change with age-related hepatic and renal changes. For example, drugs that bind to plasma proteins (for example digoxin) produce effects only from the unbound portion of the drug, so in elderly patients with malnutrition or polymorbidity, a decrease in serum albumin levels may result in higher therapeutic levels and an increased effect of the drug.

Polypharmacy has been variously defined as "the practice of administering many different medicines, especially concurrently (as in the treatment of a single disease or of several coexisting conditions)," (Merriam-Webster 2015), "the use of inappropriate medications" (Farrell and coworkers 2013) and "the use of more medications that are medically required" (Tjia and coworkers 2013).

Table 2   Examples of age-related pharmacokinetic and pharmacodynamic changes (after Nobili and coworkers 2011)

Pharmacokinetics	Age-related changes	Clinical considerations
Absorption	Decreased gastric and saliva secretion; delayed gastric emptying; decreased mesenteric blood flow, impaired absorption and active transport, reduced hepatic blood flow	Greater effect of acid labile drugs (penicillin, erythromycin) Reduced absorption of actively transported drugs (calcium folate, B_{12}); reduced rate of absorption; increased effect of drugs undergoing first-pass metabolism
Distribution	Reduction in total body water, increase in body fat. Changes in plasma-protein binding (reduced serum albumin, increase in α-1-acid glycoprotein)	Higher serum levels of water soluble drugs (digoxin, theophylline, aminoglycosides) Lower serum levels of lipid soluble drugs
Metabolism	Reduced hepatic blood flow, volume, and rate of liver phase-I metabolism (phase-II relatively unaffected)	High clearance rate drugs retained longer; reduction in phase-I metabolized drugs (SSRIs, benzodiazepines)
Excretion	Reduction in renal blood flow, (in excess of decrease in cardiac output) mass, GFR, hence a 40% to 50% decrease in renal function with age	Accumulation of drugs excreted in un-metabolized for (gabapentin, aminoglycosides); reduction in the excretion of other drug metabolites or those eliminated by tubular secretion (penicillin, cimetidine)

Pharmacodynamics	Age-related changes	Clinical considerations
Sensitivity/ tolerance	Increased sensitivity to benzodiazepines	Sedation, confusion, falls risk
Drug/receptor interactions	Increased sensitivity to anticholinergic effects	Agitation, confusion, orthostatic hypotension
Age-related change in target system	Greater inhibition of vitamin K synthesis by warfarin	Increased bleeding

The presence of concomitant multiple diseases frequently results in the provision of multiple medications, which is of course a common form of polypharmacy. However, there appears to be no currently accepted definition of the number of concurrent medications that constitute polypharmacy (Hajjar and coworkers 2007).

Regardless of the lack of consensus on definitions, the prevalence of multiple-drug regimes is indisputable. A national survey in the USA concluded that 57% of women over 65 years were taking more than 5 medications per day, and 12% of those women more than 10 medications (Kaufman and coworkers 2002). In Europe, it has been estimated that more than half of the elderly population is taking more than 6 medications per day (Fialová and coworkers 2005).

All medicines have the potential for harm as well as benefit; a medication that may be very beneficial in the treatment of one specific condition may have a less beneficial effect, or even cause harm, in a situation of multiple diseases. Multiple-drug regimes can give rise to risks such as adverse effects, drug-drug interactions, drug-disease interactions, and dose errors, any or all of which can cause additional morbidity (Gandhi and coworkers 2003). Such ADEs also have a significant impact on health-care economics.

Polypharmacy is as prevalent in the outpatient setting as it is in institutions. An elderly patient with heart failure and COPD will usually be taking at least five prescription medications (Boyd and coworkers 2005). A US-based outpatient study found that 36% of women and 37.1% of men aged 75 to 85 years took at least five prescription medications with approximately half also taking non-prescription medications (Qato and coworkers 2008).

In the hospital setting, polypharmacy may be more prevalent, with reports of up to 58.6% of patients taking one or more medications that were unnecessary (Rossi and coworkers 2007); it is possible that the number of prescribed medications for an individual will actually increase as a result of hospitalization for medical conditions (Hajjar and coworkers 2005).

There is less evidence for the occurrence of polypharmacy in the institutional setting (Tjia and coworkers 2013). Some have suggested that the prevalence may be lower (Bronskill and coworkers 2012), particularly amongst the very old (over 85 years) (Dwyer and coworkers 2010). Other research has shown that more than 90% of community-residing residents were exposed to a potential error in their medication (Zermansky and coworkers 2006).

In 2008, about 1.9 million people in England had more than one long-term condition managed with a number of different medicines (Department of Health UK 2012) and this figure is expected to reach 2.9 million by 2018, approximately one quarter of whom will be aged 65 years or older. The UK National Institute for Clinical Excellence (NICE) has published figures indicating that 30%–50% of medicines prescribed for long-term conditions are not taken as intended. The guidance notes that "when patients move from one care setting to another, between 30 per cent and 70 per cent of patients experience an error or unintentional change to their medicines." The same report found that 5% to 8% of all hospital admissions are due to preventable ADEs or interactions with other medicines (NICE 2015).

There are many unanswered questions, including benefit-to-harm ratios inherent in polypharmacy and the health priorities of an individual patient—future mortality may be of less concern to the patient than quality of life (Fried and coworkers 2011b; Kuluski and coworkers 2013).

Many prescribing guidelines are inevitably based on a disease-specific approach, and the prevalence of events associated with multiple medications is probably underestimated, since the available data reflect only recognized ADEs. Much remains unknown about the wider physical, cognitive, psychological, and other effects that may yet be unrecognized (Tinetti and coworkers 2004).

This is particularly so in elderly patients with multiple health conditions, who are often excluded from randomized controlled trials (Gross and coworkers 2002). Consequently, there is little evidence-based information on the effects of multiple drugs on adverse events, health-care economics, quality of life, and mortality, as coexisting conditions are often only considered if they have an impact on the target condition of the study (Jones and coworkers 2009; Guyatt and coworkers 1994).

However, it is recognized that the impact of polypharmacy on patients over 65 years is greater (Beijer and de Blaey 2002). Factoring in the increasing age of a patient adds further complicating issues, such as the differences in pharmacokinetics and pharmacodynamics of certain medications in the elderly, leading to increasing susceptibility and sensitivity with age (Hanlon and coworkers 2010). Inappropriate drug prescriptions are relatively common in the elderly community (Stuck and coworkers 1994). Patients frequently do not know why they are taking a particular medicine. Elderly patients are less likely to recognize insidious and slowly progressive changes in their health and report these to their physician. Missed interaction between patient and general medical practitioner, a lack of knowledge, or misunderstandings related to the complexity of the current drug regime can lead to further complications (Gandhi and coworkers 2003)—such as falls, cognitive impairment, urinary incontinence, malnutrition (Maher and coworkers 2014), or conditions that result in further prescriptions and the development of a "prescription cascade," where a drug is prescribed to treat a side effect of another (Farrell and coworkers 2013).

There is evidence to suggest that patients on combinations of drugs for multiple medical conditions only manage to take about 50% of their medications correctly as prescribed and that "medication adherence" (the ability to take the correct medications at the right time and dose) only worsens as the number of drugs increases (Haynes and coworkers 1996). Various compliance aids can be used to help reduce non-adherence (Barat and coworkers 2001; Claxton and coworkers 2001). These may include drug-list checks with a pharmacist, who can then provide a medication timetable for the patient or caregiver. The dental professional should provide clear and appropriate information on how their own prescribing should fit in with their patients' ongoing medication. However, there will be particular considerations in patients suffering from dementia or living alone. Complex prescription regimes in combination with memory loss or cognitive decline can severely affect the ability to comply with doses and frequencies or adhere to other treatment recommendations.

As a health-care professional, the dental practitioner has an important role to play in being alert for any situation that may affect patients' general health. The most common ADE are inevitably associated with the most commonly prescribed drugs. One paper identified a rate of adverse drug events of 50.1 per 1,000 person-years of exposure, of which 38% were serious, life-threatening, or fatal, and more than 25% were preventable (Gurwitz and coworkers 2003); the most common medications associated with ADEs are frequently taken by patients receiving implant therapy:

- Cardiovascular medications   24.5%
- Diuretics   22.1%
- Non-opioid analgesics   15.4%
- Hypoglycemics   10.9%
- Anticoagulants   10.2%

Antibiotics, steroids, opioids, anticholinergics and benzodiazepines are also frequently involved in ADEs.

There are important potential side effects and interactions between drugs in these groups and commonly prescribed analgesics and antibiotics used in dental implant surgery. Equally important considerations apply to the medications a patient may be taking and surgical implant procedures. For example, a survey of complications associated with the dental use of local anesthetics indicated that, while the incidence in patients with no risk factors was 3.3%, this more than doubled to 6.9% in patients taking more than two medications per day (Daubländer and coworkers 1997). Lower body weight or changes in drug metabolism in the elderly can more easily result in overdoses of local anesthetics, particularly if inappropriately long procedures are performed. It is generally recommended that maximum local anesthetic doses be halved in patients over 65 years due to reduced liver function. Other important and relevant examples of such considerations are described in each of the sections below.

It is also necessary to consider what non-prescription medications a patient may be taking in addition to the prescribed drugs—this may contribute to the rate of polypharmacy in the general public and is often not considered (Batty and coworkers 1997). Over-the-counter (OTC) medications are used more frequently by elderly patients (Sihvo and coworkers 2000), who—as previously described—frequently suffer from polymorbidity and prescription polypharmacy.

In one example of a population-based study, in older age groups (75 to 85 years) taking at least one prescription medication, 47.3% reported the use of an OTC medication, and 54.2%, of a dietary supplement (Qato and coworkers 2008). Other studies reported 90% of elderly patients taking at least one OTC drug (Stoehr and coworkers 1997); rates of use of dietary supplements approach 60%, and of herbal supplements, 14% (Kaufman and coworkers 2002).

Patients often regard OTC medications as safe, with no significant side effects (Wawruch and coworkers 2013) and regularly fail to read the package information leaflets (Hanna and coworkers 2011). However, studies have shown that up to 50% of elderly patients taking OTC medications were at risk of ADEs (Olesen and coworkers 2013).

Commonly used OTC medications in the elderly include analgesics (e.g., acetaminophen, ibuprofen, acetylsalicylic acid), which are known to significantly contribute to ADEs in the elderly. Also implicated are cold and cough medications (e.g., pseudoephedrine, diphenhydramine), dietary supplements (e.g., multi- and single-vitamin supplements, glucosamine), antacids, and laxatives. Herbal medications are also commonly taken by elderly people (e.g., ginseng, Ginkgo biloba extract, St. John's wort). All of these can have potentially significant ADEs when taken alone or in combination with prescribed medicines.

The role of community pharmacists in assisting patients with OTC medications is important; pharmacists gather specific information about patients' medication profiles, health conditions, characteristics of the problem, and past treatments in order to make a recommendation (Chui and coworkers 2013).

Some publications list drugs that are unwise to use in elderly patients and generally "safe" drugs that can occasionally cause problems, and these can be useful points of reference (Beers and coworkers 1991; Fick and coworkers 2003).

It is clear that there is a complex web of interactions between medical conditions, the medications used in their treatment, and the physiological effects of aging, with an almost infinite number of possible permutations. The situation will be dynamic; for example, given the period of time over which even a simple implant therapy may take place, there may be a change in medication or dose. This can cause significant problems in the complex management of the elderly patient for medical professionals in the primary-care setting (Del Fiol and coworkers 2014).

It is easy to consider only the possible impact of drug changes on the procedure we as dental practitioners are about to undertake. However, in doing so we may miss subtle changes in the well-being of the patient, such as increasing confusion, which could be dismissed as "getting old" but might in fact be a result of a minor prescription change or the introduction of an OTC medication. The changes could have wider consequences—which could be as straightforward as patients not understanding the postoperative instructions you have given them, with events that could potentially lead to treatment failure.

5.1.3 Frailty

The syndrome of frailty has been described as a state of increased vulnerability towards stressors in older individuals, leading to a heightened risk of adverse health outcomes (Fried and coworkers 2005). However, there is no accepted consensus on the definition of frailty.

Frailty is considered highly prevalent in old age and is associated with a high risk of falls, disability, hospitalization, and mortality. Frailty has previously been considered synonymous with disability and comorbidity, but it has been recognized that it may have a biologic basis and be a distinct clinical syndrome, with an intermediate stage identifying persons at risk of becoming frail (Fried and coworkers 2001). Comorbidity is a known risk factor in the development of frailty; together, frailty and comorbidity are strongly related to impaired immunological status and periodontal disease (Charlson and coworkers 1987).

Physiological reserves are lower in frail patients and may become inadequate for the maintenance and repair of multiple systems in the aging body (Lang and coworkers 2009). Multiple authors have identified characteristics of frailty to include wasting (loss of muscle mass and strength, with consequent weight loss), loss of endurance, decreased balance and mobility, slowed performance, relative inactivity, and potentially decreased cognitive function. Frailty is a distinct entity from aging; symptoms are multiple and may include appearance (whether or not consistent with age), nutritional status (thin, weight loss), subjective health rating (health perception), performance (cognition, fatigue), sensory/physical impairments (vision, hearing, strength), and current care (medication, hospital). Increasing frailty is considered potentially reversible. Given the need for good nutrition to combat several of the above symptoms, adequate masticatory function and good oral health are important factors in the prevention of increasing frailty (Saarela and coworkers 2014).

A combination of aging and frailty can make it difficult for patients to access conventional care (Vernooij-Dassen and coworkers 2011) in both the dental and medical fields. Misunderstanding the concept of frailty by health care providers can result in an increased level of care being required by the frail patient. Loss of hearing, visual impairment and cognitive decline can compromise compliance by the patient, as can social factors such as living alone and economic difficulty (Nobili and coworkers 2011).

Coordination between clinicians and caregivers, with clear communication of clinical and therapeutic decisions for the frail elderly patient is vitally important in successful short-term and long-term health-care efficiency (Kripalani and coworkers 2007).

Frail and vulnerable elderly people have a higher risk of oral diseases; their treatment needs are often complicated by medical, functional, and psychosocial factors. They may be unable to express their needs or the fact that they are in pain; they may be incapable of performing simple oral hygiene procedures. Care providers are often unaware of the importance of oral health and are frequently unlikely to understand the nature of even simple implant-based rehabilitations.

We should remember that the treatment of the aging, polymorbid, or frail patient is not just a consideration of whether or not to provide implant treatment. We are inexorably moving towards a population of such patients already treated with dental implants. This cohort will require maintenance therapy, replacement of prostheses, or treatment of technical and biological complications such as fractured prostheses, components, implants and the development of peri-implant disease. Such treatment is frequently not simple, and in the case of the latter conditions it may require surgical intervention.

In this patient group, it will be important to consider such factors as the timing of treatment in relation to other health-care needs, the length of the procedure (which may be directly related to the experience and proficiency of the surgeon), the ability of patient to cope with the treatment, and the balance between breaking down the treatment into shorter sessions versus considerations such as the modification of prescribed medications, or the need for anesthesia or sedation and their impact on the patient's general health.

Comprehensive medical assessment of the geriatric patient, and in particular the effects of polymorbidity, polypharmacy, and frailty, is an essential component in the provision of safe and effective dental care. Obtaining an accurate history will be essential.

5.1.4 Taking the Patient's Medical History

Patients should be assessed in the context of all their problems, including:

- Dental problems (such as pain, difficulties with function, comfort, patients' needs and wishes).
- Medical problems, polymorbidity and polypharmacy considerations, past surgical issues, etc.
- Psychosocial factors (see Chapter 3).
- Planning for decline and the effect on/impact of our treatment (see Chapter 11).

However, obtaining a clear medical history from a geriatric patient can sometimes be challenging, especially if there is a lot of history to unravel. It may be wise to plan consultation appointments of greater length, as more time will be required. In a busy primary-care setting, this may seem impractical, but time spent on getting the patient's history gives a greater chance of identifying and preventing complications later. It may be easier to be wise in hindsight, but foresight and planning make for happy patients, better economics, and fewer sleepless nights for clinicians.

Many factors could influence this process, including sensory impairment; patients with hearing loss may need induction loops to render hearing aids more effective. That soothing in-surgery music could be counterproductive, and other extraneous noise (suction, outside traffic, etc.), while merely "background" to you, may be a cacophony that prevents the patient from hearing not only what you say, but also the way you say it. Misunderstandings and confusion can result, adding to the stress and to the problem of obtaining or imparting important information. A quiet room is essential; sitting closer to the patient, ensuring they can see your face, and talking clearly and slowly in an even tone is helpful. Stop frequently to check understanding—both yours and theirs.

Another factor in getting the patient's medical history is that elderly patients may have cognitive impairments and quite simply cannot remember when their dentures were made or when a tooth first began to hurt. Elderly patients may find it difficult to describe a problem or symptom, so particular complaints may seem vague; this could be the sign of a change from their normal "baseline" and could be important.

A structured approach to getting a medical history will help both the clinician and the patient along. A template is highly recommended, as it acts as a checklist to make sure that there are no errors or omissions, particularly with patients who are poor historians, confused, or simply delighted to have a rare opportunity of social contact and will provide a verbal autobiography spanning many decades of their life. Most clinicians will have experienced the difficulty of filtering important information from a rambling but enthusiastic account of a patient's lifetime medical and dental experiences.

Designing a history template will depend a lot on the clinical setting, personal preference, culture, and many other factors. However, there are useful strategies that can be employed to obtain the required information, including:

- *Review past records in advance.* It is not possible to listen well and read old records at the same time. In addition, there may be notes in past records that may indicate a specific line of questioning that needs to be pursued.
- *Provide a self-administered questionnaire in advance.* While such questionnaires have been shown to be useful (Scully and Boyle 1983), elderly patients may have difficulty with such questionnaires due to visual impairment or memory loss (Kilmartin 1994). Providing the questionnaire in advance allows the opportunity for family members or caregivers to help in the accurate completion of the form and prevent omissions.
- *Obtain a current repeat prescription/medication list.* Perhaps from the patient, caregiver or general medical practitioner.
- *Specifically ask about "alternative" medications.* Gingko biloba, St. John's wort, Echinacea, vitamin, and mineral supplements may be considered "safe" and therefore unimportant by the patient, but they may cause interactions.
- *Bring a family member/caregiver/friend.* Elderly patients sometimes have a poor social network. Slow changes in chronic conditions will often go unnoticed in the patient, and confused patients may be unable to identify new problems. Having someone present at a consultation who knows the patient well can be very helpful in both obtaining a good medical history and in terms of imparting information, as well as facilitating the matter of consent.

- *Understand when to use open and closed questioning.* Also, understand when cognitive issues may make answers unreliable.
- *Consult with other clinicians.* Confirming important details and filling in the information gaps is achieved by communicating clearly and promptly with the patient's general medical practitioner, referring dentist, and other specialists.

The following sections will deal with considerations related to the elderly patient and, inevitably, are stratified by organ system. The irony of the classification is not lost on the author, given the previously discussed problems in adopting a disease-specific approach to patient care and the need for a wider consideration of the interactions between diseases, the medications used to treat, and the multiplicity of patient-specific factors. While aging is a term used in different ways, the occurrence of age-related changes to a specific organ system resulting in decreased efficiency is known as "senescence."

Senescence is associated with a lack of physiological reserves in the organ system, with a concomitant decrease in repair or regeneration, decreased ability to cope with stressors, and an increase in susceptibility to disease or infection. The functional decline of one organ system will lead to the decline of other organ systems and consequent further considerations in polymorbid geriatric patients.

Each section will consider:

- The medical background of the condition and normal age-related changes.
- The impact of disease on implant dentistry (both placement and long-term maintenance) and vice versa.
- Treatment considerations.
- The drugs to treat the disease and the impact of medication on implant therapy.
- Possible interactions with drugs commonly used in dentistry.

5.2 Cardiovascular System

5.2.1 Age-related Changes

Cardiovascular aging is a continuous and irreversible process, which remains the most common cause of death and is likely to remain so in the near future (World Health Organization 2011). The rate of cardiovascular decline is affected by other physiological changes that occur with advancing age, the sequelae of previous health events, and lifestyle (Ribera-Casado 1999).

Age-related changes in the heart include structural and conduction issues, such as thinning and weakening of the myocardium, increased atrioventricular conduction time, decreased resting and maximum heart rate, decreased baroreflex, and an increase in ectopic atrial and ventricular beats.

The prevalence of cardiovascular disease increases with age in both men and women. For men, prevalence increases from 3.3% at age 16–24 to 53.8% at age 85 and above. For women, prevalence increases from 4.8% at age 16–24 to 31.1% at age 85 and above (Oyebode 2012).

Cardiovascular disease includes conditions such as hypertension, atherosclerosis, coronary artery disease, atrial fibrillation, and chronic heart failure, all of which are prevalent in the elderly population (Aronow 2002).

The main age-related structural and functional changes are in the cardiac tissue, the conduction system, and the coronary arteries. However, there is a general decrease in blood supply to all tissues due to age-related vascular narrowing and peripheral vascular disease. Atherosclerotic changes result in decreased blood flow and consequent reduction in oxygenation of tissues. Wound healing is dependent on angioneogenesis, collagen formation, and macrophage activity, all of which in turn depend on good oxygenation (Gottrup 2004). Good tissue perfusion and oxygenation is also important in preventing infection (Rabkin and Hunt 1988).

Coronary artery disease is an atherosclerotic narrowing of the vessels resulting in ischemic changes in the cardiac muscle, which causes angina. It has been suggested that the prevalence of symptomatic ischemic heart disease is only 10% to 50% of the true prevalence in older patients, who may not exercise sufficiently to experience angina or dyspnea due to musculoskeletal or other medical problems (Andres and coworkers 1990).

Myocardial infarction can result from severe narrowing or can occur more suddenly if an atherosclerotic plaque detaches and forms a thrombus that blocks an artery. Ischemic cardiac tissue becomes necrotic and results in functional deficits of the muscular structure of the heart wall. Survival rates after myocardial infarction remain low but are improving, and after a period of healing and with appropriate treatment, patients can return to relatively normal function. However, approximately 75% of sufferers of a myocardial infarction (MI) have further complications in the following days or hours, such as arrhythmias, cardiogenic shock, pericarditis, myocardial rupture, or progressive heart failure (Schoen 2005)

Hypertension is a widespread form of cardiovascular disease with an increased prevalence in elderly patients due to age-related structural and physiological changes in the cardiovascular system, including arteriosclerosis and atherosclerosis. It is potentially fatal, with a 2-mmHg rise in systolic pressure being associated with a 7% increased risk of fatality. Hypertension increases the risk of ischemic heart disease and cerebrovascular events, chronic renal disease, and cognitive decline. It has been shown that blood pressure rises during or after medical or dental visits ("white-coat syndrome")—and particularly during oral surgical procedures. Baseline and intraoperative blood-pressure monitoring may be useful in the overall monitoring of the elderly surgical patient (Kilmartin 1994; Lambrecht and coworkers 2011).

Recent evidence suggests that the effect of lifestyle on the risk of myocardial infarction is more significant than genetic factors or a family history of, for example, coronary artery disease (Horne and Anderson 2015). Hypertension, hyperlipidemia, obesity, and type 2 diabetes are prevalent conditions in the aging population that are predicted to result in an increasing number of older patients with cardiovascular disease (CVD) (Pandya and coworkers 2013).

5.2.2 Treatment Considerations

There are anatomical and histological changes resulting from vascular changes in aging bone and decreased tissue oxygenation. It has been demonstrated that in the edentulous mandible there may be a significant deterioration of the inferior alveolar artery, with periosteal stripping for dentoalveolar surgery potentially compromising the predominant vascular supply, resulting in poor bony healing and a risk of osteonecrosis (Bradley 1981). Decreased oxygenation of tissues results in a reduction of fibroblast activity, collagen production, angioneogenesis, and macrophage activity, all of which may increase the risk of postoperative infection.

However, there is evidence to suggest that there is no increased risk of osseointegration failure in patients with well-controlled cardiovascular disease (Khadivi and coworkers 1999; Moy and coworkers 2005; Alsaadi and coworkers 2007; Alsaadi and coworkers 2008).

Historically, established guidance has been to delay dental treatment for six months following myocardial infarction (Hwang and Wang 2006), as it is important to avoid stress, which could trigger post-ischemic complications (Niwa and coworkers 2000). Advances in the treatment of ischemic heart disease including thrombolytic therapy and coronary artery bypass grafting, which increase the rate of reperfusion and salvage ischemic tissue, have recently improved the treatment of patients with the disease. There are indications that patients with unstable angina or a recent MI may safely undergo minimally invasive dental treatment if appropriate precautions are taken, including monitoring and anxiety management such as sedation (Niwa and coworkers 2000). However, 10% of the patients treated experienced a cardiovascular complication either during the dental procedures or in the first week thereafter.

Other studies support the opinion that it may be not be necessary to delay potentially beneficial treatment for so long and that a post-MI patient who has been medically assessed as having no risk of continued ischemia may be allowed to undergo dental surgery with the support of the cardiologist as early as six weeks after an MI. Such treatment would need to be carried out with prophylactic nitrates, continuous supplementary oxygen (in the absence of contraindicating respiratory conditions, author's comment), monitoring of oxygen saturation, blood pressure, and heart rate, adequate local anesthesia, perioperative pain medication, and stress reduction measures, in a hospital setting (Roberts and Mitnitsky 2001).

It is important to note that such studies investigate the effects of only relatively simple dental treatments of up to 30 minutes that are minimally invasive; the procedures were performed in hospitals with appropriate specialist support. The recommendation remains that more prolonged or invasive non-essential elective procedures, such as implant placement, be delayed for three to six months after an MI and planned in conjunction with the patient's physician or cardiologist.

Stress or anxiety management and adequate pain control are key factors in the safe management of patients with ischemic heart disease (Findler and coworkers 1993). Following invasive dental procedures, these patients may suffer post-infarction angina, arrhythmia, or left ventricular failure demonstrated by a reduced ejection fraction. Such events are more frequent in elderly patients (Niwa and coworkers 2000).

While elderly patients may satisfactorily tolerate normal stress, they may not cope well with severe stress because of a lack of organ system reserves. For example, although resting cardiac function in a healthy elderly patient will normally be adequate for physiological needs, normal or almost normal cardiac output in the elderly has to be maintained under stress by increasing the stroke volume and the ejection fraction—i.e. the heart is "working harder." As with any muscle working harder, increased oxygenation is required, as may be an augmented cardiac filling (preload) (Ribera-Casado 1999). The myocardial muscle responds favorably to preload up to a point, beyond which, rather than increasing cardiac output, it may fail, giving rise to an ischemic event.

The stress of treatment and related pain results in catecholamine-mediated hypertension and tachycardia, which can affect the oxygen tension in the myocardium, induce cardiac spasm, and increase platelet aggregation (Muller and coworkers 1989). Hypertensive events are the main risk factors for complications in cardiovascular events precipitated by stressors such as dental or surgical treatment, and elderly patients, particularly those who are polymorbid, are frequently high-risk cardiovascular patients. Some researchers have highlighted the value of monitoring the heart rate, blood pressure and oxygen saturation during outpatient oral surgery, finding that in 0.6% of patients (n = 3,012) the procedure had to be discontinued due to significant hypertension or cardiac arrhythmias (Lambrecht and coworkers 2011). Prophylactic anxiety control with appropriate medications may also be useful.

While there are cardiac effects associated with epinephrine-containing local anesthetics, these are usually slight. It has been argued that significant effects occur in CVD patients or those on beta-blockers, but the clinical significance of the reported effects is debatable—for example, interactions in patients on beta-blockers have only been demonstrated when excessively large doses of epinephrine-containing local anesthetics have been used. There is also evidence that inadequate local anesthesia and pain control will result in even greater endogenous catecholamine release (Scully 2014).

It is preferable to avoid general anesthesia in patients with cardiovascular disease, especially elderly patients, and intravenous sedation is commonly used for anxiety control. For the cardiac patient, such techniques can be useful and may prevent excessive intraoperative hypertension (Taguchi and coworkers 2011). However, intravenous midazolam does not prevent the occurrence of certain cardiac arrhythmias during procedures such as the placement of dental implants (Romano and coworkers 2012), although the arrhythmias noted did not present a serious clinical risk.

Hypotensive events such as syncope are also associated with dental treatment and are more prevalent in elderly patients (Soteriades and coworkers 2002), where orthostatic hypotension can occur as a result of lengthy immobility during prolonged treatment (Ungar and coworkers 2009). Hypotension reduces coronary-artery perfusion and increases the risk of thrombotic occlusion. Fainting in the elderly patient can have many causes, including cardiopulmonary or cerebrovascular events as well as pharmacological ones.

Congestive cardiac failure is the leading cause of hospitalization in people over 65 years, with a 10% mortality rate. Symptoms include dyspnea due to pulmonary hypertension and pulmonary edema. Treating such patients in a supine position for prolonged periods is inadvisable, and coughing may complicate treatment itself. Advanced congestive cardiac failure in the elderly patient can, like other forms of CVD, result in reduced cerebral perfusion and disorientation or confusion.

Appointment planning for implant treatment in elderly patients with CVD therefore has to be managed carefully and systematically, bearing in mind those risks. One possibility is to schedule appointments for the late morning, when endogenous epinephrine levels are falling, and to have the patient's glyceryl trinitrate spray readily available or even used prophylactically if necessary. Shorter appointments that are less stressful or require less chair time may be preferable to prolonged treatment sessions. The skill and experience of the surgeon performing the invasive aspects of implant treatment will of course also have a significant impact on the duration of the surgical procedure.

5.2.3 Pharmacological Considerations

There are many possible oral and systemic side effects (SE) or adverse effects (ADEs) from medications commonly used in the treatment of CVD; these are summarized in Table 3, with important considerations for the elderly patient.

As can be seen, there are some important interactions between routinely used prescription drugs and medications frequently prescribed in the dental clinic. For example, the use of non-steroidal anti-inflammatory drugs (NSAIDs) for postoperative pain relief is contraindicated in patients with hypertension or heart failure—acetaminophen may be safer. Some commonly used antibiotics are contraindicated with certain cholesterol-lowering drugs.

In addition, the clinician may need to consider the need for endocarditis prophylaxis. Valvular disease and replacement, and both congenital and surgical cardiac shunt conditions, have been considered risk factors for endocarditis where prophylactic antibiotic cover should be employed. This practice has been questioned in some countries; both guidelines and the widespread acceptance across disciplines are variable. In the UK, guidelines by the National Institute of Clinical Excellence (NICE) advise that there is no evidence to support the need for routine antibiotic prophylaxis in many situa-

Table 3   Important drug considerations in the elderly patient

Condition	Drug type	Example	Oral effects	SE/ADEs	Elderly
Hypertension	Alpha blocker	Doxasosin, tamsulosin	Xerostomia Thrombocytopenia	Orthostatic hypotension	Increased risk of orthostatic hypotension
Hypertension	ACE inhibitor	Captopril enalapril perindopril	Ulceration, dysgeusia Dysesthesia Glossodynia Xerostomia Lichenoid reactions Angioedema	Indomethacin reduces effect NSAIDs (other than acetylsalicylic acid) may increase the risk of renal damage	Worsening xerostomia, dysgeusia
Hypertension	Beta blocker	Atenolol Bisoprolol Propranolol	Xerostomia Paresthesia Lichenoid reactions	Adrenaline-containing LA	Increased risk of bradycardia
Hypertension	Angiotensin II inhibitor	Candesartan Losartan Valsartan	Xerostomia Dysgeusia Facial redness		
Hypertension	Calcium channel blockers	Amlodipine, diltiazem, nifedipine, verapamil	Gingival swelling Angioedema		
Hypertension/ heart failure	Diuretics	Bendroflumethiazide Furosemide Indapamide	Xerostomia		
Hypertension/ heart failure	Potassium-channel blockers		Ulceration		
Anticoagulation	Coumarins	Warfarin	Purpura bleeding	Increased bleeding when Ginkgo Biloba or St. John's wort are taken Interactions with azoles, macrolides, cephalosporins, metronidazole, tetracycline, doxycycline, NSAIDs, cranberry juice, St. John's wort, alcohol, dietary supplements	Increased tendency to bleed

Condition	Drug type	Example	Oral effects	SE/ADEs	Elderly
Anticoagulation	Antiplatelet	Clopidogrel	Purpura Bleeding	Erythromycin St. John's wort	Increased tendency to bleed
Anticoagulation	Direct thrombin inhibitors	Dabigatran	Purpura Bleeding	Azoles, NSAIDs, macrolides, dabigatran, clopidogrel Dexamethasone Carbamazepine Rifampicin Amiodarone, verapamil Alfalfa, bilberry St. John's wort	Increased tendency to bleed
Anticoagulation	Anti Factor Xa	Apixaban Rivaroxaban	Purpura Bleeding	Azoles, NSAIDs, phenytoin, rifampicin St. John's wort Alfalfa, bilberry, grapefruit	
Arrhythmias	Digitalis	Digoxin	Xerostomia	Adrenaline-containing LA Increase in gag reflex St. John's wort	
Atherosclerosis	Statins	Simvastatin, atorvastatin		Muscle damage increase with macrolide antibiotics and azole Antifungals; rosu-, pra-, and fluvastatin excepted.	

tions. However, the American Heart Association maintains advice to give antibiotic cover when there is a risk. As is the case with antibiotic prophylaxis for orthopedic joint replacements, guidance from both clinical and medicolegal authorities varies considerably between different countries, and a risk assessment should be undertaken and fully discussed with the patient before any surgery.

Finally, the clinician should be aware that the patient might be taking one or more medications for anticoagulation as part of the prevention of, or treatment for cardiovascular disease.

5.3 Hematological System

5.3.1 Age-related Changes

Age is a known risk factor in prolonged bleeding, together with gender, arterial hypertension, cardiac disease, cerebrovascular disease, pulmonary embolism, active cancer, chronic liver and renal disease, diabetes mellitus, a previous history of major bleeding, recent surgery, and hematological disorders such as anemia or thrombocytopenia (Leiss and coworkers 2014). Bone marrow diseases such as leukemia, immune disorders or immunosuppression, and polypharmacy may also result in a tendency to increased bleeding.

Purpura may be caused by solar exposure, diabetes, acetylsalicylic acid, steroids, thrombocytopenia, or connective-tissue disorders. Senile purpura typically affects elderly patients due to atrophy of the dermal tissue and increasing fragility of blood vessels, resulting in a tendency to bruise easily with minimal trauma. This is not necessarily a clinical sign of an increased bleeding tendency, and the same is true of intraoral purpura ("angina bullosa haemorrhagica"). However, antiplatelet drugs may exacerbate the condition.

Congenital bleeding disorders are generally diagnosed in childhood. Acquired coagulation defects, while generally less severe (with the exception of coagulation problems due to liver disease) are more likely to be prevalent in an elderly population as a result of age-related anticoagulant and fibrinolytic activities (Bauer and coworkers 1987).

Due to the increased rate of cardiovascular or cerebrovascular disease in aging patients, the clinician will often encounter the use of different individual anti-clotting medications or indeed combinations of such drugs, which can be broadly divided into antiplatelet drugs and anticoagulants.

Antiplatelet drugs

Antiplatelet drugs may include acetylsalicylic acid, monoclonal antibody drugs, phosphodiesterase inhibitors, and thienopyridines.

Acetylsalicylic acid inhibits platelet cyclooxygenase enzymes, which via further pathways irreversibly reduces platelet aggregation. It is the first line drug for prophylaxis of thromboembolic disease and MI. Acetylsalicylic acid is not only a common OTC medication in generic form, but is also an active ingredient in numerous proprietary OTC preparations, and patients who are unaware of this fact can easily consume an excessive amount. There is no evidence to suggest that cessation of prophylactic acetylsalicylic acid therapy is necessary in advance of oral surgical procedures.

Monoclonal antibody drugs used in antiplatelet therapy are GP IIb/IIIa inhibitors, which prevent platelet crosslinking and include abciximab. Such drugs are used parenterally and can have significant side effects.

Phosphodiesterase inhibitors include dipyridamole, which decreases platelet agglomeration. It is often used in conjunction with acetylsalicylic acid or warfarin in the prophylaxis of thromboembolic disease.

Thienopyridines act by inhibiting platelet activation via the ADP dependent pathway, such as clopidogrel, used to prevent post-MI atherosclerotic events or CVA. Clopidogrel is an example, commonly used in the control of CVA/atherosclerotic post-MI risk, post CABG surgery, or in established peripheral vascular disease.

The life cycle of a platelet is seven to ten days, and so cessation of therapy for drugs used as primary prevention of thromboembolic disease one week before the procedure can normally be considered safe. However, when the drug is used for the treatment of previous ischemic or thromboembolic disease, cessation should only be considered in consultation with other relevant specialists. Hemorrhage from antiplatelet drugs or platelet disorders is usually less severe than when caused by a clotting disorder. There is no evidence to suggest that continuing single antiplatelet therapies such as acetylsalicylic acid, clopidogrel, or dipyridamole significantly increases the risk of postoperative hemorrhage with dental extractions; simple implant surgery could be considered in the same way.

The risk increases with combination therapy of acetylsalicylic acid and clopidogrel, but this regime is generally used in patients at higher risk of thromboembolism and so specialist advice should be sought.

Straightforward implant placement for a patient with platelet count of greater than 100,000/µl should be possible with only local hemostatic measures and monitoring. However, procedures such as sinus lifting may require consideration of platelet transfusions and the use of postoperative tranexamic mouthwash.

Anticoagulant drugs
Anticoagulation therapies are used in the prevention and treatment of thromboembolic disease. They are also used, for example, in atrial fibrillation and other heart-valve disease/replacement, CVD, CVA, DVT, and PE. The most common drugs prescribed are warfarin for long-term use and heparin for short-term use.

Heparins potentiate the effect of antithrombin-III and thereby inhibit clotting factors II, IX, X, and XI. Two forms are used: unfractionated (UFH) or low-molecular-weight heparins (LMWH), with the latter being the more commonly used.

Heparins are used for example in the prophylaxis of deep-vein thrombosis (DVT) and for bridging therapy if it is necessary to stop warfarin for a time for surgical reasons. There is an immediate but short-lived effect on blood clotting.

Warfarin is a vitamin K antagonist whose main anticoagulant effect arises from a reduction in factor II, although it also affects factors VII, IX and X. The effect of warfarin therapy is measured by INR, the ratio of the patient's prothrombin time (PT) to an international normalized PT. A recent INR should be obtained before surgery, preferably within the previous 24 hours. It is important to be aware of the many polypharmacy considerations affecting warfarin and therefore patients' INR.

Older patients may show an exaggerated anticoagulant response to warfarin (Gurwitz and coworkers 1992). The half-life of the drug is approximately 40 hours; if the drug is stopped for surgery to take place, it may take several days for the INR to reach the pre-cessation level, during which time the patient may be at risk of a thromboembolic event. While vitamin K or fresh frozen plasma can be used to reverse the drug effect, it is generally accepted that cessation in order to reduce the risk of bleeding in dental procedures is unnecessary (Lockhart and coworkers 2003).

However, there is evidence to demonstrate a higher risk of major and less severe but clinically relevant bleeding due to polypharmacy in elderly patients due to drug interactions (Leiss and coworkers 2014), and the need for NSAIDs or antibiotics should be carefully reviewed in order to prevent life-threatening complications such as CVA.

Elderly patients may demonstrate greater inhibition of the synthesis of vitamin K-dependent clotting factors at similar plasma concentrations of warfarin, although the mechanisms are not clear (Shepherd and coworkers 1977). Such a relationship with plasma heparin concentration and anticoagulant effect does not appear to vary with age (Whitfield and coworkers 1982).

Novel oral anticoagulants (NAOCs) include direct thrombin inhibitors such as dabigatran and anti-factor Xa drugs such as rivaroxaban and apixaban, which have minimal drug interactions and which are less affected by diet; they are increasingly used as a replacement for warfarin. They do not require monitoring, are fast acting and irreversible, but have a shorter half-life of 12 – 14 hours in elderly patients.

5.3.2 Treatment Considerations

These drugs are given to prevent important, potentially life-threatening conditions. The dentist must understand that the desire for oral implants does not necessarily justify interrupting the therapy (Hwang and coworkers 2006).

Hemorrhage is a relatively common complication in dental implant surgery. However, there is no indication that a bleeding disorder is an absolute contraindication to implant surgery (Napeñas and coworkers 2009).

Immediate postoperative bleeding is more indicative of a vascular or platelet disorder; later hemorrhage is more indicative of a coagulation defect. While there is no data on the prevalence of bleeding complications in dental implant surgery, such complications have been reported (Kalpidis and Setayesh 2004), including upper-airway obstruction secondary to severe bleeding in the floor of the mouth, which is a rare but potentially life-threatening complication of implant placement (Givol and coworkers 2000).

The risk of serious bleeding complications in implant surgery is generally far less significant than the complications arising from thromboembolism, and so the decision to stop therapy should only be taken by consultation with the appropriate specialist if the risk of hemorrhage is greater than the risk of a thromboembolic event. It is also important to understand those groups of drugs where INR measurement is not possible and to be aware of appropriate local hemostatic measures that can be employed.

Heparins have a short half-life (3–4 hours for UFH, 24 hours for LMWH), and there is normally no need to stop therapy for dental procedures with a low risk of bleeding (extraction of 1–3 teeth, simple implant placement).

Simple implant surgical procedures may be considered in patients taking warfarin with an INR of less than 3.5 (extraction of up to three teeth, simple implant placement with local hemostatic measures) in consultation with the patient's physician (Madrid and Sanz 2009b; Bacci and coworkers 2011).

Procedures associated with a higher risk of bleeding (bone grafting, sinus lifts, large mucoperiosteal flaps), should be considered with appropriate specialist advice; heparin-bridging therapy may be required in some circumstances if warfarin is stopped, although this is not applicable to NOACs.

While there is no INR monitoring for patients on NOACs, the bleeding tendency will be similar to an INR of 4, although there have been no clinical studies to date. Heparinized patients have a low risk of bleeding complications (Hong and coworkers 2010).

In such patients, it may be wise to avoid regional block anesthesia and use local infiltration techniques, although lingual infiltrations would need to be considered in the same way as an inferior dental block; care should also be taken with venipuncture if intravenous sedation is used. The patient should be warned of the possibility of more significant postoperative ecchymoses.

Treatment should be planned for earlier in the day and week so that any problems can be dealt with during normal working hours when full resources are available. It may be wise to consider breaking down the surgical treatment into a multiple simple visits, although this has to be balanced with any requirement for drug interruptions. It may be useful in geriatric patients to assess the response to shorter surgical procedures, if possible, before moving on to more advanced surgery.

In general, postoperative analgesia is more safely achieved with acetaminophen or codeine. Antibiotic therapy with penicillin V or clindamycin is safe in terms avoiding anti-clotting drug interactions. Appropriate local hemostatic measures, such as microcrystalline collagen sponges or oxidized regenerated cellulose, and the availability of tranexamic acid mouthwash (10 ml of a 5% w/v solution) should be considered.

Patients with a mild to moderate bleeding tendency may be treated in the general or specialist care setting, depending on the procedure; those with a severe bleeding tendency or congenital coagulation defects should be treated in a specialist or hospital care setting and be planned in close liaison with the hematologist.

5.3.3 Pharmacological Considerations

Drugs that are commonly used in dentistry and oral surgery that can also impair hemostasis by interacting with warfarin or affecting platelet function include:

- Other non-steroidal anti-inflammatory drugs such as selective COX-2 inhibitors (celecoxib, rofecoxib), propionic derivatives (ibuprofen, ketoprofen, naproxen), and piroxicam, indomethacin, phenylbutazone, etc.
- Antifungals (gentamycin, azoles).
- Many antibiotics such as amoxicillin, ampicillin and derivatives, azithromycin, benzylpenicillin, cephalosporins, isoniazid, rifampicin, sulfonamides.
- Some antihistamines, chlorpromazine, diazepam, digitoxin, immunosuppressants, amiodarone, carbamazepine, cimetidine, omeprazole, furosemide, quinine, sodium valproate, tolbutamide, and tricyclic antidepressants may also have an effect, as may excessive alcohol consumption.

Even acetaminophen can enhance warfarin activity, and the typical regime of 500 mg four times per day for a week can result in an increased INR. Codeine may be added safely to enhance analgesia.

There are dietary effects on warfarin that may raise or lower INR. The consumption of "alternative" medications and supplements is common and compounds such as Echinacea, gingko biloba, St. John's wort, garlic and ginseng may either contain coumarins or interfere with platelet activity.

5.4 Hematopoietic System

5.4.1 Age-related Changes

The hematopoietic tissues in the marrow space undergo a progressive decline over the first 30 years of life and then stabilize before beginning to decline again from around the age of 70 years, for unknown reasons. The number of stem cells decreases with age, and there is a reduction in marrow function.

Evidence suggests that there is no change in the baseline rate of erythropoiesis in old age or in the lifespan of red blood cells, their hemoglobin concentration, and other variables. However, there may be a reduced capacity to compensate for erythropoietic stress such as hemorrhage or hypoxia, as the marrow in elderly patients appears to respond less to increased erythropoietic stimulation. There is controversy over the association between aging and anemia.

However, numerous studies indicate an increased prevalence of anemia in elderly individuals (Guralnik and coworkers 2004) and that in such circumstances there is an association with reduced bone-mineral density, skeletal muscle mass, and physical performance, as well as with frailty. Although no causal mechanisms have been defined, there is speculation that anemia may be involved in adverse outcomes (Price 2008). Anemia has also been implicated in an increased incidence of medication-related osteonecrosis of the jaw (MRONJ) (Tsao and coworkers 2013; Saad and coworkers 2012).

Senescence of other organ systems can produce changes that may result in anemia. For example, an age-related decrease in the number of nephrons in the kidneys may cause a decline in erythropoietin secretion; atrophy of the gastric mucosa reduces B_{12} absorption due to reduced secretion of intrinsic factor, which could give rise to pernicious anemia. Nutritional deficiencies may also cause anemia. Large-scale studies of institutionalized older adults in Europe and North America have indicated increases in anemia rates of up to 25% (Patel 2008).

The main causes of asymptomatic anemia in the elderly are iron deficiency and "anemia of chronic disease" (Lipschitz 1981). Iron absorption is not impaired in the elderly individual, but iron supplements taken orally are less effective (Marx 1979). It is recommended that elderly patients with signs of anemia be investigated for a cause such as deficiency of folate, iron, or vitamin B_{12}, or underlying disease such as malignancy (Baldwin 1988).

Normal bone-marrow changes in the aging patient may or may not result in a decline in the number of immune cells such as leukocytes and mature lymphocytes; considerable disagreement exists between authors over this subject. However, there is agreement that there is a progressive decline in the functionality of the immune system, leading to "immunosenescence" characterized by impaired immunity and inflammatory responses (Gravenstein and coworkers 2003).

This is thought to be primarily due to altered T-lymphocyte function, given that, in elderly patients, it will have been some time since thymic atrophy (which is complete by later middle age) (Pawelec 1998). This may affect antibody-antigen responses and cellular immune functions. This progressive decline in the immune system is implicated in several age-related diseases such as osteoporosis, autoimmune disease, Alzheimer's disease, and cancer (Hakim and Gress 2007).

Therapies such as immunosuppressants and immunomodulatory drugs are more commonly used in elderly patients and will also impair immunity, as may radiotherapy and prolonged serious illness.

Morbidity and the prolonged duration of illness also increase with age. Older individuals may not respond as well to therapy for infections and may not present with "typical signs" of infection, such as fever. Instead of pain symptoms, elderly patients may show increased signs of confusion, agitation, or withdrawal.

5.4.2   Treatment Considerations

The clinical relevance of anemia in terms of increased morbidity/mortality is unclear. There are suggestions that anemia may lead to increased cardiac output or reduced tissue oxygenation, or a decline in physical and mental function (Fried and Guralnik 1997). Anemia has also been implicated with an increased risk of osteonecrosis of the jaw in cancer patients (Saad and coworkers 2012; Tsao and coworkers 2013).

However, we should be aware of our role in the overall care of the geriatric patient and be vigilant for the intraoral manifestations of anemia such as glossitis, ulceration, burning mouth syndrome, and angular stomatitis, as well as denture comfort or any interference with effective mastication and consequent nutritional impact. The dentist should also be aware of the general signs such as lassitude, dyspnea, or tachycardia.

Age-related changes result in altered immune responses to infection, which may start early, progress in an atypical fashion, and take longer to resolve in geriatric patients. Opportunistic infections such as candidiasis or herpetic infections are more common in immunocompromised patients.

Oral signs of impaired hematopoietic function may include recurrent or unusually severe bacterial infection (in neutropenia), florid gingivitis, or oral petechiae (thrombocytopenia).

There is a greater incidence of neoplastic disease as we age. More than 50% of leukemia cases occur in patients aged 65 years and older, and myelodysplastic syndromes occur mostly in elderly patients, the most common of which is chronic lymphocytic leukemia (Baker 1987). Such patients are unlikely to present for implant treatment with active symptoms of disease, but there may be some patients with undiagnosed or low-level chronic disease presenting as complications following dental extractions or implant placement, such as an increased tendency to bleed or an unusually severe infection. We also have to consider the development of such disease and its future (unknown) impact on the management of later problems with previous implant treatment.

Sedation or general anesthesia in patients with certain types of anemia with reduced hemoglobin levels could lead to hypoxia.

Agranulocytosis has been associated with penicillin and some other antibiotics, some NSAIDs including naproxen, anticonvulsants (Andersohn and coworkers 2007), and clindamycin has been associated with pancytopenia (Morales and coworkers 2014).

Thrombocytopenia has been associated with hundreds of medications as a result of impaired platelet production or increased destruction; again, commonly prescribed antibiotics and NSAIDs are implicated, as well as anticonvulsants, oral antidiabetic drugs, antirheumatics, diuretics, and antacids such as ranitidine (Visentin and Liu 2007), all of which are common medications in the elderly patient.

The immunosuppressive effects of glucocorticoid therapy, such as the inhibition of leukocytes, macrophages, and cytokines, and further hematopoietic effects, including a reduction in eosinophils and monocytes, may affect the severity and presentation of infections, increase susceptibility to infection, or cause delayed healing.

5.5 Respiratory System

5.5.1 Age-related Changes

As in other organ systems, maximum lung function and capacity decline with age, which has an impact on physiologic reserve. A general weakening of musculature includes the respiratory muscles; the elasticity of the lungs changes and is accompanied by a reduced bronchiolar diameter and enlarged alveolar ducts. The vital capacity of the lungs is reduced with a concomitant decline in peak flow and gas exchange, with lower oxygen saturation. There is also a change in immunological lung defense mechanisms. However, in healthy elderly individuals there are few associated symptoms other than a reduction in capacity for exercise, which is more affected by cardiovascular functional decline. There is no change in tidal volume with age, as ventilatory capacity is maintained by an increase in respiratory rate.

Age-related changes in the lungs can compound heart and lung disease or the long-term effects of smoking. Older people are more at risk of complications from upper respiratory tract infections.

Chronic obstructive pulmonary disease (COPD) is the collective term for lung diseases, including chronic bronchitis, emphysema, and chronic obstructive airways disease, characterized by a persistent productive cough, shortness of breath on exertion (SOBOE) and chest infections. The condition normally presents later in life and is very common in elderly patients; like other conditions, it is often undiagnosed (Halbert and coworkers 2006). COPD also results in pulmonary hypertension and ventricular hypertrophy, causing dyspnea. It is expected to become the third most common cause of death and disability by 2030 (WHO 2000).

Asthma is common in patients over 65 years; in some patients, it may be a new development rather than a lifetime condition or a recurrence of previous asthma, although the triggers and risk factors may be similar (Gibson and coworkers 2010). The diagnosis of asthma in an elderly patient is often difficult due to the high incidence of COPD in this age group, but the prevalence of asthma in the over-75 age group has been estimated at 7% to 9% (Braman and Hanania 2007).

5.5.2 Treatment Considerations

A recent publication found that edentulism was associated with a higher frequency of COPD-related hospitalization and mortality (Barros and coworkers 2013). This was tentatively attributed to a possible link between the exaggerated inflammatory response of aggressive periodontitis and a susceptibility to inflammatory events associated with COPD. No causal link was proved, but it is interesting to consider to what extent peri-implant infections in the periodontally susceptible patient may also be a factor. Patients with COPD are more frequently mouth-breathers with concomitant gingival dryness and gingivitis.

Patients with SOBOE and poor mobility or patients who are frequently hospitalized will be less willing and able to seek dental treatment or supportive periodontal therapy.

COPD is often associated with comorbidities, including cardiovascular disease, osteoporosis, and depressive illness (Agustí 2007). Osteoporosis may result in vertebral compression, spinal kyphosis, and the typical "dowager's hump." This can impede normal thoracic-cage expansion and impair diaphragmatic efficiency. Accessory muscles of respiration are therefore often employed by such patients, but this is not possible in a fully supine position.

It is consequently advisable to treat patients with respiratory conditions upright in the dental chair in order to avoid respiratory difficulty and maintain adequate oxygen saturation. This may present marked technical difficulties, particularly in terms of access for some surgical procedures. In some patients, fluid irrigation of instruments may also compromise breathing or exacerbate coughing, requiring frequent stoppages during procedures. Such considerations have to be included as part of the decision as to what treatment may be practically achievable, as well as advisable.

Current guidelines suggest caution in the use of epinephrine-containing local anesthetics in patients with COPD, with a limit of two cartridges of 2% lidocaine with 1 : 80,000 epinephrine (45 µg epinephrine) (Brown and Rhodus 2005). Using the patient's own salbutamol inhaler immediately before treatment may be helpful.

The presence of oral pathogens, and in particular anaerobes, in sputum has long been established as connecting oral and pulmonary diseases (Bartlett and Gorbach 1975; Mojon and coworkers 1997). Dental and oral factors present a significant risk of aspiration pneumonia, especially in elderly patients with diabetes, COPD, or reduced functional status requiring assistance with eating. Both periodontal and cariogenic microorganisms have been associated with aspiration pneumonia (Terpenning and coworkers 2001; Brook and Frazier 2003).

The frequent use of broad-spectrum antibiotics in patients with COPD can lead to the suppression of normal oral bacteria and result not only in opportunistic infections such as candidiasis but also in colonization by potential respiratory pathogens such as methicillin-resistant *Staphylococcus aureus* (MRSA) and *Pseudomonas aeruginosa* (Scannapieco and coworkers 1992).

Gastric reflux is a common comorbidity of COPD and again may require treatment in a more upright position. The importance of good masticatory function to reduce exacerbation of the reflux is highlighted. Gastroesophageal reflux may also commonly cause asthma-like symptoms.

COPD is strongly correlated with smoking; to quit smoking is the single most effective therapy in the treatment of COPD, and the dental professional has an important role to play in encouraging the patient to engage in smoking cessation therapy (Devlin 2014).

The treatment of the patient with COPD under sedation will require vigilant monitoring of blood oxygen saturation with pulse oximetry. A minority of patients are acclimatized to a certain level of hypoxia and their respiratory drive may be suppressed by the use of supplemental oxygen. This may also be a consideration in the event of a medical emergency in the dental office, where the use of supplemental oxygen may result in hypercapnic respiratory failure (Jevon 2014).

5.5.3 Pharmacological Considerations

Many of the drugs prescribed for COPD can cause significant adverse effects in elderly patients. Also, because elderly patients are often on a polypharmacy of medications, management of COPD can be difficult.

The first-line drugs used in COPD are bronchodilators such as short- and long-acting β_2 agonists (short: salbutamol, terbutaline; long: salmeratol, formoterol), and inhaled muscarinic agents such as ipratropium.

The long-term use of steroid inhalers has been implicated in the development of osteoporosis in the elderly, and it is recommended that subjects be monitored for reductions in bone-mineral density.

Inhaled corticosteroids are used in the treatment of severe COPD and asthma, but only 10% to 20% of the metered dose reaches the lungs, with the greater proportion remaining in the oropharynx (Barnes 1995). The correct use of an inhaler device can be particularly challenging for an elderly patient. Inhaled corticosteroids are often associated with oropharyngeal candidiasis and have been implicated in poor intraoral wound healing. Patients should be advised to rinse their mouth after use or to use the inhaler with a spacer. As stated, elderly patients often have difficulty adhering accurately to pharmacological regimes, particularly when multiple drugs make the process complex or the patient has memory loss or cognitive dysfunction. Nasal inhalers may be used as an alternative in patients who are more at risk of oropharyngeal candidiasis, such as diabetics or immunosuppressed patients.

Oral mucosal changes resulting from the use of steroid inhalers may also include xerostomia (caused by the β_2 agonist effect on the salivary glands, anticholinergic effects of ipratropium, and steroid effects) caries (as a result of multiple effects of reduced salivary flow), oral ulceration, and dysgeusia.

It should be noted that some drugs used in nicotine replacement therapy also cause dry mouth.

5.6 Alimentary System

The digestive system has considerable physiologic reserves and is therefore functionally less affected by aging than other organ systems. However, aging can be a factor in digestive and gastrointestinal disorders, both as a consequence of primary disease and as a result of ADEs in polymorbid individuals. Furthermore, any factors that affect the ability to eat and that have an impact on nutritional status can be of greater significance in elderly individuals. It has been estimated that even in developed countries, 16% of patients over 65 years and 2% of those over 85 years are malnourished (London Office for National Statistics 2004). Polypharmacy may also have an effect on nutritional status, with reports identifying 50% of people on 10 or more medications as being malnourished or at risk of malnourishment (Jyrkkä and coworkers 2010).

Aging results in a loss of muscle mass, and this can have an impact not only on skeletal muscle function but also on smooth muscle affecting vital organs, including cardiac function. The basal metabolic rate declines, and changes in liver and kidney function can decrease protein synthesis; changes in cytokine and hormonal levels occur and fluid and electrolyte balance alters. Malnutrition in elderly people is also associated with reduced cognitive function, poor wound healing, delayed recovery from surgery, and mortality.

Elderly people tend to exhibit declining appetite, with average daily food intake decreasing by approximately one-third between the ages of 20 and 80 years (Wurtman and coworkers 1988). While this is often accompanied by a reduction in physical activity and therefore in energy expenditure, in some people this is not the case, and energy expenditure exceeds intake resulting in "anorexia of aging" (Ahmed and Haboubi 2010).

These and other changes described elsewhere in this chapter mean that effective and appropriate nutrition are essential in maintaining health in the elderly person. The importance of a healthy mouth with the ability to chew and swallow properly is clear, and the clinician has to consider many factors in both the provision of dental implants and the ongoing care of patients rehabilitated in this way.

Oropharyngeal changes. The changes in the oral mucosa that occur with age are similar to those of the skin, with a decrease in elastin and increased cross-linking of collagen. The effect on mucous membranes is somewhat reduced by the moist oral environment. However, normal age-related vascular changes reduce the mucosal blood supply, contributing to a thinning of the mucosal layer of stratified squamous epithelium, with consequent fragility and greater susceptibility to infection (De Rossi and Slaughter 2007).

Elderly patients with multiple chronic diseases are more likely to be taking medications that can cause mucosal irritation, gingival enlargement, and immunosuppression.

Older patients frequently complain of a loss of taste sensation. There is an age-related decline in olfactory and gustatory neurologic function, and it is known that the number of taste buds is reduced with age, resulting in a decline in taste sensation (hypogeusia). This chemosensory decline is also associated with a change in chemosensory preference: the thresholds for salt and bitter taste increase, although those for sweet and sour remain relatively constant. Studies have shown that changes in nutritional status can also affect taste sensation and vice versa. Further effects on taste can be caused by palatal denture coverage and reduced salivary flow, which can significantly affect food choices and the quality of life. Often older people will add salt or sugar to foods to compensate for decreased taste sensation, which can have adverse health effects.

Decreased salivary production (hyposalivation) leading to dry mouth (xerostomia) has been considered part of the normal aging process and was associated with age-related changes to the parenchymal structure of salivary glands. However, it is now thought that salivary production and composition are largely unrelated to age; there is no reduction in either resting or stimulated salivary flow rates of the parotid, although there is a reduction in other salivary glands (Percival and coworkers 1994; Challacombe and coworkers 1995). The prevalence of xerostomia increases with age; approximately 30% of individuals over 65 years are affected (Ship and coworkers 2002). Causes may include primary diseases such as diabetes, Sjögren's syndrome, secondary Sjögren's in rheumatoid disorders such as rheumatoid arthritis, scleroderma, or systemic lupus erythematosus, and radiotherapy to the head and neck region. Drug-induced xerostomia is common, with an estimated 80% of commonly prescribed medications having a xerostomic effect (Sreebny and Schwartz 1997) It has been estimated that most elderly people take at least one medication that may cause decreased salivary flow (Schein and coworkers 1999) and that polypharmaceutical regimes are a common cause of dry mouth in older people (Porter and Scully 2000). Elderly people may also present with a dry mouth and enlarged parotid glands due to chronic dehydration. Altered perception in dementia states can give rise to complaints of dry mouth even with normal salivary flow.

The major functions of saliva are lubrication, buffering and remineralization, immunological (saliva contains antifungal and antibacterial proteins), and digestive, including food breakdown with salivary enzymes, bolus formation, and gustatory function. The effects of dry mouth are many and varied: functional limitations include dysphagia, altered speech, and difficulty wearing dentures. Physiological effects include mucus/food/plaque retention and associated caries and periodontal disease with a change in oral microbiota and halitosis, neurosensory symptoms such as "burning mouth syndrome" and dysgeusia, and a susceptibility to opportunistic infections such as candidiasis. Such problems can have a significant effect on social interaction and quality of life (Turner and Ship 2007).

The generalized reduction in motor control and activity in aging individuals is reflected in reduced masticatory muscle strength and lip seal, and swallowing can take longer (Ferguson 1987). The ability to identify food textures and manipulate both food and removable prostheses may be compromised.

Other age-related changes in the oropharynx include a decline in thirst perception. Along with decreased salivary flow, chewing and swallowing capacity can be markedly impaired, causing dysphagia and nutritional defects (Ney and coworkers 2009). The elderly, polymorbid, polymedicated, and frail population is known to be at increased risk of aspiration pneumonia because of poor oral health, impaired resistance to infection, and oropharyngeal aspiration (Rofes and coworkers 2010).

Oral mucosal conditions and manifestations of systemic diseases. Examples of systemic diseases with oral manifestations include dermatological conditions, inflammatory connective-tissue diseases, hematological problems, endocrine diseases, inflammatory gastrointestinal diseases, and neurological problems. Any condition causing a sore mouth will have an impact on the ability to chew and swallow food, wear dentures, speak, etc., and this may have a greater significance in an elderly person.

Examples of systemic conditions that may present with a sore mouth in the elderly include:

- Candidiasis (immunosuppression/immunodeficiency, hematological disorders , diabetes, antibiotic usage)
- Mucosal atrophy, recurrent painful ulceration (hematological disorders)
- Sore tongue (B_{12}/folate deficiency, hematological disorders)
- Florid gingival inflammation (hematological disorders, Crohn's disease)
- Drug-related (oncology medications, immunosuppressants, calcium-channel blockers, antiepileptics)

Autoimmune skin conditions are relatively more common in the elderly population, possibly due to immunodysfunction or ADEs related to increased polypharmacy in this age group (Loo and Burrows 2004). Some of these conditions can result in oral vesiculobullous lesions, which if they burst will result in desquamation appearing as shallow ulcerating erosions. Bullous pemphigoid is the most common autoimmune blistering mucocutaneous condition that affects mainly the over-70 age group. However, oral involvement is rare. Pemphigus vulgaris and pemphigoid (both bullous and mucous-membrane subtypes) are also more prevalent in the elderly and occur more commonly as oral blistering. Oral lichen planus can also cause desquamative gingivitis; such conditions putatively present both a desire for implant-retained prostheses and a challenge for their provision.

Crohn's disease is an autoimmune chronic granulomatous inflammatory condition that can affect the entire alimentary tract. Symptoms include vasculitis, enteritis, arthritis, keratoconjunctivitis and the disease can result in nutritional deficits. Previously considered a "lifetime" disease with onset in the young, it is now recognized that this disease can initially appear in elderly people, with approximately 15% of diagnoses for inflammatory bowel disease made in the over-60 age group (Gisbert and Chaparro 2014).

In the elderly, it is more limited to colonic disease and is less severe. However, older patients with long-standing Crohn's disease may present for implant therapy when teeth are lost; in addition, the management of the disease may change as they age.

In the oral cavity, lesions appear as either linear or aphthous ulceration, with swelling of the lips and oral mucosa, which may acquire a "cobblestone" appearance. It has also been associated with periodontal lesions (van Steenberghe and coworkers 1976).

It has been suggested that dental implants may produce an antigenic response in Crohn's patients, thereby affecting osseointegration (van Steenberghe and coworkers 2002), but in this cohort there were multiple comorbid factors. Subsequent studies by the same group indicated varying outcomes for dental implants, and there is scant evidence on which to base any conclusions (Bornstein and coworkers 2009).

Other changes of the digestive tract. The strength of esophageal contractions and of the upper esophageal sphincter decreases with age. Although the movement of food seems to be unaffected, other age-related changes may combine to cause problems. Age-related decrease in salivary production with a reduced chewing efficiency may mean that food is less macerated and drier, making swallowing difficult.

Although food transport is otherwise less affected, elderly people may have difficulty in eating in a recumbent or lying position and reflux may occur. The lower esophagus may be less able to move refluxed acid back into the stomach, with resulting "heartburn." This can be complicated by the presence of a hiatus hernia in older patients.

Gastroesophageal reflux disease is present in up to 80% of older patients with asthma, although may not always be accompanied by the classic symptoms of reflux (Harding and coworkers 2000).

Older people have a reduced volumetric capacity of the stomach due to reduced smooth muscle elasticity, which also adversely affects the rate of gastric motility and emptying (Moore and coworkers 1983). Old people are consequently often unable to consume large portions of food in one sitting.

Aging of the stomach lining results in a thinner gastric mucosa that is less resistant to damage. Older people have an increased tendency to bleed from NSAID use and are at higher risk of developing peptic ulcers. Other drugs that are normally absorbed in the stomach may have altered effectiveness.

As the gastric mucosa atrophies, it produces less of the intrinsic factor needed for vitamin B_{12} absorption. This increases the risk of pernicious anemia. B_{12} deficiency is common among older people and may lead to cognitive decline.

There is little age-related change in the secretion of gastric acid and pepsin. However, conditions such as atrophic gastritis, long-term use of proton-pump inhibitors, and gastric surgery are more common in the elderly and may result in a reduction in gastric-acid secretion. The resulting increased stomach pH can reduce intestinal calcium absorption.

The small intestine undergoes little functional change with age (Fich and coworkers 1989). There is, however, a reduction in lactase secretion, which may lead to intolerance of dairy foods and contribute to calcium deficiency. Reduced gastric-acid secretion can result in bacterial overgrowth in the small intestine, which in turn can contribute to malnourishment (Parlesak and coworkers 2003).

Diverticulosis is more common in elderly patients; it is estimated that any person reaching the age of 90 has many diverticula. The cause is unknown but thought to be related to smooth muscle spasm due to a diet low in fiber. The muscle spasm causes a balloon-like distension of the intestinal wall, often near a penetrating blood vessel, and can cause painful abdominal cramps. If the diverticulum becomes inflamed, intestinal bleeding may occur and manifest itself as blood in stool.

The large intestine also changes little as we age, although constipation is more prevalent in the elderly, sometimes due to comorbidities such as diabetes, but often as a result of a low-fiber diet or due to reduced physical activity and the side effects of drugs given to treat other conditions.

5.6.1 Treatment Considerations

Older people may become insidiously malnourished due to reduced food intake for many reasons, including the physiological changes outlined above, depression-related anorexia, or apathy when living alone. Undernutrition and low intake of protein are common among older people and can lead to conditions such as sarcopenia (loss of muscle mass and strength) and osteopenia (reduced bone-mineral density), contributing to the onset of frailty. Immunity may also be impaired as calcium, vitamin E and zinc levels are all commonly reduced amongst institutionalized and homebound patients. Vitamin D levels are also reduced as a result of senescence of the skin and indoor living.

Consequently, the quality of the diet becomes more relevant, and higher levels of protein are required. The importance of a healthy and functional dentition or dental prosthesis is significant.

Oral mucosal soreness resulting from removable mucosa-supported prostheses in patients with xerostomia is a well-recognized problem, particularly in the elderly (Payne and coworkers 1997). The benefit of implant-supported prostheses in such instances has been highlighted for some time (Isidor and coworkers 1999) and can improve a patient's quality of life for many years, especially in complete edentulism (Binon 2005). Further benefits of implant-retained prostheses are discussed in Chapters 4, 6, and 7.

There is no apparent contraindication to the placement of implants in patients with Sjögren's disease; the prosthetic benefits of implant therapy are clear (Binon 2005; Isidor and coworkers 1999; Payne and coworkers 1997). However, the underlying cause should have been investigated and associated oral health issues properly assessed as part of comprehensive treatment planning, as with any oral condition.

There is little evidence related to the provision and long-term success of dental implants in patients with oral mucosal diseases, with reports being limited to case reports or retrospective analyses. In terms of oral lichen planus, reported success rates are high, and implant-retained overdentures provided benefits (Czerninski and coworkers 2013; Esposito and coworkers 2003). One prospective study to date has indicated a tendency to increased incidence of peri-implant mucositis and peri-implantitis in patients with oral lichen planus (Hernández and coworkers 2012).

There are limited reports of implant placement in other blistering conditions. Authors have reported successful outcomes in the relatively short term (up to 36 months) in epidermolysis bullosa (Larrazabal-Morón and coworkers 2009). Fixed reconstructions resulted in less mucosal irritation in terms of blistering (Müller and coworkers 2010) than when implant-supported overdentures were used, which was a problem (Peñarrocha-Diago and coworkers 2000). Scant literature is available on the incidence of surgical complications. In general, no surgical issues were mentioned in the case reports described. Peñarrocha reported "blister complications" during surgery and that one had to be careful with suction. Flap healing appears not to have been affected (Peñarrocha and coworkers 2007a).

However, this is a disease of younger people and may differ in its etiological factors from the occurrence of vesiculobullous lesions in the elderly patient. In the one available but well-detailed report on implant provision in a case of a 70-year-old woman with pemphigus vulgaris, surgical difficulties included the placement of sutures due to the friable nature of the acantholytic mucosa, but mucosal healing was otherwise uneventful.

Removable prostheses will frequently be impossible to wear with any degree of comfort under such conditions, which will adversely affect quality of life. Tooth- or implant-supported prostheses are undoubtedly preferable to minimize mucosal contact (Peñarrocha and coworkers 2007b).

However, such prostheses may require more effective oral hygiene; complex reconstructions are of course more challenging in this respect, but the presence of sore oral tissues, or associated secondary conditions such as rheumatoid arthritis, may severely limit the opportunity for effective plaque control (Candel-Marti and coworkers 2011)

There is clearly a need for well-designed systematic studies into the use of implants in oral mucosal conditions, but case reporting should not be discouraged, as they could be the only source of information at any given time.

5.6.2 Pharmacological Considerations

Anorexia and weight loss are common findings in the elderly. The physiologic "anorexia of aging" can progress to pathological anorexia in an elderly person with chronic medical or psychological illness; depression is the most common reason for anorexia in the elderly and antidepressant medication in the elderly is common (Morley 1996); this may result in hyposalivation.

As previously stated, dry mouth is most often the result of medications, especially in polypharmaceutical regimes, with the most commonly associated drugs being those with an anticholinergic effect and this includes proton pump inhibitors used in the treatment of gastric reflux. Other commonly prescribed groups of drugs causing dry mouth include benzodiazepines, opioids, many antihypertensives, and diuretics.

Lichenoid drug reactions can be indistinguishable from oral lichen planus and may be caused by many drugs commonly prescribed to the elderly, such as allopurinol, antiarrhythmics, antihypertensives, antidiabetics, antiepileptics, anti-inflammatories, some antibiotics, and lithium. Oral ulceration may also occur with many of these drugs.

The list of drugs causing hypogeusia or dysgeusia is extensive and dynamic, and a complaint of altered taste sensation should always include a drug review. In an affected patient, replacement with a different drug where possible is useful.

Mucositis can cause severe difficulty with speech, eating and drinking, swallowing, speaking and sleeping and can result from chemotherapy/radiotherapy. Maintaining adequate nutritional and fluid intake is of paramount importance. Some therapies have proved useful in treating this condition from simple measures, such as sucking on ice chips, to administration of recombinant human keratocyte growth factor (palifermin) (Keefe and coworkers 2007).

Patients with oral blistering are often long-term users of corticosteroid or immunosuppressive drugs, with a consequent risk of poor bone quality, poor healing, and susceptibility to infection. Adrenal suppression may also be a consideration, requiring adjunctive oral steroid therapy.

An age-related reduction in motility, secretion, and absorption in the various parts of the alimentary tract is slight and has little effect on drug behavior in the elderly. Liver and biliary function is of greater significance and is discussed in the relevant section below.

NSAID analgesia is best avoided in elderly patients due to the increased risk of gastric bleeding and renal injury (Wolfe and coworkers 1999). Acetaminophen is the preferred analgesic option, but may be inadequate for effective postoperative pain relief in some cases and may be contraindicated in patients with liver disease. The use of a selective COX-2 inhibitor (e.g., rofecoxib) may be considered (Malmstrom and coworkers 1999).

The combination of acetaminophen with an opioid such as codeine may be beneficial, and combination products are often considered safe. However, it should be noted that elderly patients have an increased sensitivity to opioids and lower doses should be considered. They are also more likely to be taking other medications that may interact. There is a significant increase in side effects such as constipation, sedation, confusion, and falls (Buckeridge and coworkers 2010). More potent opioids such as oxycodone may carry a significant risk of respiratory depression.

5.7 Hepatobiliary System

The liver is responsible for glucose metabolism and the conversion of excess carbohydrate and protein into fat. A greater proportion of body fat is stored in the liver of elderly people, which has been associated with insulin resistance and a higher risk of diabetes (Roubenoff 1999). Bile is manufactured in the liver and is required for the absorption of fat, vitamins A, D, E, and K. It is also important in the manufacture of albumin, complement, hormones, and proteins, including blood-clotting proteins using vitamin K and B_{12}. It has a role in immunology through the eradication by mononuclear phagocytes of bacteria, fungi, parasites, and other cellular material, and water-insoluble toxins are modified to allow excretion by the kidneys.

Hemoglobin, cholesterol, proteins, alcohol, and most drugs are metabolized by the liver; in particular, orally administered drugs absorbed by the gut are modified in a "first-pass" metabolism before they enter the circulatory system, which may activate, inactivate or change the mode of action of the drug.

There are several age-related changes in the liver, including a reduction in size and blood flow. Liver function tests generally remain normal in healthy aged individuals, with a possible rise in serum alkaline phosphatase in older women. There may be less bile formation and secretion, with an increased risk of gallstones. The capacity of the liver to metabolize many substances decreases with aging. The main effect of this is a reduction in clearance of drugs metabolized in the liver of elderly individuals and an increase in volume and distribution of drugs soluble in lipids. This is associated with a risk of side effects at lower doses than would be seen in younger persons. Doses may therefore need to be reduced (Mangoni and Jackson 2004).

Along with a general lowering of physiological stress reserve in the elderly, reduced hepatic reserves mean that the liver is also less able to tolerate increased stress; toxic substances are more likely to cause liver damage, which is also slower to repair.

Examples of drugs metabolized in the liver include:

- Analgesics such as acetylsalicylic acid, acetaminophen, codeine, ibuprofen
- Antibiotics including ampicillin, clindamycin, metronidazole
- Azole antifungals such as miconazole, fluconazole
- Benzodiazepines
- Local anesthetics

The prevalence of chronic liver disease is increasing with the aging general population. Increasing alcohol-related liver disease is seen in elderly patients (Seitz and Stickel 2007). Non-alcoholic fatty liver disease is associated with insulin resistance and diabetes. Other liver diseases that are not age-related may have more severe initial morbidity and mortality. The incidence of liver transplants in patients over 60 has also increased significantly, doubling during the 1990s (Frith and coworkers 2008).

There appears to be little effect on the osseointegration of dental implants, even in patients taking cyclosporin, which has been shown to impair the process (Sakakura and coworkers 2007). However, the evidence base is sparse (Gu and Yu 2011; Gu and coworkers 2011; Heckmann and coworkers 2004).

Liver damage and aging can have an impact on bleeding due to impairment of the vitamin K metabolism, failures in the synthesis of other clotting factors (I, II, VII, IX, X, XI) and increased metabolism of these factors. There may be increased fibrinolysis and a tendency to thrombocytopenia.

Vitamin K deficiency is rare in adults, but an elderly patient with obstructive jaundice, chronic liver disease, or malabsorption may be at risk of vitamin K deficiency, which can have both skeletal and anticoagulation effects; some authors recommend supplemental vitamin K in adults over 50 years.

Structural changes of the pancreas are seen with aging, but no functional age-related changes are seen independent of those associated with other diseases or medications.

5.8 Renal System

5.8.1 Age-related Changes

The main functions of the kidneys are in fluid and electrolyte balance, regulation of endocrine function, waste removal and drug excretion, vitamin D metabolism and stimulation of erythrocyte function.

As is seen in the liver, overall kidney size tends to decrease with age due to reduced cell counts. There is a decrease in overall blood flow though the kidneys with a reduction in the glomerular filtration rate, and this will have an effect on the excretion of drugs.

Changes to renal function caused by other systemic diseases will have an additional effect on drug elimination. Some drugs commonly prescribed in dentistry, such as penicillins, erythromycins, and cephalosporins, may have to be reduced in dose concomitant with renal function.

Hydration is of increased importance in elderly individuals, who may have a reduced sensitivity to thirst and tend not to drink enough fluids. Inadequate fluid intake is a greater problem in individuals with cognitive impairment or physical disability. Age-related physiological renal impairment results in a reduced ability with age to concentrate urine, less efficient sodium-sparing capacity, and reduced water excretion. Elders are consequently more at risk of problems caused by fluid and electrolyte imbalance such as dehydration.

Chronic kidney disease (CKD), defined as kidney disease resulting in a reduction in glomerular filtration rate for more than three months, is a common problem in people with glomerulonephritis, hypertension, or diabetes. In the older person, CKD is most often due to diabetes or renal vascular disease secondary to cardiovascular disease; it is also associated with the long-term use of NSAIDs and large doses of acetaminophen. Like many other conditions, aging of the global population and more effective treatment of associated diseases is causing an increase in the prevalence of CKD in elderly patients, which in some developed countries may be as high as 30% (Coresh and coworkers 2007).

Patients with CKD have a blunted erythropoietin response to anemia (Adamson and coworkers 1968), and the risk of anemia may be worsened by the effect of accumulated toxins on bone marrow. Nephrotic syndrome, uremia, and renal insufficiency are all important causes of secondary immunodeficiency in elderly patients as a result of defective phagocyte function; such patients are predisposed to infections, particularly oral candidiasis.

CKD is associated with an increased bleeding tendency; increased serum urea has an antiplatelet effect, and patients with renal dysfunction are often thrombocytopenic.

Vitamin D deficiency is very common in patients with CKD. This is worsened by reduced renal hydroxylation of vitamin D into the active form, 1,25-dihydroxyvitamin D_3. Impaired renal phosphate excretion and low serum calcium levels resulting from impaired calcium absorption may result in hyperparathyroidism. The interruption of normal calcium and phosphate regulation combined with osteomalacia is known as renal osteodystrophy and can have, in combination with a reduction in fibroblast growth factor 23, a significant effect on bone structure (Ott 2012). It has been reported that up to 84% of CKD patients have some histological evidence of bone disease and that 98% of renal dialysis patients have abnormal bone biopsies (CKD-MBD Work Group 2009).

New evidence has also suggested an autocrine role of vitamin D in the modulation of several systems, including the immune, renal, and cardiovascular systems (Williams and coworkers 2009).

Dialysis remains the most common treatment for patients with renal failure or end-stage renal disease, although the advances in renal transplants and concomitant immunosuppressive therapy mean that survival after a renal transplant has improved dramatically (Goldman 2006). Consequently, older patients with successful transplants are increasingly likely to present for care and treatment; transplantation in the older patient is increasingly common, and pre-transplantation dental disease control will often be required.

5.8.2 Treatment Considerations

Chronic kidney disease in later stages may be associated with oral signs and symptoms such as halitosis or a metallic taste disturbance due to uremia, xerostomia, signs of anemia, gingival bleeding and oral petechiae because of platelet dysfunction and anticoagulation therapy in dialysis patients. Gingival hyperplasia can arise secondary to drugs such as calcium-channel blockers and—less often—with cyclosporin, but is less prevalent in older people. Uremic stomatitis can occur as painful ulceration of the ventral surface of the tongue and anterior mucosa (Proctor and coworkers 2005).

Poor oral health can lead to poor health outcomes in patients with CKD and is associated with malnutrition including the protein-energy wasting syndrome, which disproportionately affects CKD patients (Ruospo and coworkers 2014).

Oral hygiene is often poor in CKD patients, particularly in those on dialysis, due to access problems (Grubbs and coworkers 2012). CKD has been associated with a higher incidence of periodontal disease in patients on renal dialysis (Davidovich and coworkers 2005), although controversy remains with regard to this link. Recent data suggest a higher incidence of mortality in dialyzed CKD patients with periodontal disease (Kshirsagar and coworkers 2009), which may have important implications for elderly CKD patients who develop peri-implant disease. To date, no prospective controlled studies have been published on these relationships, but there is at least one long-term study known to be in progress (Strippoli and coworkers 2013).

There may be a reduced incidence of caries arising from the antibacterial effect of urea in saliva (Bots and coworkers 2006). However, in patients with xerostomia, caries experience may be high. There may be an increased accumulation of calculus as a result of high salivary urea levels and changes in the calcium or phosphorus metabolism (Gavalda and coworkers 1999).

Oral infections such as dental or periodontal abscesses tend to be difficult to control in CKD patients, and in particular in patients on immunosuppressants. In addition, signs of infection may be masked by steroid therapy. Oral bacterial infections should be treated promptly and aggressively, but with due consideration for the changes in drug excretion and necessary dose modifications.

Immunosuppression in transplant patients and those on dialysis may lead to candidiasis, oral ulceration, and oral leukoplakia lesions. Lichenoid reactions occur and are not always drug-related. Hairy leukoplakia and an increased susceptibility to epithelial dysplasia may be associated with greater incidence of carcinoma of the lip (Proctor and coworkers 2005).

Bony changes may occur secondary to renal osteodystrophy, especially in the maxilla, with decreased trabeculation and cortical thickness or with ectopic calcification of the soft tissues. Tooth mobility may also occur (De Rossi and Glick 1996).

Treatment should be planned in close cooperation with the patient's physician, particularly in patients receiving hemodialysis, so that anticoagulation therapy can be managed accordingly and the need for antibiotic prophylaxis can be agreed as requirements vary from country to country.

The effect of CKD on the osseointegration of dental implants has been the subject of animal studies. In uremic mice, a reduced bone-to-implant contact compared to controls was found, but this was only observed in the early stages of osseointegration (2 weeks), and no significant differences were observed with control subjects at 4 weeks. The authors of one paper suggested that longer healing times should be considered for dental implants placed in CKD patients (Zou and coworkers 2013).

There are reports of successful implant therapy in renal dialysis and transplant patients (Dijakiewicz and coworkers 2007).

How the progression of CKD may affect the ongoing success of dental implants that have been in situ for some time is not yet known, although it seems reasonable to assume that the changes that occur around teeth because of poor oral hygiene and osteodystrophy may also be likely to occur around implant-supported prostheses. However, the treatment of such implant complications may be considerably more difficult and could present, in a patient who requires stabilization of oral disease prior to renal transplantation, significant challenges.

5.8.3 Pharmacological Considerations

Patients with renal disease are often taking antihypertensives such as ACE inhibitors and angiotensin II inhibitors. As there is an increased risk of cardiovascular disease, acetylsalicylic acid and statin use is also common.

Many drugs used in patients with renal disease may cause orthostatic hypotension, hyperglycemia, or xerostomia, and the effect may be greater in the elderly patient.

Calcium carbonate and vitamin D supplements/analogs are used to prevent the loss of bone mass. Secondary hyperparathyroidism resulting from renal osteodystrophy may mean the initiation of bisphosphonate therapy.

Patients on renal hemodialysis are often anticoagulated and liaison with the medical team will be required. Adjunctive corticosteroids may be required for those patients on prolonged corticosteroid therapy.

Many drugs prescribed by the dentist may require dose modification. For a review of drugs that are safe, need dose modification, or should be avoided, see Scully 2014. Due to the rapidly changing range of therapeutic drugs, reference to a national formulary should always be made, and consultation with the patient's physician is recommended.

5.9 Endocrine System

5.9.1 Age-related Changes

Changes that occur with age include a decrease in the vascularity of organs and an increasing fibrous or connective-tissue replacement of normal glandular structures. This may affect the production and secretion of hormones, with a potential effect on normal bodily function. A typical example is menopause, where a decrease in overall mass of the ovaries combined with a reduction in ovarian response to gonadotropin leads to a significant decline in ovarian function and the production of progesterone and estrogen. This may then lead to the development of osteoporosis (discussed in the section on musculoskeletal changes), hyperlipidemia, or atherosclerosis.

Elderly individuals will commonly exhibit reduced muscle mass as a result of decreasing vascularity of the anterior pituitary gland, which causes reduced secretion of growth hormone. Age-related disability, exhibited by generalized weakness, impaired coordination, balance, and mobility, with reduced endurance, defines physical frailty and will affect a person's continuing independence into advanced years.

Thymic involution—shrinkage of the thymus with age— is a progressive decline in the size of the thymus that begins during the first year after birth and has been linked to the previously discussed age-related decline in immunological function in the elderly.

One of the most important age-related endocrine changes is a reduction in thyroid function and an increased incidence of thyroid disorders, which are often subclinical. Overt hypothyroidism can be associated with a decline in physical and cognitive function, but it appears that subclinical hypothyroidism in the elderly is not. Subclinical hyperthyroidism in the elderly may be associated with abnormalities in bone microarchitecture and fragility fracture, cognitive impairment, coronary heart disease, and atrial fibrillation (Gesing and coworkers 2012).

There are some important oral findings in hypothyroidism. Given the high rate of undiagnosed disease, especially in the elderly, the dental professional may have an important role to play in detection. Common oral findings include poor periodontal health, enlarged salivary glands, macroglossia, dysgeusia, and delayed wound healing, although there does not appear to be an increased susceptibility to infection. Hyperthyroidism may arise from iatrogenic overprescription of replacement therapy or from a tumor, which may be detected during a routine head and neck examination. Elderly hyperthyroid patients may present with burning-mouth syndrome, mandibular or maxillary osteoporosis (Pinto and Glick 2002).

Hypothyroidism has been shown to result in delayed bone remodeling and repair in rats (Fadaei Fathabady and coworkers 2005) and has been implicated in non-union of mandibular fracture (Loftus and Peterson 1979). It is important to note that this appears not to be related to low TSH levels—these may be normal—but to low circulating T3 levels (Bassett and coworkers 2008).

Other studies have demonstrated a link between hypothyroidism and delayed cortical bone healing around dental implants. However, cancellous bone appeared to be less sensitive to T3 and T4 levels (Feitosa Dda and coworkers 2008).

Secretion of parathormone is known to increase in aging men and women (Chapuy and coworkers 1983). The reason for this is unclear, but may be a reaction to reduced plasma calcium levels associated with reduced calcium intake and sun exposure, resulting in reduced calcium absorption in the small intestine, with secondary hyperparathyroidism occurring as a compensatory measure. The principal effect of parathormone is to increase plasma calcium levels by stimulating the release of calcium and phosphate from bone matrix, as well as increasing calcium reabsorption by the kidney, and by increasing the renal production of 1,25-dihydroxyvitamin D_3 (calcitriol), the effect of which is to increase intestinal absorption of calcium.

Consequently, the elderly are at high risk of calcium deficiency, which in turn contributes to a loss of bone mass as well as muscle weakness, impaired glandular secretion, and degraded synaptic transmission.

The adrenal glands become increasingly fibrous with age; production of aldosterone (and, to a lesser extent, cortisol) diminishes, although epinephrine and norepinephrine levels remain unchanged. Aging appears to be associated with a reduced tolerance to physiological stress and an increasing vulnerability to illness and infection (Kale and Yende 2011). Glucocorticoid production appears to decline, although the circulatory levels appear to remain the same in normal homeostasis. Responses to stress may, however, be blunted in older people, who are more likely to develop infections after stressful events as a result of reduced neutrophil function (Vitlic and coworkers 2014). Sepsis can rapidly develop into a serious problem in an elderly patient, with significant mortality rates (Starr and coworkers 2014). Healing is slower, there is increased morbidity, and infections tend to start early, be late in causing symptoms, and be slow to resolve.

A reduction in the secretion of the mineralocorticoid aldosterone can result in changes in electrolyte and fluid balance, to which elderly patients may be more sensitive.

The glucocorticoid hormones secreted by the adrenal glands have important effects on glucose metabolism and it has been shown that stress hormone responses can induce hyperglycemia (O'Neill and coworkers 1991). Age-related decline in levels of the adrenal hormone dehydroepiandrosterone (DHEA), an important hormone for the central nervous system, is linked to declining cognitive performance (Valenti and coworkers 2009).

Increasing age is a known risk factor for the development of diabetes and related complications. Diabetes accounts for significant morbidity and mortality in elderly individuals, although the impact of diagnosis in later years is not clear (Bethel and coworkers 2007; Barnett and coworkers 2006).

The global incidence of diabetes mellitus (DM) and in particular type 2 DM is rapidly increasing (Shaw and coworkers 2010). For example, between 1997 and 2010 the number of diagnosed cases in the US increased from 5.1% to 9.2%, and this trend is expected to continue even faster, especially in the elderly (Boyle and coworkers 2010). The International Diabetes Federation estimates that the global prevalence may be 8.3%, but with 46.3% of cases undiagnosed; by 2030, almost 10% of the world's population will be diabetics (International Diabetes Federation 2014).

Some studies have shown that up to 40% of elderly individuals exhibit impaired glucose tolerance, which can be a precursor to diabetes (Harris and coworkers 1998). Blood sugar levels increase more rapidly and take longer to return to normal, which together with a decline in cell sensitivity to insulin can result in the development of diabetes.

Aging is often accompanied by reduced physical activity, decreased lean body mass, and increased fat deposition, leading to defective peripheral insulin tolerance; coupled with relatively decreased insulin secretion from the pancreas, large numbers of elderly individuals may have undiagnosed diabetes mellitus. Dietary changes in elderly patients reflecting masticatory difficulty, a reduced taste sensation, eating prepared meals, and other factors can result in an increased intake of refined carbohydrates; combined with age-related decreases in glucose tolerance, type 2 DM can develop insidiously in elderly individuals.

Diabetes is associated with many complications, including myocardial infarction/heart failure, peripheral vascular disease, and stroke. Research has indicated that patients with diabetes mellitus have a similar risk of myocardial infarction as a healthy person ten years older (Lindhardsen and coworkers 2011). Diabetes has also been implicated as a risk factor for renal disease, retinopathy, neuropathy, depression, and dementia and can be a cause of secondary immunodeficiency.

DM and fragility fractures due to osteoporosis are two of the most important causes of mortality and morbidity in older subjects. There appears to be a correlation between fragility fracture risk and DM of both type 1 and type 2. Because thiazolidinedione drugs used in the treatment of diabetes may influence a greater differentiation of adipocytes than osteoprogenitor cells, elderly patients with type 2 DM and particularly women may be at increased risk of reduced bone-mineral density (BMD). Good glycemic control, adequate intake of calcium and vitamin D, screening for low BMD, and the prevention and treatment of diabetic complications are key elements in the management of osteoporosis in both type 1 and type 2 DM (Montagnani and coworkers 2011).

Diabetes has also been implicated as a comorbid risk factor in medication-related osteonecrosis of the jaw (MRONJ) (Tsao and coworkers 2013; Saad and coworkers 2012) and the more rapid progression of oral infections to serious deep neck space infections in diabetics (Boscolo-Rizzo and coworkers 2011).

It is recognized that DM is an important complicating factor in implant therapy. Oral symptoms associated with DM include xerostomia with parotid swelling, increased levels of salivary glucose and an increased incidence of caries and periodontal disease. Chronic hyperglycemia is associated with a reduction in bone formation by impeding osteoblast formation and interfering with bone response to parathormone (Santana and coworkers 2003). There are also effects on the production of extracellular matrix and osteoid (Nyomba and coworkers 1989; Weiss and coworkers 1981).

Wound healing is slower, and there is an increased susceptibility to implant loss (Fiorellini and Nevins 2000). Implant survival rates appear to be lower in diabetic patients, even those with good glycemic control (Moy and coworkers 2005). Despite other review studies reporting a lack of evidence for such an association (Chrcanovic and coworkers 2014; Kotsovilis and coworkers 2006; Al-saadi and coworkers 2007), there is evidence that poor glycemic control is associated with higher rates of implant failure (Ferreira and coworkers 2006).

It is easily conceivable that an elderly patient, perhaps with other comorbidities, may present as an undiagnosed diabetic. Clinicians should be aware of the signs and symptoms of poorly controlled or undiagnosed DM. We have an active role to assume in diagnosing and treating oral signs or symptoms of systemic disease, and in doing so we contribute to the overall health of our patients.

5.9.2   Pharmacological Considerations

Hypothyroid patients with atrial fibrillation may be on anticoagulation therapy and may require antibiotic cover for valvular disease. Such patients may be taking replacement therapy in the form of l-thyroxine, which can interact with warfarin to produce an enhanced anticoagulant effect. INR monitoring of such patients is of increased importance. Thyroxine may also be affected by indigestion remedies, iron supplements, antiepilep-

tic drugs such as phenytoin and carbamazepine, tricyclic antidepressants, and rifampicin. There is also an increased sensitivity to CMS depressants and barbiturates.

The main drugs used for the treatment of hyperthyroidism are carbimazole/methimazole, and, less commonly, propylthiouracil. These drugs can cause agranulocytosis or leukopenia; this may present as an apparent exaggerated periodontal/peri-implant inflammation or oral ulceration.

Patients on cortisone replacement therapy may require additional doses to prevent adrenal insufficiency and given the reduced stress tolerance in elderly patients, this may be of greater significance.

Diabetic patients may require special management, particularly for surgical procedures and point-of-care blood glucose testing devices can be useful. With good glycemic control with a normal diet/injection routine having been taken, insulin-dependent diabetics can be treated within 2 hours with no adjunctive therapy. Protracted procedures should be performed in a hospital setting.

Medications to be avoided if possible include corticosteroids, which increase blood glucose levels; ciprofloxacin, doxycycline, and tetracyclines can enhance insulin mediated hypoglycemia. NSAID use may not be appropriate, as diabetic patients often take acetylsalicylic acid for the prophylaxis of ischemic heart disease. NSAIDs also present a risk of renal damage in diabetic patients. Many other classes of drug can affect glycemic levels, including antiepileptics, antidepressants, diuretics, quinolone antibiotics, herbal supplements, alcohol, and OTC medications for allergies and head colds/coughs.

Infections in diabetic patients should be aggressively managed due to the risk of diabetic immunosuppression and rapid progression of infection.

Thiazolidinediones (TZD) such as rosiglitazone and pioglitazone appear to cause bone loss and are included in medications known to cause secondary osteoporosis (Lecka-Czernik 2010).

5.10 Musculoskeletal System

5.10.1 Age-related Changes

Age-related decline in muscle mass (sarcopenia) is a common finding in the geriatric patient (Evans 1995). Reduced muscle mass is associated with a lack of physical activity, which in itself can result in muscle disease and loss of muscle tissue. Hormonal and neurologic alterations can also be involved in loss of muscle mass—sarcopenia—as a result of reduction in the number of muscle fibers.

Sarcopenia affects the hand muscles in particular, with a concomitant effect on manual dexterity. Coordination is reduced, with extended motor reaction times due to slowed peripheral nerve transmission.

Musculoskeletal disease is very prevalent, being the second highest cause of the morbidity-related global burden of disease (Vos and coworkers 2012). Almost all old people will experience one or more forms of musculoskeletal disorder, often concurrent, and potentially due to many different reasons. Osteoporosis, Paget's disease, osteoarthritis, inflammatory rheumatoid conditions and associated connective-tissue disorders (CTDs), endocrine disease, or metastatic carcinoma are all possible causes, as are localized conditions such as fibromyalgia.

Osteoarthritis. Osteoarthritis is very prevalent in the over-75 age group, affecting more than 80% of this population. It is rarely seen in patients under 40 years (Sharma 2001). Osteoarthritis of the hands, hips, knees and spine are increasingly prevalent with aging and can progress to a severely debilitating condition.

Rheumatoid conditions. Autoimmune diseases affecting the soft tissues and bone, such as rheumatoid arthritis, and chronic connective tissue diseases such as Sjögren's syndrome, may develop in isolation or in conjunction but share similar features in pathogenicity, symptoms, and diagnosis; patients requiring implant treatment may require special considerations. These conditions are not the preserve of the geriatric patient and most commonly present earlier in life at around 30 to 40 years; however, being progressive, the effects of the disease may be more severe and of increasing significance in the elderly patient.

The presence of rheumatoid arthritis has been associated with alterations in skeletal bone mass in 30% to 50% of individuals, whether or not they are prescribed steroidal anti-inflammatory medication (Haugeberg 2008), and muscle wasting. Rheumatoid arthritis can be associated with other conditions affecting the heart (conduction defects, myo- or pericarditis), hematopoietic system (thrombocytopenia, anemia, leukopenia), renal, hepatic, neurological (trigeminal neuralgia), and respiratory systems. Research has indicated that patients with rheumatoid arthritis have a similar risk of myocardial infarction as a healthy person who is 10 years older, as is the case for example with diabetes mellitus (Lindhardsen and coworkers 2011).

Sjögren's syndrome is the most common oral complication in rheumatoid patients and is discussed in the section dealing with oral medicine.

There are studies that have indicated favorable implant success rates in patients suffering from autoimmune rheumatoid arthritis, whether or not accompanied by associated connective-tissue disorders. However, in those patients with an accompanying connective tissue disorder, there may be an increased incidence of peri-implant inflammation (Weinlander and coworkers 2010; Krennmair and coworkers 2010; there is significant cohort overlap between these two studies).

Some connective-tissue disorders are only found in aging individuals. Polymyalgia rheumatica is a rheumatoid disease that is found only in patients over 50 years, with the average age of sufferers being 70 years; it is mainly found in northern European Caucasian populations and is twice as prevalent in women as in men, causing muscular pain, particularly in the shoulders or thighs. Treatment is with oral corticosteroids. The disease may "burn out" after a few years, but approximately 20% of cases are complicated by giant-cell arteritis ("temporal arteritis"), with a risk of ocular complications. Anemia is a common finding in patients with polymyalgia rheumatica.

Alterations in skeletal bone

Calcium and vitamin D are elements of bone physiology that become increasingly important in the maintenance of healthy bones in elderly individuals. It is recognized that many of them have a "negative calcium balance" and are losing bone mass. Although this may in part be due to a lack of weight-bearing activity, there is evidence that inadequate calcium intake is a contributory factor (Heaney and coworkers 1982).

Calcium uptake is mediated by 1,25-dihydroxyvitamin D_3 (also known as 1,25-dihydroxycholecalciferol, or calcitriol), which is the hormonal form of vitamin D_3 (cholecalciferol). There is a natural decline in calcium absorption from around the age of 50 years. Furthermore, as a consequence of increasing lactose intolerance in elderly people, dietary calcium intake may be reduced if they avoid dairy products, a major dietary source of calcium along with green vegetables. Senescence of the skin has far-reaching effects on other organ systems, with cutaneous vitamin D production from exposure to sunlight declining in old age by as much as 75% in northern European populations; a compounding factor can be the reduced amount of time spent outdoors by elderly people. Dietary deficiencies can also play a part—vitamin D can also be obtained from cereals, eggs, meat, and oily fish. Chronic renal disease can also result in severe vitamin D deficiency (Williams and coworkers 2009).

The effect of hyperparathyroidism on bone has been discussed in the section on endocrine disorders. Parathyroid function increases with age, possibly as a response to reduced dietary calcium and less effective vitamin D production; oversecretion of parathormone results in elevated levels of bone resorption, to restore normal plasma calcium levels. This age-related hyperparathyroidism emphasizes the importance of calcium and vitamin D supplements, especially in elderly European populations, in preventing loss of bone-mineral density. This is the case not only in long-stay patients but also in ambulatory individuals over 60 years.

Skeletal tissue loss due to age is more rapid in women, who typically lose 30% to 50% of their bone mass during their lifetime, compared to 20% to 30% in men. This is characterized histologically by a thinning of the cortical bone layer, a decrease in the density and thickness of

trabeculae with an increase in trabecular space, and an increased number of empty osteocyte lacunae. The percentage of dead osteocytes in bone increases with age from less than 1% at birth to 75% after age 80 (Tomkinson and coworkers 1997). Osteocyte apoptosis may be related to the development of osteoporosis (Heino and coworkers 2009) as a result of RANKL-mediated osteoclast recruitment (Bonewald 2011). The progressive mineralization of lacunae around dead osteocytes spreads to the canaliculi in the immediate vicinity, with the result that the bone becomes sclerotic and brittle. The reduction in vascularity caused by sclerosis of the canaliculi leads to decreased oxygenation, which may be important in the process of osseointegration (Van Steenberghe 2003). The implication of these histological findings on the osseointegration of implants in the elderly is unclear, as multiple studies have not shown any tendency to increased failure rate of implants with age, even in medically compromised patients (de Baat 2000, Op Heij 2003). However, there are significant potential consequences of the medications used to treat declining bone mass, as will be described later.

A reduction in overall bone mass can be due to two metabolic bone disorders: osteomalacia and osteopenia/osteoporosis. Reduced bone mass may also be a consequence of drug therapy with, e.g., corticosteroids.

There is also evidence that RA patients have a higher bone turnover and show an increased incidence of osteoporosis and vertebral fracture (Nakayama 2007); the prevalence of osteoporosis in RA patients may be double the incidence in non-rheumatoid individuals (Haugeberg 2008).

Osteomalacia

Osteomalacia is a condition characterized by defective mineralization of organic bone matrix (collagen) and is frequently associated with hypocalcemia due to vitamin D deficiency. Hypocalcemia results in increased secretion of parathormone (PTH), and this in turn causes increased renal excretion of phosphorus. Low intraosseous phosphorus concentration impairs the normal processes of bone mineralization. Osteomalacia is therefore characterized by a reduction in bone mass and the ratio of bone mineral to bone matrix.

Radiographic changes characteristic of osteomalacia are thinner cortical plates and decreased trabecular density. Since osteomalacia therefore causes bone characteristics typical of Type IV bone, it is possible that such patients may be characterized as merely having "poor bone quality," which has been associated with an increased rate of implant failure by some authors (Goiato and coworkers 2014; Alsaadi and coworkers 2007).

Osteoporosis

Osteoporosis is a decrease in bone mass due to a reduction in both mineral and organic bone structures, but the ratio of the two remains constant, which is what differentiates osteoporosis from osteomalacia. Osteoporosis arises from an imbalance between bone resorption and deposition; it results in thinner cortical plates and a decrease in trabecular density and diameter. Trabecular remodeling is normally faster than cortical remodeling, and so a decrease in cancellous structure is seen well before any reduction in cortical plate thickness, although radiographic changes are unlikely to be seen before approximately one-third of the bone mass has been lost. Special radiographic techniques such as dual-energy x-ray absorptiometry (DEXA) or quantitative CT are therefore required for a definitive diagnosis.

A diagnosis of osteoporosis is made when the T-score (the number of standard deviations from the normal bone density value of an average 25-year-old woman) exceeds −2.5, with osteopenia being diagnosed when the T-score is in the range of −1.0 to −2.5 (Glaser and Kaplan 1997).

Primary osteoporosis accounts for approximately 95% of cases in women and 80% of cases in men and is related to family history, racial phenotypes, gender (as a result of hormonal factors), and age. Peak bone mass occurs in an individual's late twenties and decreases thereafter. Secondary osteoporosis accounts for less than 5% of cases but is more prevalent in men than in women and may occur as part of disease processes such as malignancy, COPD, CKD, hepatic disease, and certain endocrine disorders, or through the use of certain medications, for example corticosteroids and certain anticonvulsants. Risk factors such as smoking, excessive alcohol intake, dietary deficiencies and chronic inflammatory conditions such as ulcerative colitis or rheumatoid arthritis may also have an adverse impact (Beikler and Flemming 2003).

An increased incidence of osteoporosis is seen in the over-50 population. The condition is more prevalent in the elderly individual due to accelerated normal age-related bone-tissue loss as outlined above as a consequence of decreased calcium intake and reduced vitamin D levels, or for example hyperparathyroidism. It affects nearly half of men and women over 75 years, with women being five times more likely to develop this disease. Postmenopausal women may lose up to 20% of their bone mass in 5 to 7 years after the menopause, but by 70 years, men and women lose bone at approximately the same rate.

An important consideration in osteoporotic individuals is the increased incidence of fragility fractures of the wrist, hip, and spine, leading to loss of independence and hospitalization. In elderly patients, this has been associated with significantly increased fatality rates. Indeed, the prevention of fragility fractures is one of the major indications for the prescription of antiresorptive medications.

Implant survival in "poor bone quality" is a widely discussed topic. Several classifications have been suggested for bone quality based on bone type (ratio of cortical bone to cancellous bone, types I to IV (Lekholm and Zarb 1985), type V bone with no cortical plates (Bahat 2000) and density (hard or soft) (Trisi and coworkers 1999), although the most common assessment is one made subjectively at the time of implant surgery.

In fact, quality of bone is not merely related to density or type; it will also depend on histological attributes such as vascularity, oxygen tension, cell vitality, and associated systemic health factors that will affect the healing capacity of the bone.

There are publications that show little difference in the survival of implants placed in "poor-quality" or "good-quality" bone, particularly when using implants with a microrough surface (for a review see Stanford 2010), although the level of evidence in all of these situations is weak. The level of evidence relating to implant failure in individuals with a diagnosis of osteoporosis is similarly low (Bornstein and coworkers 2009), with most reports showing no relationship between osteoporosis and implant failure (Slagter and coworkers 2008) even in highly osteoporotic patients (Friberg and coworkers 2001; Eder and Watzek 1999).

There may be a similar lack of association between peri-implant disease and osteoporosis (Dvorak and coworkers 2011).

Treatment of osteoporosis

HRT (estrogen). Studies have reported conflicting findings regarding implant loss in postmenopausal women related to hormone replacement therapy (Minsk and Polson 1998; Moy and coworkers 2005). In one study directly comparing implant failure rates in postmenopausal women with or without HRT and premenopausal women, there was no difference between the groups for mandibular implants. For maxillary implants, the postmenopausal non-HRT group had a significantly higher implant failure rate than the premenopausal and postmenopausal HRT-treated group (August and coworkers 2001).

Antiresorptive medications. While osteoporosis as such may be of questionable concern to clinicians involved in dental implant and related surgery, the potential consequences of medications used to treat the condition are significant. Antiresorptive medications may be used for the treatment of osteoporosis/osteopenia, metabolic bone disease (Paget's disease, hyperparathyroidism), or in the treatment of malignancy such as multiple myeloma or metastatic bone disease (such as breast or prostate cancer); there are different forms of medications in current use.

One of the most widely used groups of drugs is that of the bisphosphonates, of which there are two main types: nitrogen-containing (alendronate, risedronate, ibandronate, pamidronate, zoledronate) and non-nitrogen-containing (etidronate). Nitrogen-containing bisphosphonates are more potent, as they are not metabolized and are concentrated in the bone, where the drug bonds to hydroxyapatite (Russell and coworkers 1999) and has been associated with osteonecrosis of the jaw after many years of use (Wang and coworkers 2007).

The primary mode of action of bisphosphonates is by targeting osteoclastic activity and reducing bone resorption. Oversuppression of bone turnover has previously been postulated as a possible mechanism in the pathophysiology of osteonecrosis due to bisphosphonates being concentrated in the jaws, where bone turnover is more active (Masarachia and coworkers 1996; Huja and coworkers 2006). However, recent research suggests that there is no significant change in bone turnover in the jaws with either bisphosphonates or denosumab (Ristow and coworkers 2014; Malan and coworkers 2012).

There are clinical reports of a possible toxic effect on other cell types, including oral epithelial cells (Reid and coworkers 2007), which could in theory contribute to soft-tissue breakdown. While unbound bisphosphonates are present in tissues other than bone for only a short time, being renally excreted within a few hours, in-vitro studies report toxicity affecting oral mucosal cells (Landesberg and coworkers 2008). Common ADEs of oral bisphosphonates are gastric or esophageal ulcers, further supporting the theory of possible soft-tissue toxicity (Lanza and coworkers 2000).

The most widely discussed issue of concern to dental implant surgeons is bisphosphonate-related osteonecrosis of the jaw (BRONJ). Given the increasing use of alternative antiresorptive medications, the alternative suggested term is MRONJ—medication-related osteonecrosis of the jaw. While the term has been updated, there is still some uncertainty over the pathophysiology of the disease (Ruggiero and coworkers 2014).

Literature reviews have supported the opinion that dental implants can osseointegrate and remain in good function in patients receiving bisphosphonate therapy (Javed and Almas 2010). Systematic reviews of the literature commonly find insufficient high-level evidence to estimate the risks associated with implant therapy in patients receiving oral bisphosphonates (Bornstein and coworkers 2009; Chamizo Carmona and coworkers 2012).

However, it is apparent that the type of medication and route of administration, dose, and duration are all important factors. Clinicians involved in implant therapy should therefore be aware of the different medications and their potential impact on the placement or presence of dental implants, particularly given the increased likelihood of their use in the aging patient. The combination of bisphosphonates with medications used for comorbidities, such as chemotherapy or corticosteroids, has been implicated in the incidence, severity, and progression of MRONJ in animal models (López-Jornet and coworkers 2011; Ali-Erdem and coworkers 2011).

It is increasingly recognized that long-term bisphosphonate use can result in atypical fractures of the mid-femoral shaft, which may be preceded by thigh pain (Thompson and coworkers 2012; Schilcher and coworkers 2014). No pharmacological therapy should be considered indefinite and the efficacy of bisphosphonate therapy beyond 5 years use is limited. Given that adverse events, including atypical femoral fracture, become more prevalent beyond 5 years of therapy, bisphosphonate holidays have therefore been suggested after 5 years in patients with a DEXA-confirmed diagnosis of osteoporosis and no other risk factors, and after ten years where additional risk factors are present (Cosman and coworkers 2014).

As a consequence, the safety of long-term bisphosphonate use is being questioned for reasons other than MRONJ, and alternative medications for the prevention of fragility fractures are increasingly common. Strontium ranelate was a common alternative, but is now under review due to possible adverse cardiovascular effects.

Newer drugs developed for the treatment of osteoporosis include monoclonal antibodies (RANKL inhibitors such as denosumab) and antiangiogenic drugs. Denosumab is used six-monthly as a subcutaneous injection for prophylaxis against fragility fractures and monthly in cases of metastatic bone cancer. RANKL inhibitors do not bind to bone and their effect is substantially diminished within six months of treatment cessation. However, MRONJ has been associated with the use of denosumab (Aghaloo and coworkers 2010).

Antiangiogenic drugs inhibit the formation of new blood vessels and are used in the treatment of cancers of the gastrointestinal and neuroendocrine systems. These drugs have also been implicated in MRONJ, given the avascular necrotic nature of the condition. Inhibition of angiogenesis or interference with the VEGF pathway has been demonstrated, for example, with bisphosphonates such as zoledronate (Wood and coworkers 2002; Santini and coworkers 2003) and has been reported with novel antiangiogenic medications such as monoclonal antibodies targeting VEGF (bevacizumab) and tyrosine kinase inhibitors (sunitinib) (FDA 2014a; FDA 2014b). Such effects have not been reported with RANKL inhibitors such as denosumab.

The most recent update (2014) of the American Association of Oral and Maxillofacial Surgeons position paper on medication-related osteonecrosis of the jaw (Ruggiero and coworkers 2014) highlights the low incidence of the condition, given the small number of reported occurrences and the large number of patients prescribed intravenous/oral bisphosphonates or denosumab for osteoporosis.

It now appears to be generally accepted that the risk of MRONJ in patients receiving oral bisphosphonate therapy for osteoporosis is low (Lo and coworkers 2010; Mavrokokki and coworkers 2007; Ruggiero and coworkers 2009). However, when such medications are prescribed for patients with a relevant comorbidity such as cancer and associated therapy, the risk is higher. Table 4 shows the risk associated with the various drug types and the related factor of whether the medication is used to treat osteoporosis or malignancy.

Reported risk rates vary from 0.00038% (Felsenberg and Hoffmeister 2006) to 0.1% (Lo and coworkers 2010), with the latter group reporting an increased incidence of 0.21% in patients who had been on oral bisphosphonates for more than 4 years. Other authors indicated a lower rate of less than 0.4 cases per 10,000 patient-years of exposure (0.004%) (Malden and Lopes 2012).

The use of intravenous bisphosphonates or denosumab for the treatment of osteoporosis seems to give rise to similar rates of MRONJ, in the region of 0.017% to 0.04% (Grbic and coworkers 2010).

As a comparison, studies investigating the risk of ONJ in osteoporosis patients who were treated with placebo medications showed a risk of up to 0.02% (Grbic and coworkers 2010 and 2008).

The risk of MRONJ in patients taking antiresorptive medications as part of cancer treatment is about 100 times greater than those who are taking the medication for the treatment of osteoporosis alone. The MRONJ risk in cancer patients treated with zoledronate is in the region of 1%, according to systematic reviews and randomized controlled trials (Mauri and coworkers 2009; Qi and coworkers 2014). There are increasing case reports of MRONJ in oncology patients treated with denosumab (O'Halloran and coworkers 2014).

Again for comparison, the incidence of MRONJ in cancer patients receiving a placebo is in the region of 0.02%.

Combining bisphosphonates with antiangiogenic agents appears to result in an increased risk of MRONJ (Saad and coworkers 2012; Guarneri and coworkers 2010).

Table 4 MRONJ risk with different antiresorptive medication (Ruggiero and coworkers 2014)

Drug type	Osteoporosis	OP placebo	Cancer	Ca placebo
Oral BP	0.004%–0.21%		Not applicable	
Intravenous BP (zoledronate)	0.017%		0.7%–6.7% (1% from SR/RCT data)	
RANKL inhibitor (denosumab)	0.04%	0%–0.02%	0.7%–1.9%	0%–0.019%
Antiangiogenic (bevacizumab)	0.2%		0.2%	

The duration of medication also seems to be a risk factor in the development of MRONJ. Lo and coworkers (2010) reported a low risk of MRONJ in patients on oral bisphosphonates (0.1%) that increased to 0.21% in patients who had been taking oral bisphosphonates for more than 4 years, demonstrating a potential increase in risk related to duration of medication that has been highlighted by other authors (Dello Russo 2007; Marx 2008).

This would seem logical, given that oral bisphosphonates have a long half-life (up to 10 years) and are concentrated in bone, creating a cumulative effect.

For intravenous bisphosphonates there seems to be a plateau effect, with no significant increase after three years of administration (Black and coworkers 2012), an effect that is also seen with denosumab (Saad and coworkers 2012).

Other newer antiresorptive medications in current use include teriparatide, a form of recombinant human parathormone and raloxifene, which is a selective estrogen receptor modulator effective in preventing vertebral, but not hip fractures, also used in the treatment of breast cancer. There are currently no studies investigating the impact of these drugs on dental implant survival or maintenance.

5.10.2 Treatment Considerations

Sarcopenia can cause a reduction in masticatory strength, and elderly individuals commonly have longer chewing cycles related to reduced muscle activity. Edentulous patients often have a more significant reduction in masticatory muscle mass and maximum bite capacity, although they may find their function adequate as long as their dentures are effective and comfortable (Mioche and coworkers 2004; Newton and coworkers 2004).

We should not merely view our patients as "a set of jaws" with a potential risk of osteonecrosis. The dentist can play a role in the overall care of the patient by being vigilant to both the signs and symptoms of osteoporosis, which may be undiagnosed until the patient suffers a fracture. Chronic back pain may be due to osteoarthritis, but a vertebral compression fracture can present as an acute exacerbation with spinal tenderness in the dental chair. Patients with osteoarthritis may be unable to lie comfortably in a supine position, particularly for long appointments; the use of cushions or knee/neck supports may assist. Arthritic joint pain stiffness is usually worse in the early morning and improves during the day, so scheduling appointments for the early afternoon may be helpful.

Given the high mortality rate in geriatric patients who have suffered a hip fracture, it is also important to be vigilant for a history of falls, which may be part of the reason for seeking treatment (fractured teeth or dental prostheses). Elderly people commonly suffer from confusion, poor coordination, poor vision, and muscle weakness, or orthostatic hypotension as a result of medication, all of which can be reasons for falling. It may be appropriate for the clinician to assist referral to a falls prevention service or other relevant community care.

The available studies, mostly restricted to case reports or retrospective case series, suggest that implant placement in patients with rheumatoid arthritis (with or without concomitant osteoporosis or connective tissue disorders) is not contraindicated and not associated with a higher implant failure rate, particularly when surface-modified implants are used (Oczakir and coworkers 2005; Alsaadi and coworkers 2008; Krennmair and coworkers 2010). However, attention must be paid to medication with corticosteroid or immunosuppressive therapy (Mombelli and Cionca 2006). It is important to consider how different diseases may have an impact on treatment, given polymorbidity and associated pharmacotherapy.

There may be a risk of increase peri-implant mucosal inflammation and marginal bone loss in patients with rheumatoid arthritis and an associated connective-tissue disorder, notably Sjögren's syndrome (Krennmair and coworkers 2010).

Musculoskeletal disorders are the second most common cause of disability (Vos and coworkers 2012) and patients with impaired mobility may find difficulty in accessing dental maintenance care.

Rheumatoid or osteoarthritis can have an effect on manual dexterity and strength (Sheehy and coworkers 2013). There have been studies showing an increased incidence of inflammation and periodontal attachment loss in patients with arthritic hands (Gleissner and coworkers 1998; Wolff and coworkers 2014). We should therefore consider how well the patient will be able to perform the necessary oral hygiene procedures to care for any implants and dental prostheses. It may be possible to provide augmented handles for toothbrushes; electric toothbrushes may be of significant help. But what chance would a patient with rheumatoid arthritis of the hands, with swan-neck deformity and ulnar deviation, have with small interdental brushes or floss? Daily plaque control at home is of course of paramount importance in the maintenance of adequate peri-implant health; a patient with a complex fixed rehabilitations may be physically unable to perform the necessary procedures and may require assistance from caregivers or more frequent professional dental maintenance.

We may consider that removable implant-supported overdentures present a "better" option, but will such a patient be able to grip the denture well enough and have the ability to unclip the denture from the bar or Locator attachments? We may have to consider progressive changes to the attachment system and the degree of retention.

Such considerations should be assessed at the outset of treatment, perhaps as simply as offering a handshake to the patient and testing coordination and muscle strength (Incel and coworkers 2009) or observing a tremor. Wheelchair patients may exhibit a weakening of the extensor muscles of the wrist and fingers as a result of radial nerve compression caused by resting on the arms of their wheelchair.

Osteoarthritis can affect the temporomandibular joints, but is rarely of clinical significance, even if radiographic evidence of the disease is marked or where the individual has more severe disease of other joints.

Patients with a history of joint disease will often have received a joint prosthesis. There is no good evidence for prophylactic antibiotic therapy before implant placement in most patients with artificial joint replacements. It has been estimated that the risk of antibiotic adverse events such as gastrointestinal upset (which may include a risk of more severe complications in the elderly), ana-phylaxis, or development of *Clostridium difficile*, especially in the elderly patient, with a risk of severe morbidity and mortality. However, patients with a recently placed joint prostheses (< 2 years) or a comorbidity affecting immune status, such as corticosteroid therapy, diabetes, rheumatoid arthritis, or chemo- or immunosuppressive therapy, may be at a greater risk of prosthesis infection, and consultation with their orthopedic surgeon on the provision of antibiotic cover is necessary (AAOS/ADA 2014).

As is the case with antibiotic prophylaxis for cardiac conditions, guidance from both clinical and medicolegal authorities varies considerably in different countries, and a risk assessment should be undertaken and fully discussed with the patient before any surgery. An important recommendation of several publications is that patients have good oral health before joint replacement surgery and that good oral hygiene is maintained.

Implant placement in osteoporotic patients. The relationship between skeletal bone loss due to osteoporosis and loss of mandibular or maxillary bone is unclear. Researchers have previously suggested that there is no link (von Wowern and Melsen 1979; von Wowern and coworkers 1988; Jacobs and coworkers 1996). However, some recent studies have found a correlation between reduced skeletal bone-mineral density and reduced mandibular alveolar bone mass, such that dental radiographs could be an important tool in the detection of osteoporosis (Amam and Rustom 2014). This has been confirmed by DEXA measurements of the jaw, which show a high degree of correlation between reduced mandibular bone--mineral density and typical scan sites such as the proximal radius and lumbar spine (Horner and coworkers 1996). Some authors have noted implant failure in low-density (type IV) bone; they considered whether this might be related to osteoporosis but found no significant correlation (Alsaadi and coworkers 2008). Dental implant integration can be successful even in the mandibles of highly osteoporotic individuals (Fujimoto and coworkers 1996; Eder and Watzek 1999; Degidi and Piattelli 2003; Friberg and coworkers 2001).

However, there have been reports of a greater degree of peri-implant marginal bone loss in osteoporotic patients compared with non-osteoporotic patients after 5 years of functional implant loading (von Wowern and Gotfredsen 2001). It is of course important to consider the risk of mandibular fracture when implant surgery is performed in atrophic mandibles (Mason and coworkers 1990).

Risk of MRONJ. MRONJ is undoubtedly a significant complication of dentoalveolar surgery that is difficult to manage and has considerable morbidity. Clinical studies have shown that MRONJ can arise spontaneously in patients on antiresorptive medication in the presence of inflammation or infection as a result of bacterial disease (Hoff and coworkers 2008). Animal studies have indicated that this may be one of the possible factors in the pathogenesis of MRONJ (Aghaloo and coworkers 2011; Aguirre and coworkers 2012; Kang and coworkers 2013).

Consequently, while extractions and bony surgery in patients taking such medications carries a small risk of MRONJ, ignoring a periodontal or peri-implant infection may also carry the same or greater risk. The role of complex biofilms that are adherent to exposed bone presents further questions in the treatment of established MRONJ (Sedghizadeh and coworkers 2008 and 2009). It may therefore be useful to consider risk-reduction strategies when considering dentoalveolar surgery in such patients.

Although the usefulness of dental assessment and completion of dental treatment before starting oral bisphosphonates is questioned by some authorities as the risk of MRONJ is low (Raj and coworkers 2014), in patients who are to be prescribed intravenous bisphosphonates or antiangiogenic medications there is evidence to support pre-medication dental assessment and treatment (Ripamonti and coworkers 2009; Dimopoulos and coworkers 2009; Vandone and coworkers 2012).

Based on current evidence, the risk of MRONJ after dentoalveolar surgery in patients taking oral bisphosphonates or denosumab for osteoporosis is small, being in the region of 0.45% (Kunchur and coworkers 2009). However, there is considerable variation in opinion. A recent case-control study reports that there may be an increased incidence (odds ratio 13.1; 95% CI 4.4 – 39.3; p < 0.001) of delayed healing after extractions in patients taking oral bisphosphonates, which may progress to osteonecrosis (Borromeo and coworkers 2014).

There is limited data on the risk of MRONJ following the placement of dental implants, or after periodontal or endodontic surgery. Expert advice is that the risk associated with flap elevation and bone manipulation approximates the risk associated with dental extractions (Ruggiero and coworkers 2014). The placement of implants in osteoporosis patients taking oral bisphosphonates for up to 3 years appears to carry little risk of MRONJ (Jeffcoat 2006; Grant and coworkers 2008; Madrid and Sanz 2009a).

However, as stated, there is a significantly greater risk in patients with comorbidities or those on intravenous antiresorptive therapy. Although there is little data relating to implant placement in patients on intravenous bisphosphonate therapy, most authors believe that given the risks, implant placement is contraindicated (Dello Russo and coworkers 2007; Bornstein and coworkers 2009). Relevant comorbidities may include simultaneous medication with corticosteroids, diabetes, or in cancer patients possibly anemia (hemoglobin < 10 g/dl) (Tsao and coworkers 2013; Saad and coworkers 2012). Smoking may also be considered a relevant factor due to reduced tissue oxygenation.

It is therefore important to consider social issues, polypharmacy, and polymorbidity as individual "warning lights," with the risk increasing as the number of warnings increases.

The incidence of MRONJ following a dental extraction in cancer patients on intravenous bisphosphonates is higher, with one prospective study showing a rate of 2.8% (Mozzati and coworkers 2012). Overall, it has been estimated that up to 61% of MRONJ cases in cancer patients on intravenous bisphosphonates (Vahtsevanos and coworkers 2009) were precipitated by dental extractions.

Dentures have also been associated with MRONJ in cancer patients treated with intravenous bisphosphonates (Vahtsevanos and coworkers 2009; Kyrgidis and coworkers 2008).

Drug holidays. At present, it is not clear whether cessation of oral antiresorptive medication before dentoalveolar surgery is beneficial. It is important to consider the medical risks to the patient of not taking the medication for some time. It has been reported that there is no evidence to support cessation of oral bisphosphonate therapy in osteoporosis patients before dentoalveolar surgery (FDA 2011). A recent consensus conference concluded that a "drug holiday" might be beneficial in high-risk patients with long-term exposure to antiresorptive medication or in patients with comorbidities such as smoking, diabetes, steroid therapy, or rheumatoid arthritis (Khan and coworkers 2015).

The question of cessation of drug therapy in cancer patients on antiresorptive medication in combination with other pharmacotherapy is unlikely to be of relevance in terms of dental implant surgery. Such procedures are unlikely to be appropriate in oncological patients. These patients may require extractions, but elective invasive dental treatment should only be considered as part of a multidisciplinary approach with the specialists involved in the care of the patient. Given the growing elderly population, in which many may have had implants placed earlier in life—before developing a condition that requires the use of antiresorptive medications—it is conceivable that we will face problems in the future as we treat patients suffering from MRONJ associated with peri-implant infections. The challenge of a situation where implant removal may be required but will carry a significant risk of serious complications could present the clinician with difficult decisions regarding the optimal treatment for the patient.

Regularly updated guidelines list details of useful resources, the staging of treatment strategies, preventive measures, and algorithms for the management of patients with MRONJ. Implant practitioners should ensure that they are aware of the current guidelines, as there can often be significant changes over relatively short periods as new knowledge becomes available (Ruggiero and coworkers 2014).

Paget's disease (osteitis deformans). After osteoporosis, Paget's disease of the bone is the second most common bone disorder in elderly patients, with an incidence of 10% in patients older than 80 years. It is characterized by an imbalance in the bone-remodeling process: while osteoclastic resorption increases, new bone formation increases even more. However, the newly formed bone is highly vascularized woven bone with enlarged trabecular space, meaning that it is weaker and more susceptible to fracture. There appears to be a genetic and environmental component, and the condition is more prevalent in Caucasian populations of Europe, North America, and Australasia, with the axial skeleton, including the bones of the skull, being the most common site affected.

Most patients with Paget's disease are asymptomatic. However, as the disease progresses, bone pain is common and the increased vascularity may lead to overlying erythema. Cranial Paget's disease may lead to cranial nerve damage due to compression, and malocclusion, optic changes, vertigo, and tinnitus. Antiresorptive medications such as bisphosphonates are the first-line treatment; patients may be hyperresponsive to vitamin D and calcitonin. Sarcomatous change is possible, although rare, in the jaws and may be treated with radiotherapy.

Implant placement in patients with Paget's disease is not extensively documented. The above considerations regarding antiresorptive medications apply. However, the guidelines relating to implant placement for patients on intravenous bisphosphonates are generally derived from research where cancer is a comorbidity. Paget's disease is often managed with a single infusion of intravenous zoledronate, and it has been reported that such a dose may equate to similar accumulative concentrations of bisphosphonates as five years of oral therapy (Madrid and Sanz 2009a). Reduced bone density may present difficulties, but there are a few reports of successful implant placement under these conditions (Rasmussen and Hopfensperger 2008; Pirih and coworkers 2009; Torres and coworkers 2009; Mattheos and coworkers 2013).

5.10.3 Pharmacological Considerations

Many drugs used to treat rheumatoid arthritis can have oral adverse effects, such as lichenoid reactions, ulceration, and dysgeusia, all of which may be worse in an elderly patient with reduced salivary flow.

Non-steroidal anti-inflammatory drugs are commonly used in the treatment of inflammatory musculoskeletal diseases, with a concomitant increased bleeding effect. To prevent gastric bleeding, proton pump inhibitors such as omeprazole may be prescribed and have been associated with an increased incidence of fragility fractures in at-risk groups (Eom and coworkers 2011). Patients who take other antacids (e.g., aluminum hydroxide) may be at risk for hypophosphatemia, which is a more uncommon cause of osteomalacia.

The main therapeutic agent in osteoarthritis is acetaminophen due to the risk of upper gastrointestinal tract bleeding with NSAIDs, especially in polymorbid patients with, for example, COPD, heart disease, or diabetes. Acetaminophen doses need to be reduced in patients with chronic renal disease.

Corticosteroid therapy is also employed in the treatment of rheumatoid arthritis and musculoskeletal inflammatory conditions and can be associated with oral candidiasis.

Secondary osteoporosis may also occur as a side effect of glucocorticoid therapy. It is recognized that corticosteroid therapy is a major risk factor for osteoporosis (NICE CKS 2014) Corticosteroids reduce intestinal calcium absorption and increase renal calcium excretion; there is a compensatory increase in parathormone (PTH) secretion and an increased bony response to circulating PTH, resulting in reduced bone mass. Corticosteroids are associated with an increased risk of MRONJ (Saad and coworkers 2012; Tsao and coworkers 2013). However, more recent studies suggest that the use of polypharmaceutical regimes including calcium and vitamin D supplements with antiresorptive medications such as bisphosphonates, may reduce the incidence of steroid-induced osteoporosis over a two-year period (Jacobs and coworkers 2015).

Data from observational studies and ADE reporting suggests that although there is no high-quality evidence, long-term use of anticonvulsant drugs such as carbamazepine, phenytoin, and sodium valproate may be associated with decreased bone-mineral density. Patients taking these drugs may consequently also be prescribed vitamin D (Lee and coworkers 2010).

Diabetes- and osteoporosis-related fractures are two of the most important causes of mortality in elderly patients. There is clinical evidence that bone-mineral density is decreased in type 1 diabetes and increased in type 2 diabetes mellitus, although even type 2 diabetic patients appear to be at a higher risk of fracture (Montagnani and coworkers 2011). In addition, thiazolidinediones (TZD) such as rosiglitazone and pioglitazone appear to cause bone loss and are included in medications known to cause secondary osteoporosis (Lecka-Czernik 2010).

Thyroid hormone affects the rate of bone replacement; hyperthyroidism can result in normal osteoblastic function being unable to compensate for excessive bone resorption and can result in osteoporosis, especially in postmenopausal women. It has been shown to result in fragility fractures. While hypothyroidism is not associated with osteoporosis, excessive replacement therapy with thyroxin can result in depressed TSH secretion and has been implicated in osteoporosis. Subclinical thyroid dysfunction has no effect on bone-mineral density (Grant and coworkers 1993), but there is evidence of an increased incidence of hip fractures in patients over the age of 70 years who are taking high doses of levothyroxine (Ko and coworkers 2014).

Long-term heparin-induced osteoporosis can result in up to 30% of patients displaying a subclinical reduction of bone-mineral density and 2% to 3% experiencing a fragility fracture (Muir and coworkers 1996), with vertebral fractures being the most common (Handschin and coworkers 2005).

Unfractionated heparin remains in the bone, and the consequent reduction in BMD may be irreversible (Rajgopal and coworkers 2008).

HIV infection is no longer considered a life-shortening disease. Antiretroviral therapies can now provide patients with normal life expectancy, meaning that these patients are more likely to reach advanced age. However, HIV patients are more likely to suffer a disease-related loss of bone-mineral density, and antiretroviral treatment may contribute to a reduction in BMD (McComsey and coworkers 2011).

Cigarette smoking is an established risk factor in osteoporosis. Its cumulative effects on many aspects of bone metabolism and healing can be significant in elderly individuals with a long history of smoking (Yoon and coworkers 2012; Abate and coworkers 2013). Tobacco use is controversial as a risk factor for MRONJ, with some authors finding tobacco use approaching near statistical significance as a risk factor for ONJ in cancer patients (Kyrgidis and coworkers 2008). Other studies have not found an association between tobacco use and ONJ (Vahtsevanos and coworkers 2009; Tsao and coworkers 2013).

Intranasal calcitonin is used in the treatment of osteopenia/osteoporosis and for short-term pain relief after osteoporotic fracture, as it produces an endorphin effect. Reported side effects have included oropharyngeal burning or tingling sensation and jaw pain.

5.11 Neurosensory System

5.11.1 Age-related Changes

There is a progressive loss of brain neuronal tissue throughout life. Although the amount and location vary, this loss is principally of grey matter rather than white matter (Lim and coworkers 1992). Short-term memory loss and a reduced capacity to learn new things occur relatively early, with a decline in verbal ability beginning from approximately the age of 70. In the absence of neurological issues, intellectual ability will not usually begin to decline until age 80. The resulting forgetfulness, reduced reasoning ability, and declining neuroplasticity (adaptability) are generally termed "cognitive decline" and may progress to depression, dementia, or Alzheimer's disease, although there is considerable individual variation in the degree and rate of decline due to many medical, social, and environmental factors.

Some of these risk factors include chronic inflammation, insulin resistance, endothelial dysfunction, and oxidative stress from free radicals. Declining hormone levels affecting androgens, thyroid hormones, dehydroepiandrosterone (DHEA), and other neurohormones are also implicated.

Blood flow to the brain decreases by around 20% with age, but may be greater in atherosclerotic patients with cerebrovascular disease, which is more common in smokers, diabetics, or those with hypertension or hypercholesterolemia. Large cohort studies suggest a relationship between an increased risk of cognitive impairment and dementia in patients with cardiovascular disease, perhaps as a result of cerebral hypoperfusion or embolic stroke (Abete and coworkers 2014).

Aging brings impaired neuronal function due to myelin degradation and reduced synaptic transmission, resulting in impaired neuromotor function and increased reaction times. A generalized decrease in peripheral sensory nerve cells means that sensory impairment is also a normal part of aging (Hubbard and Squier 1989).

In elderly people, the sense of smell markedly decreases because of a reduction in the number of olfactory neurons. The incidence of upper respiratory tract infections over a lifetime and other factors such as allergic rhinitis can also contribute; consequently, there is an alteration in taste sensation, which can also be worsened by complete denture wearing, xerostomia, or medications. All these factors can have a negative impact on nutritional status in the elderly (Winkler and coworkers 1999).

Hearing and visual impairment are more a result of age-related changes in the eyes and ears than a change in nerve pathways. A decline in visual acuity occurs as the lens of the eye becomes less flexible with age due to fluid loss, making it less able to focus, particularly on close objects. Pupillary size is also reduced, and the pupillary light reflex may be slower; upward gaze is limited, and to a lesser extent downward gaze. Eye movements may be jerky when tracking an object. Macular degeneration may result in a significant reduction in the central vision necessary for more delicate tasks, such as oral hygiene procedures or accurate denture placement, while adequate peripheral vision may be maintained for walking, sitting, etc.

Visual impairment can be a significant handicap in the elderly, who may then consequently be unable to detect and recognize early oral disease. The performance of normal oral hygiene procedures, the insertion and replacement of dentures, and even the perceived need for treatment are all affected. Access to dental care may be difficult due to mobility, access issues, and fear, as well as cost. It has been reported that although over 80% of a cohort of blind patients stated that they needed no help in tooth brushing, 21% had dental pain or denture problems, and 32% had denture-related pathology (Schembri and Fiske 2001).

Cranial nerve evaluation in the elderly may be difficult because of non-neurologic age-related changes, such as diabetes, which also affects peripheral nerves. Facial pain may affect up to 50% of the elderly population (Madland and coworkers 2001).

Oropharyngeal dysphagia is prevalent in elderly people and may be a risk factor for other diseases (Charlson and coworkers 1987). Studies on otherwise healthy patients over 80 years found that aging impaired the swallowing response (Nagaya and Sumi 2002). It may be further impaired by certain neurological disorders such as stroke or dementia (Logemann 1998), or it may be medication-induced (for example by neuroleptic drugs) or a side effect of drugs. As previously stated, this presents a risk of aspiration pneumonia in the elderly (Cabre and coworkers 2010; Almirall and coworkers 2013).

Stroke. A "stroke" (cerebrovascular accident, CVA) can be due to embolism, thrombus, or hemorrhage (subarachnoid or cerebral). Subarachnoid hemorrhages are more commonly found in younger age groups.

Hypertension and atherosclerosis, which are frequent in the elderly population, are common causes of CVA such as cerebral thrombosis. Embolitic CVA can arise from an embolus formed on a damaged cardiac wall following a myocardial infarction or on a heart valve in atrial fibrillation. Clinicians should be aware of the signs and symptoms, as urgent medical attention will be required; 15% of patients die within the first three months of a CVA.

Post-stroke complications include unilateral limited mobility and, if the left hemisphere is affected, speech difficulties. Oral complications include sensory deficits and motor impairment with possible loss of gag reflex, functional difficulty with chewing and swallowing, reduced denture tolerance and inability to perform adequate oral hygiene (Ostuni 1994).

Transient ischemic attack (TIA) is a known precursor to stroke and is often a result of carotid artery stenosis. TIA's will present as a short-lived and more focal neurological disturbance, often in the form of a temporary "vacant" episode. Any neurological deficit is usually recovered within days or hours.

Parkinson's disease. Parkinson's disease is caused by dopamine deficiency due to degeneration of the pigmented cells in the substantia nigra and can be age-related or a consequence of cerebral damage from trauma or a

CVA; it not just a disease of the elderly. It is characterized by muscle rigidity, tremor of the arms and hands, gait disturbances such as shuffling or rigidity, bradykinesia (slower movement), and akathisia (restlessness). It may result in sialorrhea (Chou and coworkers 2007) and hypotension due to impaired autonomic function. Dysphagia can arise in up to 80% of Parkinson's patients, who may also experience other gastrointestinal problems such as reflux, nausea, and anorexia (Edwards and coworkers 1991).

Dementia. The likelihood of developing mental illness increases with age (Berr and coworkers 2005), with dementia affecting approximately 7.1% of the above-65 age group, approximately 20% of the above-80 age group, and 32.5% of the above-95 population in the UK. The main cause of dementia is Alzheimer's disease, with vascular and other forms of dementia such as those associated with Parkinson's disease being less prevalent (Alzheimer's Society 2014).

Dementia is not a normal part of aging and can be due to cerebrovascular disease or pathological processes such as Alzheimer's disease.

Alzheimer's disease initially manifests as temporal and spatial disorientation with memory loss. As the disease progresses the patient develops intermittent problems with speech and verbalization; apraxia (loss of coordination) and the ability to perform activities of daily living, including oral hygiene declines. In the final stages, the patient becomes disoriented, apathetic, and bedridden.

Confusion in the elderly patient can be due to these processes or a result of chronic disease such as diabetes, acute illness, infection, or dehydration, which can produce behavioral changes. It can be difficult to distinguish between the different causes of confusion; for example, in elderly patients with dementia, confusion may arise from that condition or from advanced aging. However, it may be due to an unrecognized infection and if left untreated for too long, such infections may spread to septicemia more rapidly than in a less old person.

Depression is common in elderly people, variably as a result of bereavement, Parkinson's disease, stroke, chronic pain, and changes in life patterns brought on by aging and illness.

5.11.2 Treatment Considerations

Reduction in food and fluid intake contributes to further neurologic deterioration, so maintaining oral comfort and the ability to process food is the prime objective in caring for patients with neurological disorders and aging patients in general. Patients with Parkinson's disease as well as post-stroke and dementia patients may have great difficulty even in managing dentures that were previously comfortable, and more so in adapting to new dentures. A gradual decline in neuroplasticity associated with aging can create problems in otherwise healthy elderly patients tolerating new dentures, even those dentures that are technically perfect.

Many patients with neurological diseases will not have any form of cognitive impairment; they can be greatly helped by the improvements in oral comfort and masticatory function offered by implant-supported prostheses. However, special considerations will inevitably have to be made in terms of treatment and ongoing maintenance, particularly in relation to any future progressive deterioration in the patient's condition. Treatment planning and decision-making may need to involve not only the patient but also family members or caregivers. Close cooperation between the dental professional and the psychogeriatric team is needed in achieving successful outcomes (Welsh and coworkers 2000).

Visual impairment and deafness as well as cognitive decline, confusion, and the complexity of a lifetime of medical issues can make communication and understanding more challenging in elderly patients. A patient who appears confused or mentally impaired in conversation may actually be deaf or dysphasic because of a stroke. A patient with dementia may be able to maintain adequate social graces from instilled long-term practice to give plausible answers to certain conversational questions and appear unaffected. When speaking with patients, it is important to sit in front of them, not wear a mask, and speak slowly and clearly. Advocacy and consent are discussed in the chapter on psychosocial challenges.

It is important to realize that patients with Parkinson's disease may not have any form of cognitive decline and are otherwise fully functioning individuals. This can often be forgotten, given the inexpressive facial tone that is characteristic of the disease. They will be slower to perform normal tasks as a result of the disease and can become frustrated. Dental implants may provide significant benefits in both mastication and predigestion capacity (Heckmann and coworkers 2000). However, patience and compassion are necessary when providing treatment, as emotional stress can exacerbate the symp-

toms. Parkinson's patients often suffer from sialorrhea (excess saliva production), which can make treatment difficult. They are also at risk of hypotension with postural implications, and the characteristic head position or dyskinesia in orofacial musculature can cause treatment problems.

Patients who have suffered a CVA may have reduced swallowing or gag reflexes, which has implications not only for the treatment but also for the safety of removable appliances or small components. Sensory or motor defects affecting the oral cavity may result in food accumulation and poorer plaque control on the affected side. Post-stroke patients often suffer from depression (Gupta and coworkers 2002), which may affect motivation, attendance, and compliance, with a consequent adverse impact on treatment objectives.

Access and mobility may be impaired in stroke patients; communication can be affected by the presence of dysarthria, and aphasia can give the impression of confusion or memory loss. It is often recommended that elective dental treatment be avoided in the first six months following a stroke. Such patients will be anticoagulated and interference with this regime may be inadvisable. In addition, avoidance of stressful procedures is advisable (Little and coworkers 2002), so shorter appointments are preferred. Patients are susceptible to further events as a consequence of hypertension; blood pressure should be monitored, and it is important to use minimal doses of epinephrine-containing local anesthetics. If complex interventions are necessary, the use of conscious sedation may be considered with appropriate medical advice and monitoring, given the risk of respiratory depression. In cases of marked impairment of gag reflex, coughing, and swallowing, it may be necessary to consider inpatient general anesthetics with airway protection via intubation.

There are no specific oral manifestations in Alzheimer's disease or other dementia conditions other than those related to drugs that may be taken. However, such patients are increasingly unable to manage self-performed oral hygiene, and special precautions are necessary (Fiske and coworkers 2006).

Implant treatment in patients with neurodegenerative disease can provide benefits and problems (Faggion 2013).

Treatment can be challenging; these patients prefer known people and places and are easily disoriented and upset. While there is no absolute contraindication to implant placement, careful consideration is required as to the appropriateness of introducing complex treatment, particularly surgical, in a situation that will only decline further, making care and maintenance ever more difficult.

The effective use of intricate oral hygiene aids such as floss or small interdental brushes may be impossible in many of these conditions. When planning treatment, the ability of the patient (or caregiver) to perform adequate plaque control is a basic tenet in all individuals. But it is particularly important in elderly patients with visual impairment, cognitive decline, dementia, sarcopenia-related weakness of the hand muscles, or reduced manual dexterity, perhaps due to Parkinson's disease, where a significant impact on peri-implant health parameters may arise. Of course, such handicaps may develop after placement of a complex prosthesis earlier in life, and custom maintenance plans involving the patient and caregivers will need to be prescribed. Professional maintenance will be required more frequently and managed in the most accessible setting. Finally, revision of the prosthesis in good time to a simpler form, while such therapy is still practicable, may be advisable in certain cases.

Depression itself can present challenges for dental treatment, in particular complex treatment that requires many appointments over a long time. Oral complaints such as facial pain, dysesthesia, perceived mysterious fluid or slime secretions, and dysgeusia have all been attributed to depression and treated with antidepressants, although with variable success. The appreciation of outcomes of treatment or progress made may not always be present in depressed patients and meeting patients' expectations may be very difficult.

5.11.3 Pharmacological Considerations

The oral effects of many drugs used in the treatment of neurological disorders have been discussed in the section on the alimentary tract. Xerostomia and dysgeusia may result from anti-Parkinson drugs, antidepressants, sedatives and tranquilizers.

Stroke patients may be hypertensive or may be taking anticoagulant medication.

Parkinson's disease patients are often treated with levodopa, which can interact with the epinephrine in dental local anesthetic and induce cardiac arrhythmias or tachycardia, and hypertension. Non-epinephrine containing local anesthetic should be used in these patients.

Macrolide antibiotics can interact with bromocriptine, also used in the treatment of Parkinson's disease.

Tricyclic antidepressants (TCAs) such as amitriptyline, imipramine, and dosulepin cause xerostomia. They can also cause severe hypotension in the elderly, especially orthostatic hypotension and other side effects such as arrhythmias, neurological disturbance, neutropenia and jaundice are more serious in older people. Acetaminophen can inhibit the metabolism of TCAs. Selective serotonin reuptake inhibitors (SSRI) such as sertraline may be used as an alternative to TCAs, but may still cause a side effect of dry mouth.

Monoamine oxidase inhibitors (MAOIs) used in the treatment of depression are now rarely used due to many, often dangerous, side effects.

St. John's wort has been shown to be effective in the treatment of mild depression. However, if taken with serotonin reuptake inhibitors, there is an increasing risk of serotonin syndrome in older adults. As previously mentioned, this can also interfere with warfarin and digoxin.

Elderly people generally require less sleep but often suffer from chronic insomnia. Barbiturates may be used to treat insomnia or anxiety in the elderly. Diazepam is lipid-soluble and has a long half-life. In older patients, the effect may be enhanced, leading to a risk of dependency, confusion, or falls and related fractures. Presurgical anxiety control should employ alternatives with a shorter half-life, such as midazolam.

5.12 Cancer

The most common malignancies affecting the elderly population are pulmonary, gastrointestinal, and genitourinary (Hansen 1998). Oral manifestations of these cancers are not seen, but the treatment of malignancy can have effects in terms of chemotherapy and radiotherapy. Oral cancer is primarily a disease of the over-50 population in developed countries (Koch and coworkers 1995).

Successful implant placement has been described and may be very useful in the reconstruction of deformity and morbidity caused by resective treatment for oral cancer. However, implant survival rates may be significantly compromised by comorbidity, and implant loss is more frequent (Barrowman and coworkers 2011; Nelson and coworkers 2007; Kovács 2000). As always, careful and comprehensive planning of treatment, taking into account the medical, surgical, and psychosocial factors relating to the individual patient, is mandatory.

Chemotherapy causing bone-marrow suppression may cause thrombocytopenia and have an impact on hemostasis, and leukopenia, resulting in an increased tendency to infection. Proper preoperative assessment will be required. Radiotherapy may cause xerostomia, hypogeusia, dysgeusia, trismus, and osteoradionecrosis (Rankin and Jones 1999).

Approximately 80% of patients undergoing radiotherapy to the head and neck region and 40% of patients in chemotherapy will experience oral mucositis as a consequence (Dodd and coworkers 1996).

5.12.1 Osteoradionecrosis

While not the preserve of the elderly, and with increasing incidence in younger patients in some countries such as Scotland—perhaps due to social factors such as smoking and alcohol use—rates of oral cancer are still significant in elderly people (Cancer Research UK 2014). Survival rates following treatment of head and neck cancer with resective surgery, chemotherapy, and radiotherapy have improved slightly over the past decade in developed nations—from approximately 50% to 57% in the USA, for example (Oral Cancer Foundation 2012).

However, quality of life may be adversely affected by resective surgery, and radiation treatment can have an adverse effect on the salivary glands, oral mucosa and the bones of the jaws. The clinician has to consider not only the provision of dental implants in irradiated bone, but also the effect that radiotherapy may have on implants placed before radiotherapy, even many years previously. Damage to salivary tissue, in particular the parotid glands, can lead to hyposalivation and increased dental caries; this increases the potential need for dental extractions, with a concomitant risk of ONJ. Post-radiation periodontal attachment loss may occur (Epstein and coworkers 1998; Marques and Dib 2004) and may be exacerbated by difficulty in performing effective oral hygiene, due to trismus, soreness of tissues and a lack of motivation. All these can increase the risk of tooth loss. A combination of oral mucosal damage and hyposalivation can lead to patients then experiencing great difficulty in wearing conventional removable prostheses.

Radiotherapy for head and neck oncology typically consists of a dose of 60–70 Gy over a four- to six-week period, in five daily doses with breaks of two days. Radiotherapy can cause damage to the microvasculature of the bone, with a consequent reduction in tissue oxygenation and nutrition, and deficiencies in cellular repair capacity. This can result in the development of osteoradionecrosis (ORN), which has a specific pathophysiologic sequence (Harrison and coworkers 2003). Radiation-induced tissue damage results in oral soft tissues that are highly susceptible to trauma, for example from denture wearing. Non-healing ulceration of tissues results in areas of exposed, necrotic bone that can become secondarily infected, as is the case with MRONJ. ORN is thought to occur in approximately 3% to 35% of patients undergoing radiation therapy to the head and neck (Marx and Johnson 1987).

The risk of ORN increases with both radiation dose and with time as a result of progressive deterioration in tissue oxygenation following irradiation. Consequently, ORN may arise many years after radiation therapy following dental extractions, in periodontal disease, or from denture pressure sores; it may also arise seemingly spontaneously (David and coworkers 2001; Meraw and Reeve 1998; Marx and coworkers 1987).

The onset of ORN may be affected by the site of the tumor and the irradiated region, as well as other systemic and social factors such as chemotherapy, smoking and alcohol intake. The mandible appears to be more susceptible to ORN as a result of its reduced vascular supply compared to the maxilla and a consequential increased susceptibility to endarteritis obliterans. Consequently, implant placement in an irradiated area carries a risk of defective wound healing due to osteoradionecrosis.

There is evidence to show that radiotherapy can significantly affect successful dental implant healing (Linsen and coworkers 2012), and that the long-term impact of radiotherapy on bone quality and implant failure may be unfavorable (Alsaadi and coworkers 2008). A retrospective study found that implant failure rates in irradiated bone might be approximately double that of implant placed in non-irradiated bone (Granström 2005). Failure rates may also increase in the years after implant placement in irradiated bone (Jisander and coworkers 1997), reflecting the increased incidence of ORN with time since radiation therapy, presumably due to the aforementioned progressive degradation of tissue oxygenation. The occurrence of ORN after implant surgery is a complication with equally significant morbidity as MRONJ and may be underreported (Granström 2003), although some studies report no increased incidence of ORN with implant placement (Wagner and coworkers 1998).

The available literature should be interpreted with caution; success rates ranging from 40% (Ali and coworkers 1997) to 100% (Esser and Wagner 1997) have been reported, but significant confounding variables are frequently left unconsidered.

Just as intraoral implant failure varies according to the characteristics of the bone at the implant site, the same is true of implants used to retain extraoral prostheses (Granström and coworkers 1992; Granström and Tjellström 1997).

Hyperbaric oxygen therapy (HBO) has in the past been claimed to assist in the treatment and prevention of ORN by increasing oxygen tension in wounds and, as a consequence, also increasing the rate of angioneogenesis and fibroblast proliferation; implant placement has been successful when such a protocol was employed (Larsen 1997). However, recent research questions the clinical benefits of HBO (Keller 1997; Donoff 2006; Esposito and Worthington 2013).

Recent evidence supports the established belief that head and neck radiotherapy may be linked to an increased failure rate of implants, compared to failure rates in patients who had not undergone radiotherapy. Failure rates may be higher in the maxilla and HBO therapy does not appear to improve implant survival. A systematic review of 15 trials, comprising 13 case series and 2 RCTs, produced 10,150 implants, with 1,689 (14.3%) placed in irradiated mouths. Mean survival rates of implants ranged from 46.3% to 98% with pooled estimates indicating implant failure to be statistically significantly higher in irradiated patients, compared to patients who had not undergone radiotherapy (an increase of 174%) with a risk ratio of 2.74 (95% CI: 1.86, 4.05; p < 0.00001). In maxillary sites, the risk ratio was 5.96 (95% CI: 2.71, 13.12; p < 0.00001) with the risk of loss increasing to 49.6%. There were three studies with patients receiving HBO finding that HBO did not reduce the risk of implant failure, with a risk ratio of 1.28 (95% CI: 0.19, 8.82). However, the authors pointed out the low level of evidence; neither of the RCTs was rated as at low risk of bias, and none of the observational studies were of high quality; in addition, many of the papers included examined machined surface implants. The authors were therefore unable to state whether HBO has a meaningful effect on implant survival (Chambrone and coworkers 2013).

Successful implant integration will depend on many factors, such as the radiation dose, comorbidities and associated polypharmacy, smoking, implant site, and the timing of surgery relative to the radiation therapy. Studies assessing the relative failure rates for implants placed before and after radiation therapy report difficulties in differentiating heterogeneous factors such as these and the type of prosthesis used. The failure rates of implants placed before and after irradiation appear similar, although outcomes were less favorable in the maxilla than in the mandible (Colella and coworkers 2007).

Some authorities recommend waiting for at least 12 months after radiotherapy to the head and neck region before considering implant placement, despite recognizing the lack of reliable evidence (Claudy and coworkers 2015). Other authors examined the difference in implant failures when implants had been successfully integrated for a time before radiotherapy compared to implants in irradiated bone. They concluded that while the site of placement may be relevant, there appears to be no significant difference related to timing. In patients with previously placed implants, radiotherapy performed from 4 months to 19 years later appeared to have a similar ultimate effect on the implants (99.2% survival rate) as pre-implantation radiotherapy (88.9%). Maxillary sites exhibited lower success rates than mandibular or grafted sites (78.9%, 93.3%, and 87.5%, respectively). In grafted sites, vascularized free flaps appeared to have better implant survival (89.3%) than non-vascularized grafts (87.1%). HBO did not appear to make a difference to overall implant survival. None of these differences was statistically significant (Nooh 2013).

There does appear to be a correlation between total radiation dose and implant failure with doses of higher than 45 – 55 Gy (Harrison and coworkers 2003; Colella and coworkers 2007; Nooh 2013) with an increased risk of ONJ at doses above 66 Gy (Harrison and coworkers 2003).

As can be seen, findings for ORN following dental implant surgery and for the integration of the implants are variable. Long-term implant survival may also be affected by other effects of radiotherapy such as reduced salivary flow and increased plaque deposits. However, implant placement may significant improve the quality of life outcomes following resective surgery, as implants may be used to retain both intraoral and extraoral prostheses. Conventional tissue-supported intraoral prostheses are often unable to provide adequate function due to altered anatomy, mucosal fragility, or reduced salivary flow (Weischer and Mohr 1999).

Deformities caused by major resective surgery coupled with deficiencies in speech, function, and comfort can all adversely affect quality of life and may have an impact on mental and physical health. Despite lower implant survival rates, implants may therefore be an appropriate option for rehabilitation in oral cancer patients who have been treated with radiotherapy (Mancha de la Plata and coworkers 2012).

Caution should be exercised when considering implant placement in patients who have received radiotherapy in the head and neck region, with appropriate specialist advice being sought. Although there is no current consensus, some authors have recommended defined protocols (Granström 2003):

- Implant surgery is best carried out > 21 days before radiotherapy.
- Total radiation dose should be < 66 Gy if the risks of ORN are to be minimized or < 50 Gy to reduce osseointegration failure: avoiding implant site/ portals.
- Hyperbaric oxygen should be given if > 50 Gy radiation is used.
- No implant surgery should be carried out during radiotherapy.
- No implant surgery should be carried out in the presence of radiation mucositis.
- Defer implant placement for 9 months after radiotherapy.
- Use implant-supported prostheses without any mucosal contact.
- Avoid immediate loading.
- Ensure strict asepsis.
- Consider antimicrobial prophylaxis.

Newer radiotherapy techniques may offer the opportunity to reduce undesirable collateral tissue damage. Intensity-modulated radiation therapy (IMRT) is a computer-controlled RT modality with more accurate targeting of rapid beams of different intensity radiation. This can offer better parotid tissue preservation and prevent hyposalivation, thereby reducing the incidence of "radiation caries." Altered fractionation schedules are also under investigation, but different schedules appear to have widely varying risks and benefits in terms of ONJ incidence after dental extractions (Nabil and Samman 2011).

5.13   Conclusions

Improved management of medical conditions and greater longevity mean that aging patients can enjoy better health for longer.

The purpose of this chapter has been to highlight the effect of advancing age on implant treatment planning in elderly patients. It can be seen that people "age" at different rates. Combining the many general health variables outlined above with the varying needs and expectations of patients makes treatment planning very difficult in many cases.

Indeed, the needs of the patient may well change with further aging or medical issues. The "idealistic" treatment plan may not be the ideal treatment plan in an aging patient, particularly one who is, or will likely become, more frail. Furthermore, what appears to be an ideal treatment plan at the time of treatment delivery may result in considerable difficulty in dealing with complications that arise many years later, when that patient is elderly and polymorbid or frail.

For most medical conditions, it is the degree of systemic disease control rather than the presence of the condition itself that is the most relevant consideration in implant therapy and in implant success or survival (Seymour and Vaz 1989; Diz and coworkers 2013). However, implant treatment is elective, non-essential, invasive surgery, and to perform surgery on a patient with an active and uncontrolled disease process carries a risk of more serious complications. In elderly patients, the margin between safety and danger can be eroded by the individual and compound effects of polymorbidity, polypharmacy, and frailty.

A careful risk-benefit analysis is required before complex and stressful procedures are undertaken. In older patients with good disease control, the considerations may not be very different from younger patients. In more medically compromised elderly individuals, the consideration of the large number of additional factors outlined above may mandate significant compromise in the treatment plan that has to be accepted by clinicians and patients alike. Simplification may be necessary to ensure that the treatment remains the most suitable as patients age further or become frailer.

We have an ultimate duty of care to ensure that we do not employ a technique-driven focus in the treatment of our patients. Everything we could do will have both advantages and disadvantages. There is no more important reason to ensure a patient-driven care plan than the proper consideration of the present, and likely future, medical condition of our aging patients, where progressive decline is the only certainty. Our task is to ensure good dental quality of life, to maintain self-esteem, and facilitate proper nutrition, without unwittingly adding problems that could adversely affect our patients on a daily basis.

We do not have a crystal ball, and hope is not a strategy; a comprehensive assessment of both the immediate and future needs of elderly implant patients with careful, meticulous planning—not only of the treatment, but the manner in which it is provided—is essential in a successful outcome. Only in this way can we be sure that the functional, esthetic, and quality-of-life benefits that may be provided by implant treatment will outweigh the potential risks in the provision of treatment.

6 Features of Removable Prostheses for the Old

F. Müller

Prospective planning

Dental prostheses for geriatric patients should not generally be designed any differently from those for younger adults (Müller 2010a). Of course, the general rules and guidelines for the construction of removable prostheses also apply to dentures for elderly and geriatric patients.

However, we should also consider the patient's general health and any physical or cognitive impairment. Of similar importance are the patients' autonomy in performing essential oral hygiene and their ability to manage removable dentures. Unfortunately, nursing staff has often had very little if any training in handling what they consider "high-tech" dentures—and even a mandibular two-implant overdenture may fall into this category.

The following testimony from the daughter of a patient who had recently received an implant-supported overdenture and who was hospitalized for stroke recovery highlights this situation:

> "… I had also asked why Dad has lost so much weight, and the doctor explained to me that this is due to the low-calorie diet and his lack of appetite. But that is not so bad, because it would facilitate his ability to move. But then Gertrud told me that she often noticed that his "new teeth" were not seated well, and I could imagine that he cannot chew properly. On the new ward, there is only one caregiver who knows how to handle "high-tech" dentures. Anna had asked him several times to train the others, but it seems that it has not worked out…"

Even for fit and active elders, prospective planning is important. While anyone can have an accident or a stroke any day, there is still a stronger likelihood for an 80-year-old to become dependent in the following 15 years than for a 50-year-old patient. Of course, 80- and even 95-year-old fit patients can be provided with fixed implant-supported prostheses, but these should allow for a "back-off" strategy when the onset of dependency requires simplification. Fixed implant-supported bridges should preferably be screw-retained to allow replacement by a removable prosthesis later in life. Implants should be placed where they could be useful when the fixed implant-prosthesis is converted to an implant-supported overdenture.

The choice of implants is equally crucial. A two-piece system with a choice of available overdenture abutments is preferable, as these abutments are easier to retrieve and replace with another version.

In short, dental prostheses for elderly adults should have the following attributes:

- Easy to insert and remove
- Easy to clean
- Freedom in centric occlusion with shallow cuspal inclines
- Polished surfaces without too much detailing that creates niches and fosters plaque adhesion
- Age-appropriate dental appearance
- Highest retention that still permits autonomous handling by the patient

Table 1 lists possible age-appropriate features from which practitioners may adopt those they consider appropriate for a particular patient.

As aging and functional decline are very individual and may vary from patient to patient, it is important to note that this list does not apply to all old patients equally and categorically. There is no specific age after which a patient is considered "geriatric" and will need a removable prosthesis!

Table 1   Possible age-appropriate features for a partial or complete removable denture for geriatric patients.

Denture design	Simple and flexible, allowing modification in case of potential future tooth loss or the onset of dependency for activities of daily living (ADLs)
Denture stability	Solid, resisting clumsy handling without a need for immediate repair
Denture-base material	Polymethyl methacrylate (PMMA) to allow for repair, addition of teeth or other parts, as well as relines
Retention components	Use only the best and well-documented materials and components to reduce material failure and wear in late life
Denture surface	Polished surfaces to facilitate cleaning and avoid adhesion of biofilm and food debris (no surface details, no papilla recession)
Palatal plate	Polished, unless problems with speech or taste are present
Denture management and retention	"Removal aids" to help the removal of the prosthesis if manual dexterity is reduced. Retention only as strong as can be managed by the patient themselves Retention should be "weakened" progressively along with functional decline
Occlusal plane	Should be on or below the equator of the tongue. As for the length of the incisors, bear in mind that the upper lip becomes longer with age and the edges of the incisors should not be longer than the upper lip. Occlusal breakdown with a loss in vertical dimension has to be corrected for a coherent occlusal plane
Vertical dimension	The less coordinated and controlled the mandibular movements, the lower the occlusal vertical dimension
Occlusion	"Freedom in centric" concept to accommodate the increased freedom of the temporomandibular joints and poorer motor coordination Canine guidance or group function for partial dentures; balanced occlusion for complete dentures and implant-supported overdentures In difficult anatomical situations, the central bearing point method should be used for the registration of centric relation
Denture teeth	Cuspal inclination of 20° or less, preferably acrylic teeth
Abutment teeth	"Bikini design"—cover as little tooth structure as possible to allow access of saliva to the enamel Abutment teeth with severe attachment loss should be endodontically treated and decoronated for a more favorable crown/root ratio Where possible, keep healthy filled roots as overdenture abutments (except for molars)
Denture kinetics and occlusal load	The mandibular denture should be "stronger" and more stable than the maxillary denture Make an effort to keep strategically important teeth, especially mandibular canines Plan occlusal load to be transferred to denture saddles rather than abutment teeth to keep the latter for as long as possible Adopt a fail-safe principle for clasps to protect abutment teeth
Appearance	Age-appropriate appearance with abraded incisal edges and a shade of 3 or above
Labeling	Individual labeling of denture with name (and matching set of dentures) for the institutionalized patient
Comfort	Oral comfort should be assured even when the denture is not worn during the night (e.g., no sharp edges from attachments)

Denture design

Any removable denture such as conventional partial, implant-overdenture or conventional complete should be designed to be as simple and adaptable as possible. Although tooth loss is not part of physiological aging, the statistical likelihood is high that oral hygiene deteriorates along with functional decline, the immune defense weakens and tooth loss occurs. Often this coincides with the transition from the third to the fourth stage of life, where dependency for normal activities of daily life (ADL) becomes evident. In this context, it is important to be able to adapt the existing denture to accommodate impaired function, rather than provide a new prosthesis. Neuroplasticity may already be diminished, and the patient should not have to endure multiple long and invasive clinical sessions. Avoiding major changes in occlusal vertical dimension, intercuspation, the shapes of the dental arch and denture body, lip support, and overall appearance makes accommodating to a new denture a smooth and atraumatic process for the patient.

Denture stability

Removable prostheses replace not only the lost teeth, but also lost hard and soft tissues. As atrophy of the alveolar crest progresses with age, most geriatric patients present with a noticeable degree of atrophy and consequently require a denture body that presents very little fracture risk. Partial dentures should also have a robust design that resists occasional clumsy handing by an elderly patient. Dental technicians often take pride in manufacturing delicate and elegant cast-metal framework. Although such efforts are to be admired, they are not adequate for elderly patients with reduced manual skills and vision. The tactile sensitivity of the mucosa diminishes with age. Elderly patients are less sensitive to bulky clasps or lingual bars and often do not mind a "solid" framework for a partial denture.

Denture-base material

Although polymethyl methacrylate (PMMA) denture bases provide the greatest flexibility for repairs, relines, and additions, a chromium or titanium base may provide more comfort and restore the sensation of heat and taste. If needed, it could later be replaced by a PMMA denture base.

While providing advantages concerning PMMA allergies, vinyl chloride and vinyl acetate denture materials (Luxene; Astron Dental, Lake Zurich, IL, USA) do not allow modifications and are therefore less favorable for elderly patients.

Retention components

Elements such as precision attachments or implant components should be of the best quality and have scientifically well-documented designs. Biological complications may still occur later in life, but mechanical failure and wear should be prevented as far as possible. It is also important to have replacement components at hand for the future, and so the choice of implant system is important. Material failure may profoundly disrupt elderly patients and impair their confidence in both the denture and the dentist.

Denture surface

Although enormous efforts are made in prosthetic dentistry to copy nature, surface details such as stippling, interproximal spaces, or gingival sulci usually exceed the elderly patient's ability and willingness to clean. Removable dentures for geriatric patients should therefore be well polished and present no niches for the adhesion of biofilm and food debris. Although recession of the interdental papilla with "black triangles" is frequent in an aged natural dentition, it is also not recommended to imitate this in a removable denture. There is perhaps nothing worse for an interlocutor than a residual leaf of spinach stuck between two incisors! Therefore, the denture papillae should be of a more juvenile form, filling the available space apical to the proximal contacts, providing a morphology where food glides off rather than being stuck. As the pink acrylic risks showing between the anterior teeth, most denture teeth are now manufactured with long proximal contacts to lower the level of visible denture resin. Polished surfaces are not only useful for avoiding food retention but also to provide greater ease of biofilm removal. Deposits of biofilm on a removable prosthesis may present a considerable risk for aspiration pneumonia, especially in elderly patients with swallowing disorders and compromised health (Quagliarello and coworkers 2005).

Palatal plate

Most dentures with full palatal coverage have a polished palate without rugae. This is appropriate for elderly patients, as it is easy to clean. However, the addition of palatal rugae may be helpful to improve taste, because it facilitates pushing the food to the taste receptors located deep down in the papillae of the dorsum of the tongue (Fig 1). Individual palatal features of a patient to a removable denture base can easily be added by taking a silicone impression of the edentulous palate, pouring this silicone key with pink wax, peeling the sheet of wax off the silicone, and adding it to the denture palate. What an experience for the patient to discover the familiar palatal pattern on the denture plate! Another addition to the palate may be indicated when pronouncing the "S" sound becomes difficult because the thickness of the artificial palate precludes a sufficient airflow in the "S canal." The addition of an acrylic incisal papilla to the denture palate helps lower the tongue during phonation and creating space for the airflow necessary for the "S" sound. Both the palatal rugae and an incisal papilla can be well polished, so they do not increase the risk for plaque adhesion.

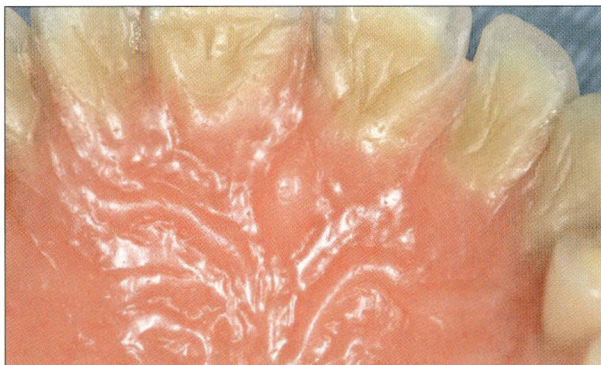

Fig 1   Palatal rugae are only applied to improve taste and speech.

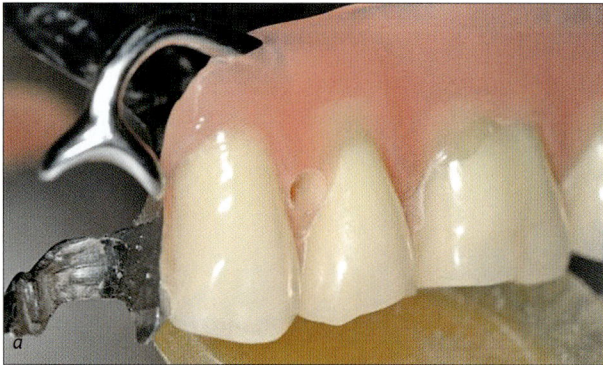

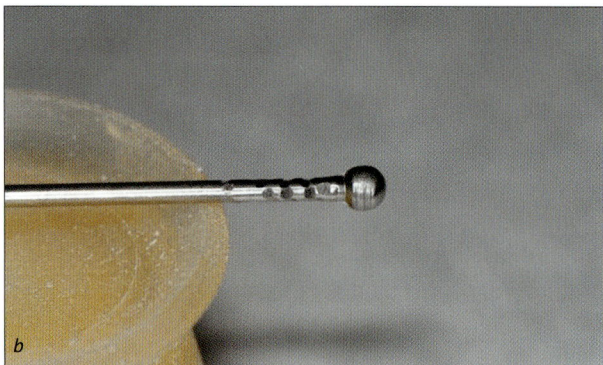

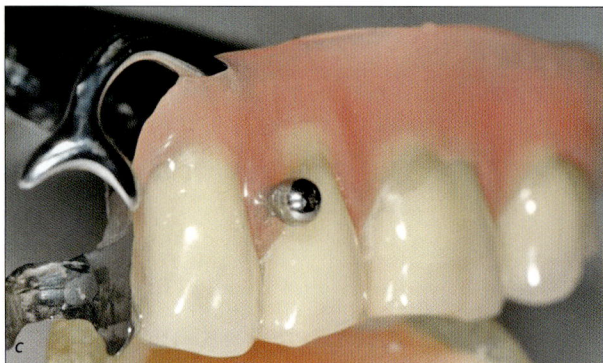

Figs 2a-c   An orthodontic ball clasp may serve as a removal aid if manual dexterity is compromised in an elderly patient.

Denture management and retention

Impaired vision, reduced tactile sensitivity, and failing manual dexterity may render the removal of a partial or implant-supported overdenture difficult. Furthermore, the fingernails of elderly patients become brittle and ill suited to insert under a metal clasp for denture removal. Removal aids may be a welcome feature to facilitate denture management. These can be fabricated using an orthodontic ball clasp polymerized into the papilla between the premolars, but could also be just a simple notch a finger is able to grip (Figs 2a-c). Whereas a younger patient might be disturbed by such an addition, elderly patients are less aware of these features, as the tactile sensitivity of the mucosa reduces with age. Special tools like DentureLifter are available for those who do mind removal aids (Fig 3). An overly retentive denture may cause considerable panic in an elderly denture wearer, especially when accustomed for many years to a prosthesis lacking in retention.

> Denture retention must be no stronger than to allow the patient to insert and remove the denture autonomously. The weaker the hand force and dexterity, the lower the maximum denture retention.

As a rule, the older the patient, the less denture retention is required. This is of particular importance for implant-supported dentures, where the strength of retention is a choice rather than a given feature of the available abutment teeth. Of course there are individual exceptions.

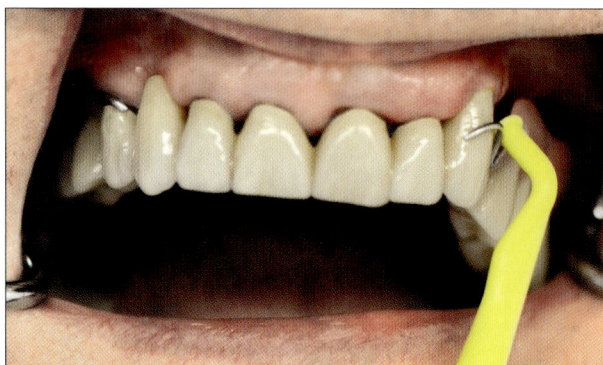

Fig 3   A removal aid (GeriaDental, Borken, Germany) may be a useful tool for patients whose fingernails are too brittle to remove a partial denture with clasps.

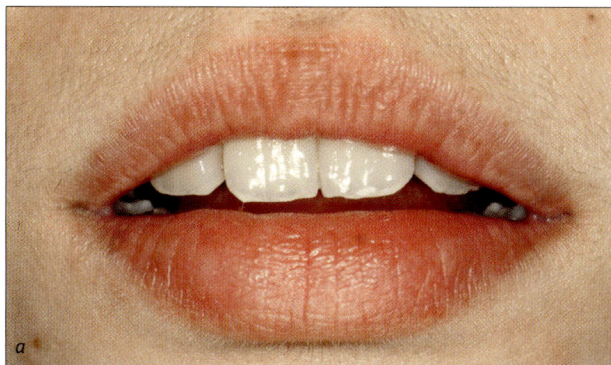

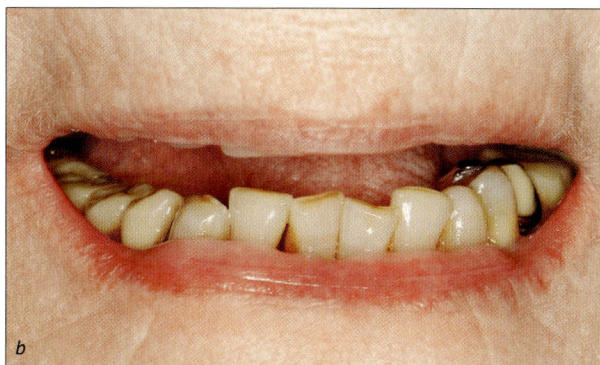

Figs 4a-b   The upper lip loses elasticity and lengthens with age. Maxillary incisors are therefore mounted without exceeding the length of the lip in a relaxed position.

Occlusal plane

When determining the occlusal plane for an elderly person's complete or implant-supported prosthesis, it is important to remember that the upper lip loses elasticity and the front teeth wear with age (Figs 4a-b). In the horizontal plane, the incisors should therefore not exceed the length of the upper lip. In the sagittal plane, the occlusal plane is still parallel to the Camper plane, the equator of the tongue, and the bipupillary line.

Where natural teeth are still present, it is very important to re-establish a coherent occlusal plane when tooth loss has created a collapsed vertical dimension. Elderly patients often present with overerupted teeth and a locked occlusion, leaving little space for a prosthetic restoration and preventing a dynamic occlusion without interference.

Vertical dimension

The rule that a complete or implant-overdenture should provide the patient with 2 to 3 mm freeway space also applies to elderly patients. Yet in a geriatric patient with poor motor control, we may want to choose a reduced vertical dimension of occlusion with increased freeway space. The risk of overload and injury to the denture-bearing tissues and pressure spots is lower, and unfavorable sounds from unintentional tooth contact during dyskinetic mandibular movements are avoided.

Occlusion

Along with age-related slackening of the ligaments in the temporomandibular joint and atrophy of the articular tubercles, the precision of mandibular guidance decreases. At the same time, motor coordination diminishes, so that the mandibular closing trajectory of geriatric patients is much less precise than in adults. A "freedom in centric" concept is more forgiving of the increased range of mandibular movements (Fig 5).

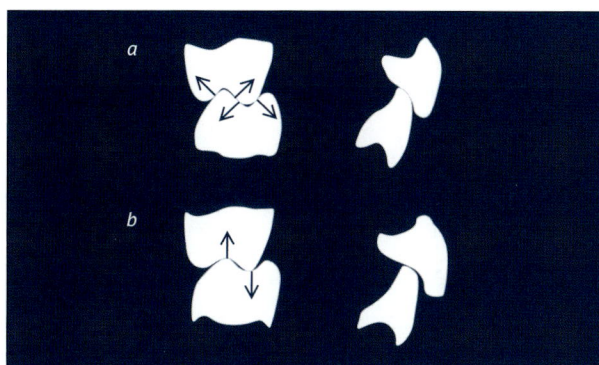

Fig 5   Rather than a locked occlusion with tripod contacts for supporting cusps (a), the occlusion for an elderly patient's prosthesis should adopt a "freedom in centric" concept (b) to meet the needs of the aged temporomandibular joint and the deteriorated motor coordination.

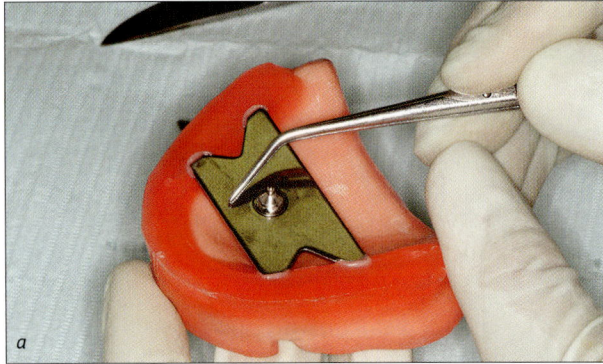

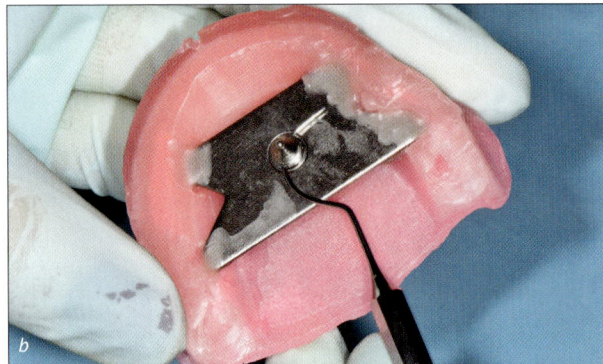

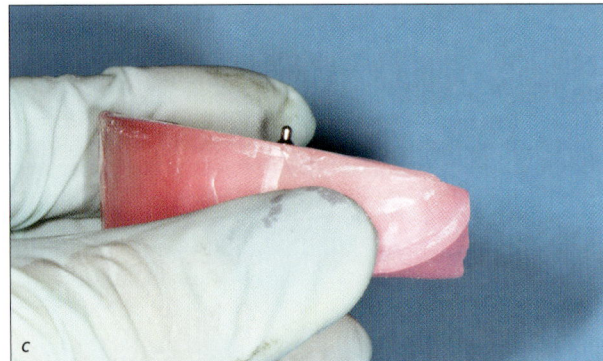

Figs 6a-c   The upper template is prepared with a writing pin plate that is heated and melted into the wax rim (a). The height of the pin can be adjusted, as it is threaded into the plate (b). For registration, the pin should exceed the upper wax rim by about 2 mm (c).

As in younger patients, the centric relation (CR) is the position of choice for reconstructing the dentition. However, in patients with Parkinson's disease, mandibular dyskinesia, or severe dementia, a "comfort occlusion" in a slightly more anterior position can be adopted without apparent problems. If no CR can be determined (as may happen in geriatric patients) or if patients cannot "find" their CR position, monoplane teeth may be the last resort to provide a functional denture. Although the chewing efficiency is less favorable than with anatomical teeth, they provide stability in almost every occlusal position the mandible "happens to adopt" (Abduo 2013).

As for a dynamic occlusion, a bilateral occlusion is adopted for implant-supported overdentures, just as for conventional complete dentures, and a canine-guided or group function is adopted for partial dentures with or without implants.

The more advanced the atrophy of the alveolar ridges, the more difficult it is to perform a centric relation registration because the bases of the occlusal rims are not seated firmly. A manually guided registration may create different pressures on each side and the templates may even dislodge horizontally. Loading the templates centrally by means of a "central bearing point" method has some "self-centering" effect, not only for the denture-bearing tissues but also for the condyles. The more difficult the anatomical situation of an edentulous patient, the more advantageous is the technique of registering the CR using the central bearing point (Figs 6a-j). If implants are present, they may of course be used to hold the templates in place. Temporary female parts or simply a silicone rubber or tissue conditioner may be used to stabilize the registration templates (Figs 7a-d).

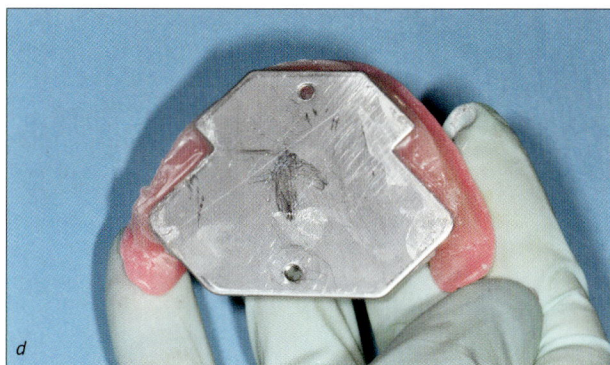

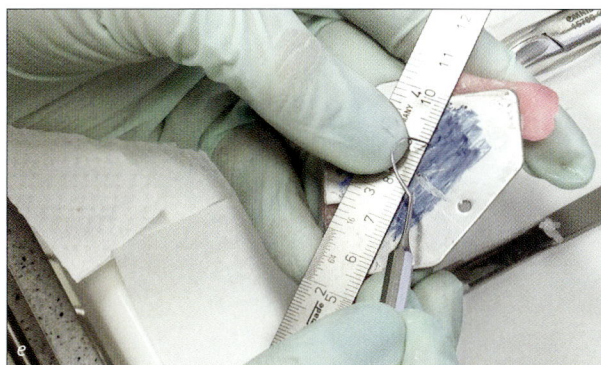

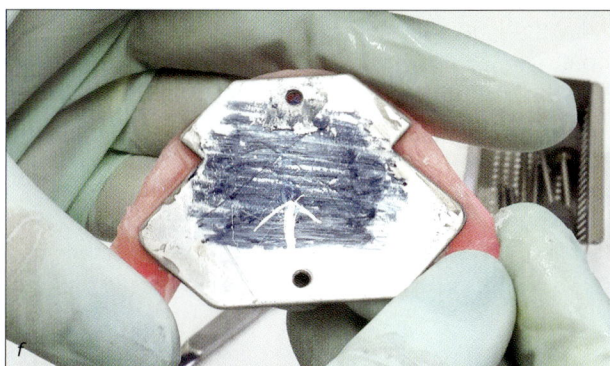

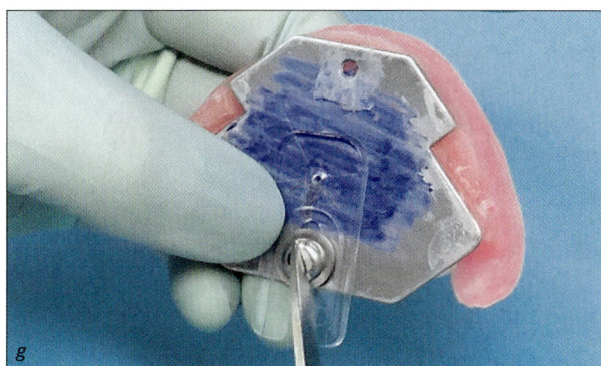

Figs 6d-g   The lower writing plate is melted onto the wax rim, slightly below the occlusal plane so that lateral movements can be performed (d). The patient performs the mandibular border movements, and the Gothic arch is traced. The tip of the arch is marked with a cross (e), and the procedure is repeated (f). The CR is located and a plastic plate determines where the upper writing pin should be situated (g).

Figs 6h-j   The patient closes with the writing pin at the tip of the Gothic arch (h). Plaster or silicone keys are manufactured and both templates are retrieved, preferably as one block. It must be verified that there is no contact between the upper and lower wax rims, other than via the pin and the plaster key (i). Finally, the casts are mounted in the articulator (j).

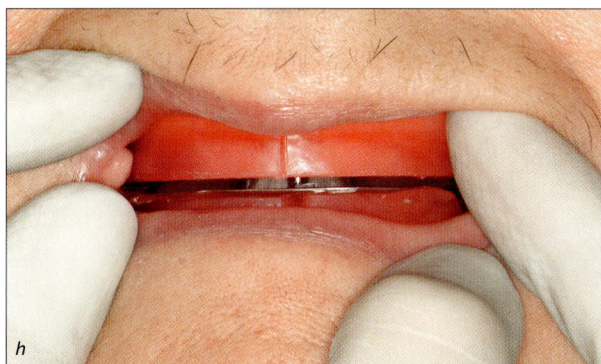

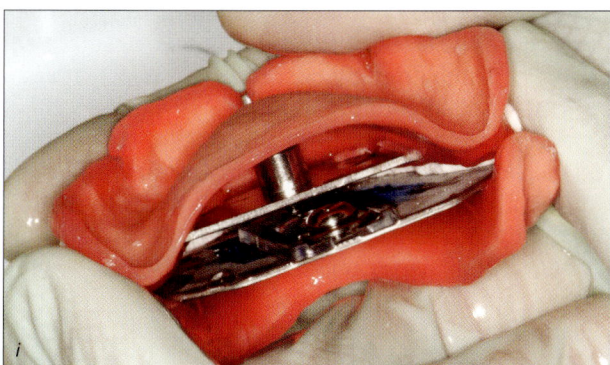

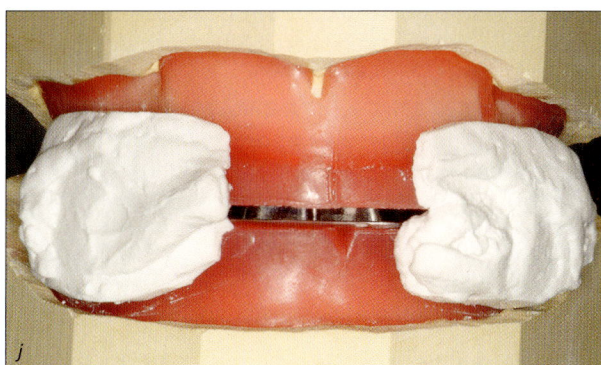

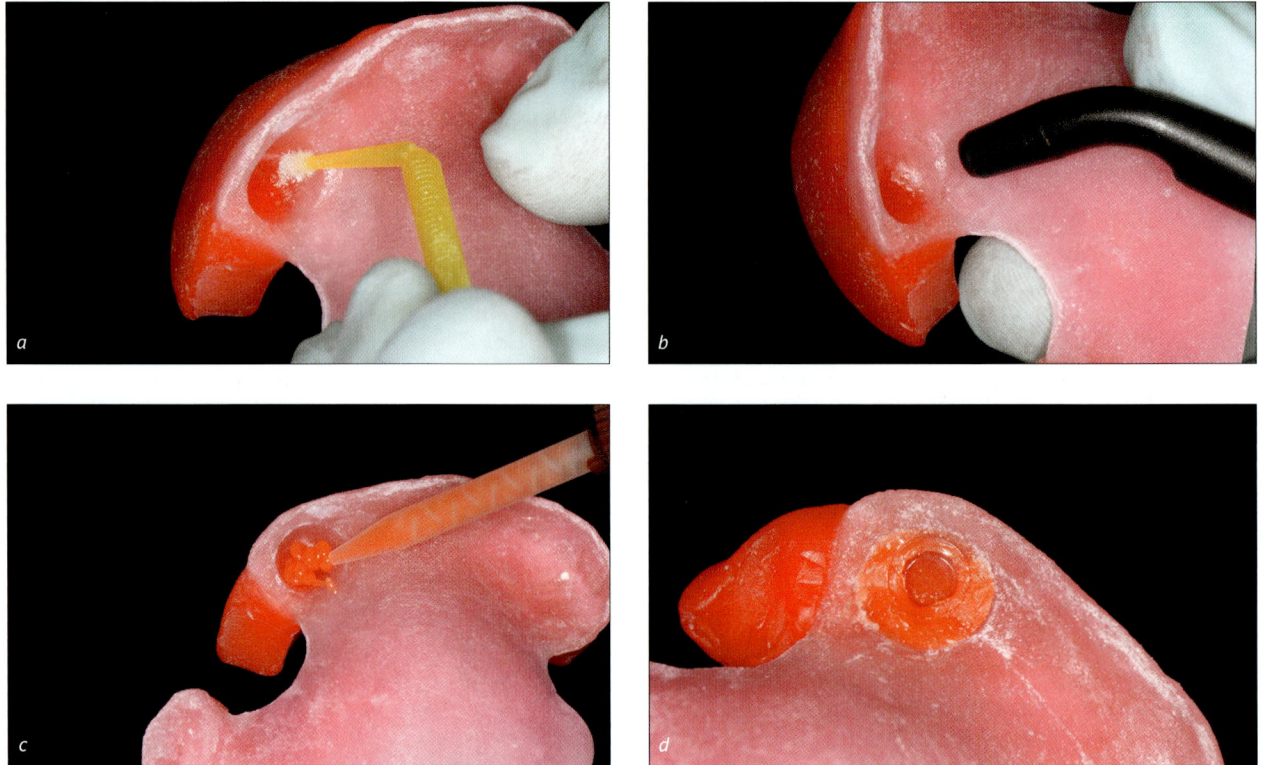

Figs 7a-d   To facilitate the retention of the registration templates, provisional female housings may be created in silicone (Retention Seal; Bredent, Senden, Germany).

Denture teeth

The above-mentioned atrophy of the articular tubercle in the temporomandibular joint leads to a flattening of the condylar path. Therefore, the denture teeth should not have a cuspal inclination of more than 20°. Acrylic teeth are preferable if the mandibular movements are poorly coordinated. As an added advantage, the fracture risk is lower when the denture with acrylic teeth is accidentally dropped during cleaning.

Abutment teeth

If natural abutment teeth are present, they present a valuable source of partial-denture retention; all efforts should be made to retain these teeth for as long as possible. The "bikini design" concept for cast chromium frameworks is adopted—the natural tooth structures are covered as little as possible to provide access for saliva and to prevent caries.

Abutment teeth often present substantial attachment loss and very long clinical crowns, which is unfavorable for partial dentures. The final impression for the prosthesis may be extremely retentive. In the mandibular anterior region, there is often very little space for a lingual bar. Furthermore, there will be "black triangles" between the abutment teeth and the denture teeth, which may severely compromise esthetics. In the phonetic zone, these spaces may even compromise speech and create occasional "spitting." Lastly, the high crown-to-root ratio presents an unfavorable lever for tooth survival.

A reduction of the clinical crown height after root filling may reduce the leverage on these abutment teeth. Periodontally healthy but endodontically treated teeth can be kept as overdenture abutments, providing occlusal support, tactile sensitivity, and physiological stimulation for the bone tissues. The root canal should be sealed with a plastic filling or a cast root coverage with or without retentive elements, the latter options usually being limited to premolars, canines, and incisors.

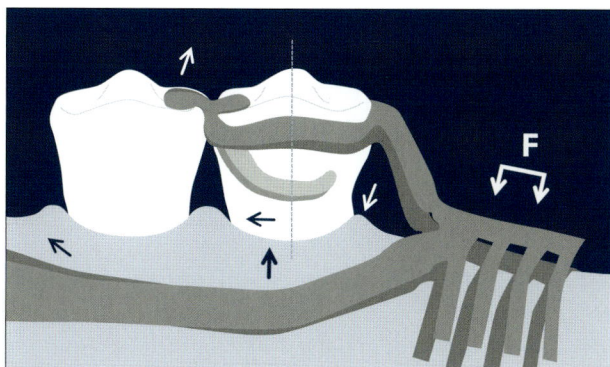

Fig 8   The "fail-safe" principle protects the abutment tooth, as the retentive part of the clasp is closer to the distal-extension saddle than the direct rest seat. On occlusal loading, the clasp disengages and protects the abutment tooth from extrusive forces.

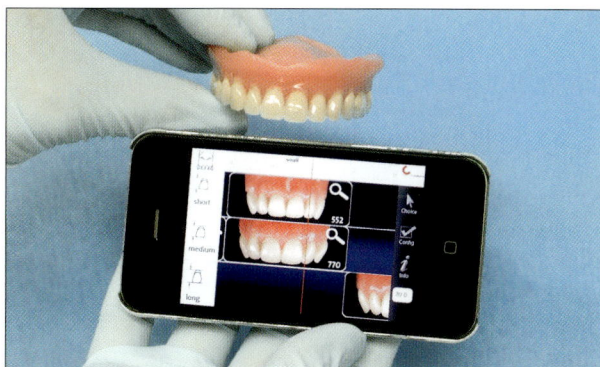

Fig 9   The tooth shade should be 3 or above, and the tooth shape could be chosen according the old denture or a photo of the patient's own natural teeth.

Denture kinetics and occlusal load

Although evaluating the prognosis of every single tooth is an essential exercise in treatment planning, it is even more important to judge the overall distribution of occlusal forces in the entire dentition. Overerupted maxillary molars, for example, may apply unfavorable loads on a mandibular distal-extension saddle.

As a rule, the mandibular prosthesis should be sturdier and stronger than the maxillary one.

Maxillary dentures have a better prognosis and are better tolerated by patients. The load distribution for a maxillary removable denture is more favorable, as the available surface for denture support is 1.5 times larger than for the mandibular denture. This concept may be difficult for the patient to understand, and it is frequently necessary to explain that it is wiser to invest in implants for the mandibular than for the maxillary denture. Strategic planning is the key for balanced force distribution in a dental restoration, and efforts should be concentrated on strategically relevant teeth, such as the mandibular canines.

In partial dentures for younger patients, the occlusal load is preferably transferred to the abutment teeth via rigid connections such as precision attachments or telescopic crowns. This concept protects the bony tissues from occlusal loads and provides high chewing efficiency and denture comfort. With no visible clasps and very good denture retention, these prostheses provide substantial esthetic and psychosocial advantages.

The abutment teeth in elderly patients are often too fragile to carry the occlusal load. To protect the abutment teeth, dentures are preferably constructed with a rotational axis, transferring the occlusal load on distal-extension saddles to the denture-bearing tissues rather than the abutment teeth. For further protection, the clasps adjacent to an extension saddle should be planned according to the "fail-safe" principle, which implies that its retentive part should be located closer to the denture saddle than the direct rest seat that accounts for the fulcrum line (Fig 8). When the denture saddle is loaded, the clasp disengages and protects the abutment tooth from extrusive forces. Despite the atrophy of the masticatory muscles, the occlusal load on an extension saddle may harm the fragile mucosa of the denture-bearing tissues. Hence, implants play an important role in converting a partial denture with a rotational axis to an entirely tooth/implant-supported partial denture.

Appearance

Age has a significant impact on dental appearance, as described in Chapter 3. An age-appropriate dental appearance may adopt one or several of the following features:

- Tooth shade of 3 or above (Fig 9)
- Abrasion of the incisal edges
- Large proximal contacts
- "Crowded" mandibular incisors
- Stronger visibility of mandibular rather than maxillary incisors

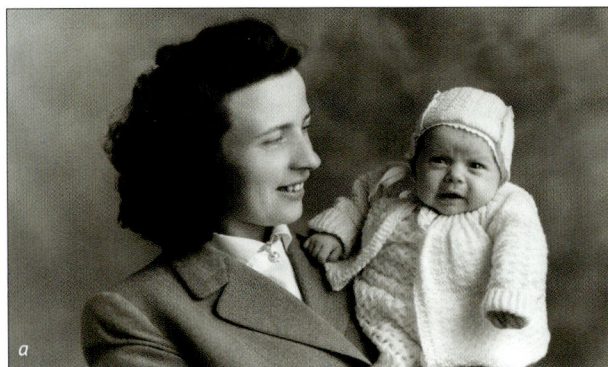

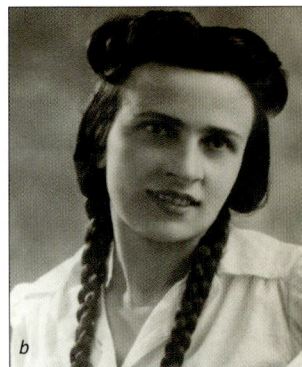

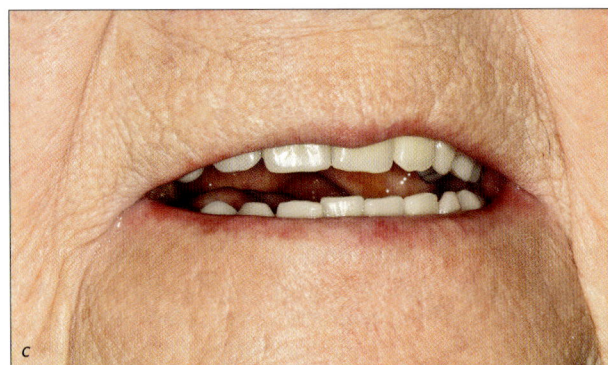

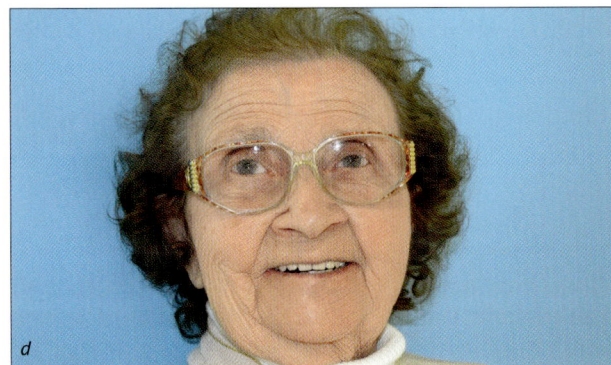

Figs 10a-d   A photograph from the "old days" on which the teeth can clearly be seen helps incorporating individual features in the anteriors of a complete denture. It also helps understanding the patient's life and background (a, b). By the way: the grumpy baby has grown into a very gentle adult daughter who regularly accompanies her mother to the dentist (a). The new denture was designed with age-appropriate and individual features according to the photograph (c) and gives the patient a happy smile (d).

A photograph of the natural dentition or a plaster cast are the most valuable records to customize tooth shapes and positions (Figs 10a-d). Lacking these documents, the old denture may serve as reference for the desired dental appearance. It would seem pragmatic to apply visible changes only in agreement with the patient and their close advisors. Further individual age-appropriate features may be added at the patient's request.

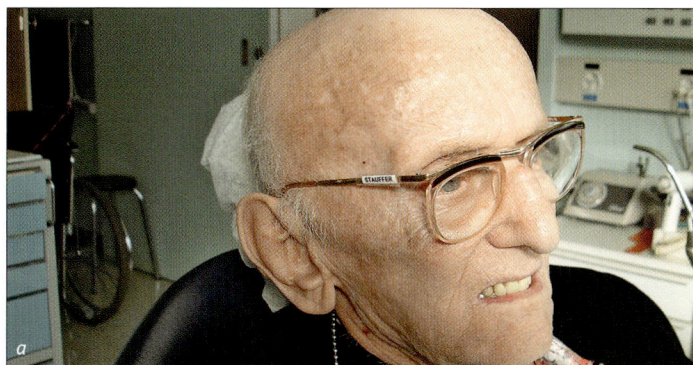

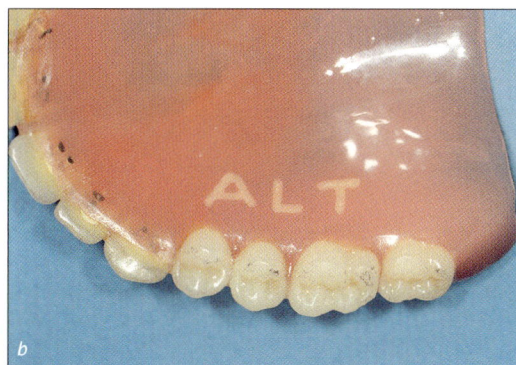

Figs 11a-b   In the case of institutionalized patients, most personal items that may get lost, for example glasses (a), are labeled, but dentures are rarely marked with the patient's name (b).

Labeling

In the context of an institution, most personal belongings such as glasses (Fig 11a), walking sticks, and wheel chairs are labeled, allowing easy return to their owner once lost. However, dentures are rarely marked with the patient's name, although this is very easy to do (Fig 11b). Also, sets of matching maxillary and mandibular dentures could be marked if the patient has several pairs of dentures (e.g., old or new). When providing an elderly patient with implant-supported dentures, it seems helpful to provide the patient with the exact type of implant and abutment used, in case they are moved to a different domicile and have to be treated by a different dentist.

Comfort

One important issue in the design of removable prostheses for elderly persons is the matter of comfort when the denture is not worn. We surely cannot expect patients to sleep without their dentures if they feel uncomfortable with this in the presence of their partners. In this case, the patient must be aware that maintaining meticulous oral hygiene is essential. Most elderly patients, however, would not mind sleeping without their dentures. A recent study revealed that nocturnal denture wearing doubles the risk of pneumonia in very old persons (Iinuma and coworkers 2015). As for the denture design, there should be no sharp edges from precision attachments or implant abutments, which may cause injury to the unprotected oral tissues while the denture is not worn during the night.

7 Implants and Partial-denture Design

F. Müller

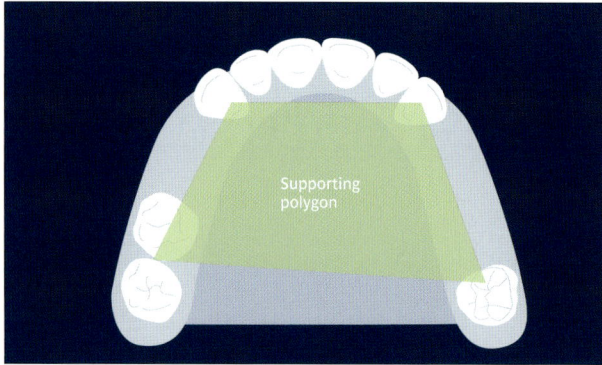

Fig 1   Basic principle: The supporting polygon.

Implants and partial dentures

At first glance, combining implants and removable partial dentures (RPDs) may not seem logical. If you have abutment teeth, why place implants? And if you place implants, why not opt for a fixed reconstruction rather than a removable dental prosthesis (RDP)?

Furthermore, the "shortened dental arch" (SDA) concept suggests that not all lost molars need to be replaced in elderly patients (Kayser 1981). However, the possibilities introduced to partial denture design by dental implants are tempting, as the treatment adopts minimally invasive and preventive paradigms widely established in other dental disciplines. Basically, dental implants can be used for three purposes: to *provide support* for improved denture kinetics, to *improve retention*, and to *enhance esthetics* by avoiding visible clasps.

Very little high-level scientific evidence exists concerning the design of RDPs. This subject taught to dental students largely based on tradition, and basic principles

and subjective beliefs are passed from one generation to the next.

Large differences in RDP design exist between countries and schools. The major shortcoming of all concepts is that they are dominated by predominantly mechanical paradigms, which take little note of the biological structures of the orofacial system. Before discussing the use of dental implants in RDP design, it is therefore expedient to outline some of the basic principles of RDP design (Budtz-Jørgensen and Bochet 1998).

Given the lack of scientific evidence for either concept, we do acknowledge that other concepts of partial-denture design may perform equally well in a clinical context.

Supporting area

> **Basic principle:** The denture-supporting polygon should be as large as possible, and ideally "frame" the prosthesis (Fig 1).

If abutment teeth are available adjacent to an edentulous space, these will support the denture saddle. If no abutment tooth is available at one end of the edentulous space, a cantilever saddle will be necessary to replace the lost teeth. This may also be the case in tooth-delimited edentulous spaces if some parts of the denture will be outside the supporting area due to curvilinear ridges, for example in a Kennedy class IV situation with missing anterior teeth. The supporting area will therefore no longer "frame" the denture, compromising stability by creating a cantilever in an orofacial direction.

Because the cantilever saddle is not supported by teeth but by resilient mucosa, any occlusal load will compress

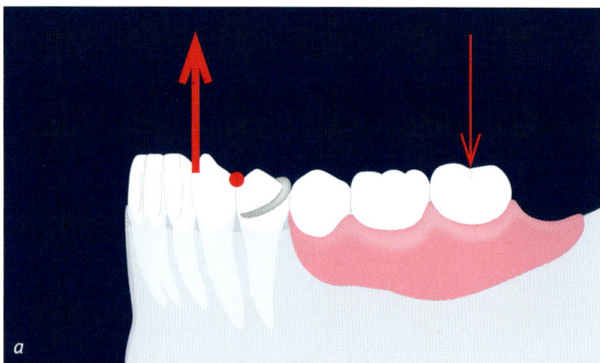

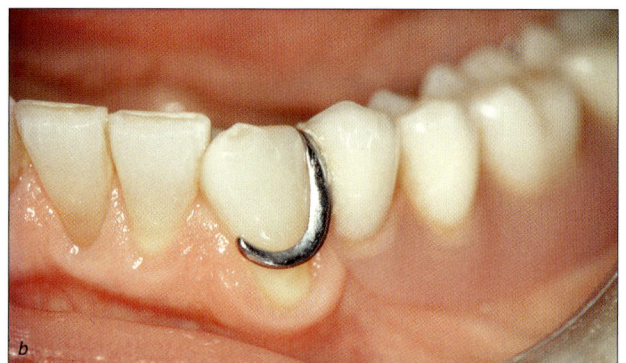

Figs 2a-b   Occlusal loads on the cantilever saddle introduce a fulcrum line on the nearest abutment tooth with a "direct rest seat."

the denture-bearing tissues, causing the denture to rotate around a fulcrum line defined by the closest "direct" rest seats on the abutment teeth. The length of the cantilever saddle has an inherent influence on the rotation torque. The lever principle states that the longer the force lever, the lower the force needed for compressing the cantilever saddle (Figs 2a-b). The surface area of the latter is also part of the equation, in that a larger surface is good for pressure distribution (a principle well known from skiing or snowshoeing). The length of the denture saddle (force arm) also plays a role. Shrinking the distal occlusal table, for example by not setting up a second molar on the cantilever saddle, may reduce the torque on the abutment tooth.

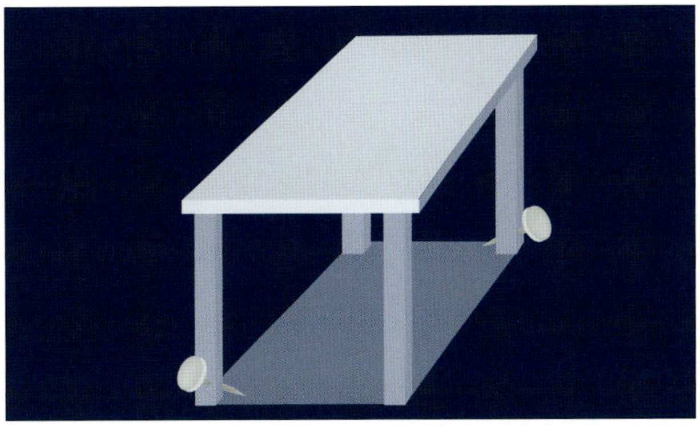

Retention

A RDP will be retentive if clasps or other retentive elements are placed at either end of the supporting area, like a four-legged table with two of its legs nailed to the floor (Fig 3). This also applies to RDPs with a fulcrum line, such as in Kennedy class I, II, or IV. Where a fulcrum line exists, clasps at the corresponding site of an indirect retainer (rest seat) on the opposite side of the fulcrum line should be avoided (Budtz-Jørgensen 1999). Such clasps would quickly exhibit material fatigue and finally fracture. This could cause additional wear on enamel of the abutment teeth or on the restoration.

> **Basic principle:** The line connecting the retention elements (the retention diagonal) should run across the RDP and ideally divide the surface of the supporting area into two equal parts (Fig 4).

A favorable distribution of abutment teeth on both sides of the dental arch is therefore a prerequisite for

Fig 3   Two clasps provide sufficient retention for an elderly patient's RPD, provided that the diagonal of retention crosses the area of support. The example illustrates that the table cannot be moved once two table legs have been secured in place.

good denture retention. In a severely reduced dentition, where the abutment teeth are only located on one side, no supporting area can be defined, and therefore the retention diagonal will not be very effective.

> **Basic principle:** In RDPs with mixed tooth/mucosa support, the retention diagonal should be closer to the cantilever saddle than the fulcrum line (Fig 5).

This principle is called "fail-safe" (Budtz-Jørgensen 1999) and is meant to protect the abutment tooth from extrusion and to minimize clasp fatigue from loads on the denture saddle. At the same time, the "fail-safe" principle ensures that the clasp protects the denture from displacing forces.

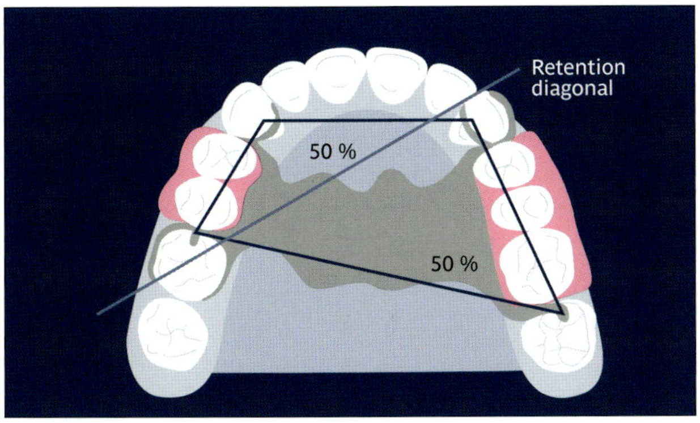

Fig 4   Basic principle: The retention diagonal (blue) should divide the supporting area into two. Two clasps are sufficient to retain a partial denture for an elderly patient.

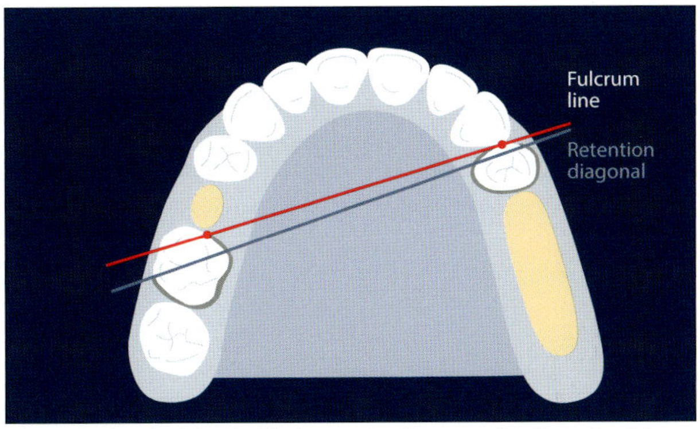

Fig 5   Basic principle: An ideal retention line runs distally to the fulcrum line (closer to the cantilever saddle) to protect the abutment tooth from extrusion forces during loading. However, for esthetic reasons, the clasp may also be placed in the mesiovestibular undercut. As long as the tip of the clasp stays distally of the fulcrum line, the basic rule is not violated.

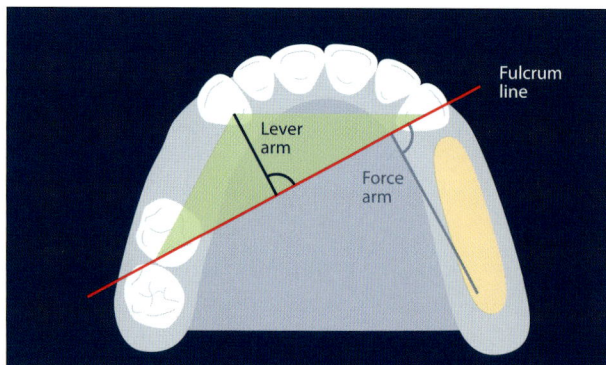

Fig 6 Basic principle: As soon as one corner of the supporting polygon (blue) is missing, a cantilever saddle is created, which will compress when loaded. The two direct rest seats (16 and 23) will create a rotational axis (red). The length of the load arm (green) should be opposed by a lever arm (yellow) which is at least as long as the load arm or longer. The lever arm is created by placing an indirect rest seat on the canine (13) and provides indirect retention of the denture saddle is displaced, for example when chewing sticky food.

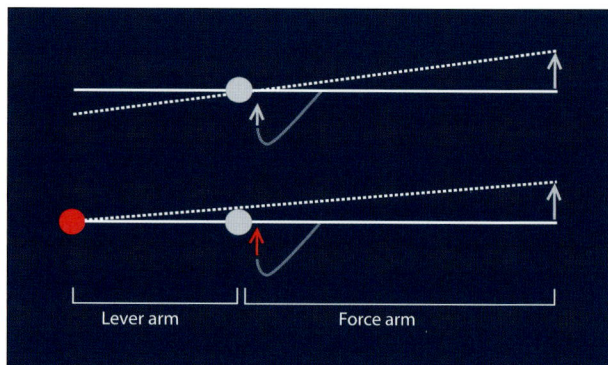

Fig 7 Basic principle: Indirect retention. The retention of a RDP with a cantilever saddle can be improved by placing indirect rest seats at the opposite side of the fulcrum line. The longer lever renders the clasp more effective against pull-off forces during mastication.

Applying this basic principle to a Kennedy class I or II situation, the clasp connector would ideally cross the interproximal area mesial to the abutment tooth as the clasp travels to retention in the distobuccal undercut. Obviously, a visible clasp often means poor esthetics, which can, however, be improved without violating the basic "fail-safe" principle by designing the clasp retention to be located in the mesiobuccal undercut, but still distally to the fulcrum line (Fig 5). Ideally, the fail-safe principle requires a reciprocal plate, which may unintentionally provide direct support when placed above the prosthetic equator. Hence, the fail-safe principle is impossible to apply to canines and incisors due to their morphology.

In the severely depleted dentition, if the distribution of the remaining abutment teeth is such that there is only a supporting line rather than a supporting area (e.g., with abutment teeth on only one side of the jaw), the retention elements should be placed on the palatal/lingual side of the abutment tooth.

Basic principle: If the retention diagonal cannot cross the supporting area, the retentive part of a clasp should be placed as close as possible to the "center" of the RDP.

This type of clasp performs so poorly in a clinical context that most clinicians would opt for other types of retention elements, such as telescopic crowns or implants. Only when the general health of the patient, functional or cognitive decline, reduced motivation, or financial aspects preclude the preparation of abutment teeth or

the placement of implants, this type of clasp may be a "last resort" for partial-denture retention. In maxillofacial-surgery patients who have undergone mandibular hemisection and radiotherapy, unilateral palatal/lingual clasps may be used temporarily until the patient's general health has improved.

Indirect retention
The retention of a RDP with a cantilever saddle can be improved by placing indirect retainers (rest seats) at the opposite side of the fulcrum line. Ideally, the force arm created by the cantilever saddle should be opposed by a lever arm, defined as the perpendicular distance of the most distant "indirect rest seat" to the fulcrum line.

Basic principle: In partial dentures with a fulcrum line (Kennedy class I, II, or IV), the lever arm should be as long as or longer than the force arm (Fig 6).

The lever arm renders the clasp more effective against displacing forces (Fig 7). Indirect rest seats provide retention to the denture when the retention of the cantilever saddle is challenged, for example when chewing sticky food such as bread or chewing gum. The longer the lever arm, the more effective it will be from a mechanical point of view. As mentioned before, indirect retainers should not be combined with a retentive clasp.

Enlarging the supporting area with implants
In terms of denture kinetics, dental implants must be considered additional abutments that enlarge the supporting area of a RDP and can significantly improve the kinetics of dentures on occlusal loading. Consequently,

these implants will change the RDP's Kennedy class (Kennedy 1928). It has been suggested to add the number and exact location of the implants to the original Kennedy class and its modifications and call this the "implant-corrected Kennedy" (ICK) classification (Al-Johany and Andres 2008).

However, given that implants and abutment teeth behave similarly in terms of denture kinetics, for the purposes of this chapter we prefer to treat the supporting implants as abutment teeth and stay with the original Kennedy classification and its modifications, in order to facilitate immediate identification of the denture kinetics. For example, by placing two distal implants, a Kennedy class I can be converted to a class III or VI (Fig 8). These distal implants may serve as rest seats, but they may at the same time serve as attachments and provide retention, as in the clinical example shown in Figures 8 and 9a-b. A three-year multicenter study indicated improved patient satisfaction and denture stability as well as masticatory performance after placing distal support implants with ball attachments to support cantilever saddles in Kennedy class I cases (Wismeijer and coworkers 2013). Furthermore, the mechanical stimulation of the bone may also lead to increased bone mineral density (El Mekawy and coworkers 2012). When planning distal implants for an RDP with a Kennedy class I or II, the mandibular deformation during chewing or wide opening has to be borne in mind. In those rare cases where such distal attachments cause discomfort, the posterior implants may serve as simple rest seats without retention (Mitrani and coworkers 2003; Fig 10). Bench experiments and finite element analyses have confirmed lower stress concentrations and mucosal loads when distal implant support is provided for class Kennedy I RDPs (Maeda and coworkers 2005b; Ohkubo and coworkers 2007; Xiao and coworkers 2014). Long-term clinical studies are scarce and usually limited to case reports or small patient cohorts. However, they confirm clinical success, increased bite forces, comfort, and patient satisfaction (Bortolini and coworkers 2011; El Mekawy and coworkers 2012; Ohkubo and coworkers 2008).

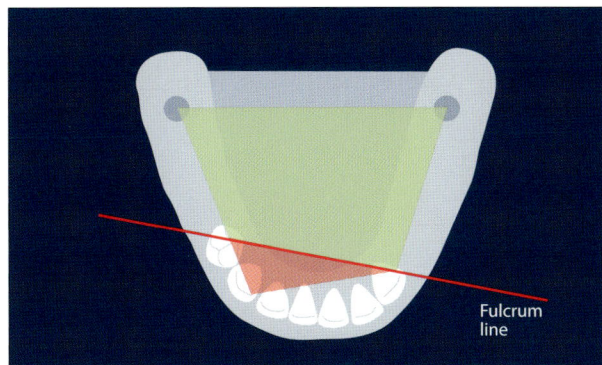

Fig 8 Implants can be used to extend the supporting polygon to meet the basic principle that the denture should be "framed" by tooth/implant support. In this example, a Kennedy class I is converted to a class V, and the initial fulcrum line no longer exists.

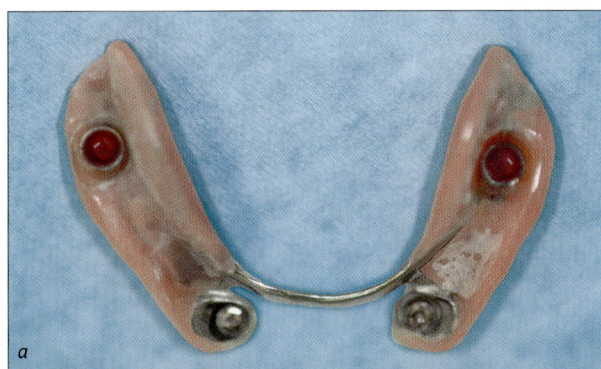

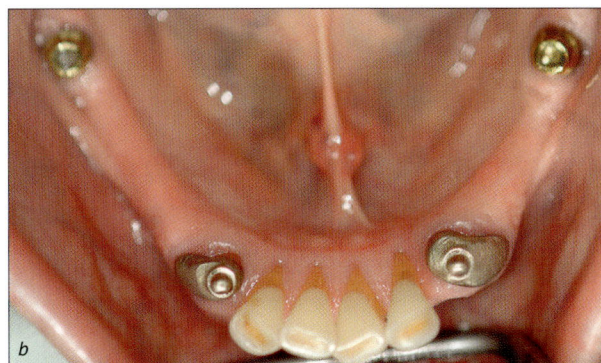

Figs 9a-b The distal supporting implants were provided with Locator attachments. Although the RDP splinted large sections of the mandible, the patient did not perceive discomfort.

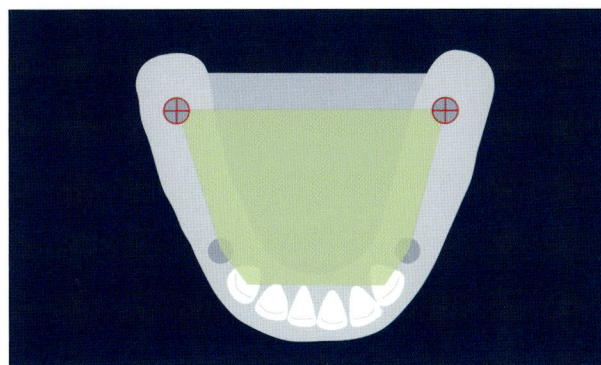

Fig 10 The concept of full tooth/implant support for a RPD with residual anterior teeth seems attractive, but mandibular deformation during chewing or wide opening may cause discomfort in some patients. In those (rare) cases, the posterior implants may serve as rest seats without retention.

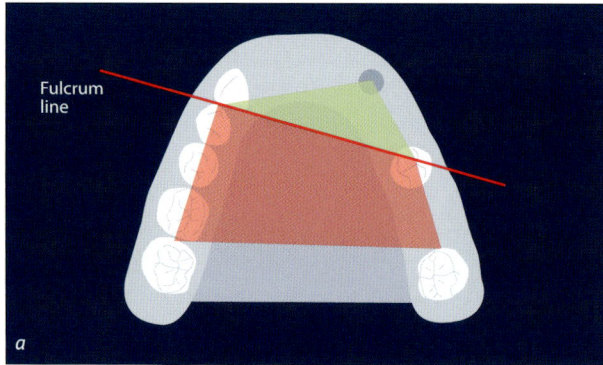

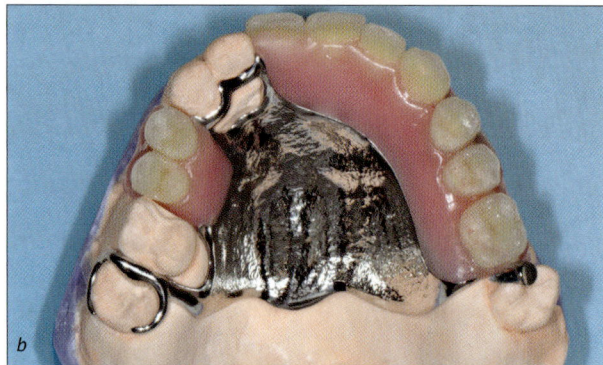

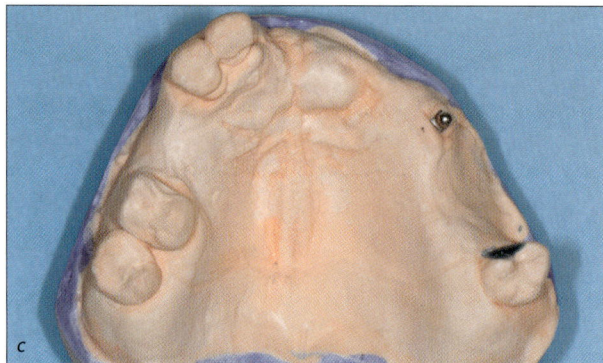

Figs 11a-c A curvilinear interdental edentulous space can be supported by an implant, eradicating the fulcrum line.

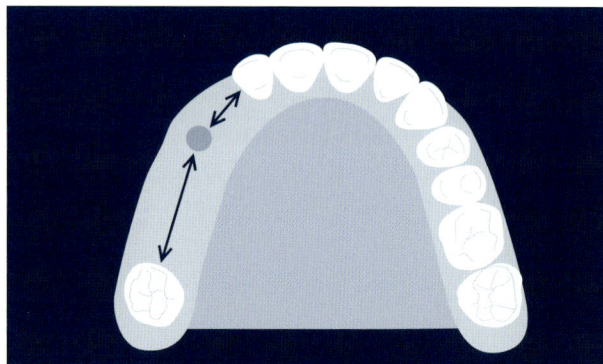

Fig 12 Support can also be increased with implants in long tooth-bound edentulous spaces when one of the abutment teeth has an unfavorable shape for a direct rest seat: for example incisors.

In the presence of a curvilinear edentulous space, implants may also be helpful in providing support, ideally at the most distant site relative to the fulcrum line (Fig 11). Even partial dentures for long edentulous spaces could benefit from a supporting implant, especially in a Kennedy class V situations where one of the abutment teeth is not suitable for a rest seat (Fig 12). However, in these situations a fixed dental prosthesis may also be a suitable restoration.

Abutment implants may even be beneficial for improving denture support and kinetics when a conversion to a more favorable Kennedy class or a fixed reconstruction cannot be achieved. By shortening the force arm and lengthening the lever arm, the RDP may still have a fulcrum line, but with a larger supporting area (Fig 13a). Several implants may even avoid the fulcrum line completely (Fig 13b). This would improve denture stability, and in the present case, the implant would eliminate the need for a visible clasp on the lateral incisor. Ideally, such implant abutments should be placed where the newly created fulcrum provides a force arm of less or equal length than the lever arm. The rest seat on the distal abutment (here, the lateral incisor) will therefore be an indirect retainer.

Exceptions from this rule may become necessary when the anatomical condition would require a major surgical intervention such as bone augmentation or a sinus lift in order to place the implant in the ideal position. The invasiveness of such intervention would largely outweigh the mechanical advantage for the RDP. In the mandible, for example, it often seems preferable to place implants distally to the distalmost abutment tooth by at least one premolar width to obtain a larger supporting area and indirect retention via a longer lever arm. However, this concept is often impractical in the mandible where the implant has to be placed mesial to the mental foramen. Thus, both the retention polygon and the lever arm remain very small (Figs 14 and 15a-c). In RDP cases with mandibular anterior natural teeth, the RPD often has an only slightly more distal fulcrum line when implants are placed. Their main advantage in this situation is the possibility of avoiding visible clasps.

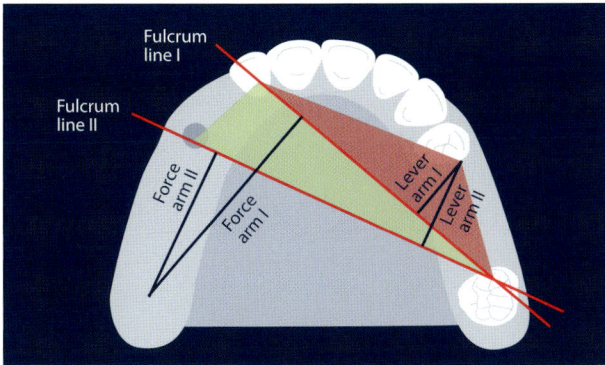

Fig 13a   Implant 14 replaces the clasp on tooth 12, which was esthetically poor and provided little retention. The implant was not placed adjacent to abutment tooth 12 but at site 14 to extend the supporting polygon and distalize the fulcrum line (II) so that the force arm for the cantilever saddle is shorter and the rest seat on tooth 12 can provide indirect retention via lever arm II. This design more closely follows the basic principle of the force arm and the lever arm ideally being of the same length.

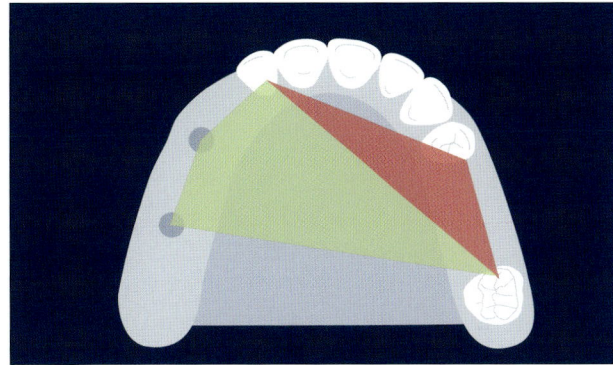

Fig 13b   If, in the same situation, two implants could be placed, there would no longer be a fulcrum line, and this Kennedy class II would be converted to a class V.

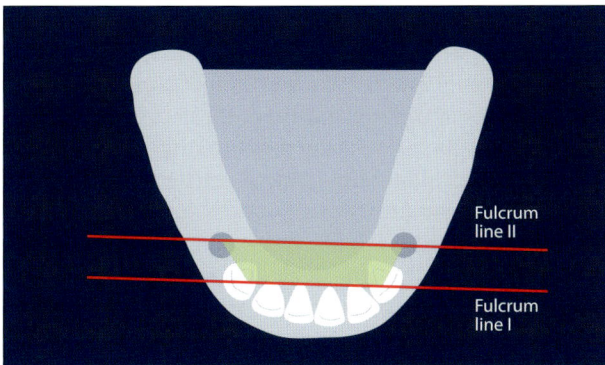

Fig 14   In the mandible, the concept of distalizing the implant by at least one premolar width to create a larger supporting area and indirect retention via a longer lever arm is not applicable if the implant has to be placed anterior to the mental foramen. Thus, both the retention polygon and the lever arm remain very small. The RPD still has a fulcrum line, but it is just slightly more distal and hence more favorable for the kinetics of the denture.

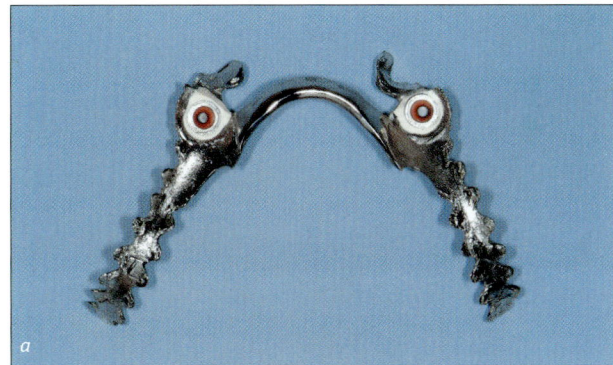

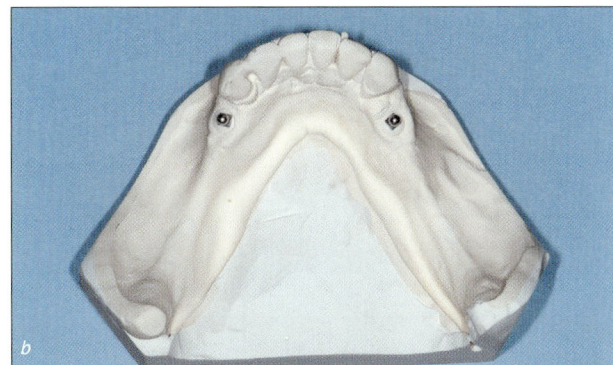

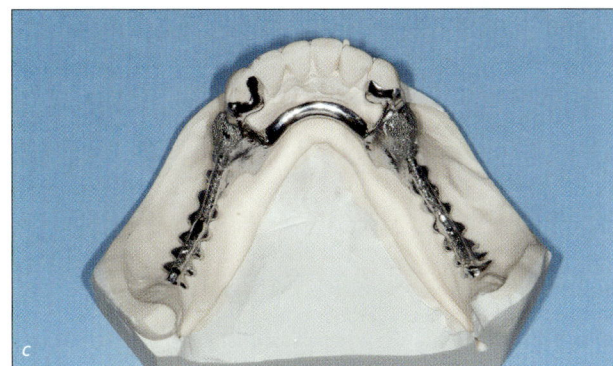

Figs 15a-c   Although implants 34 and 44 provide support, a rest seat is placed on both canines to provide indirect retention.

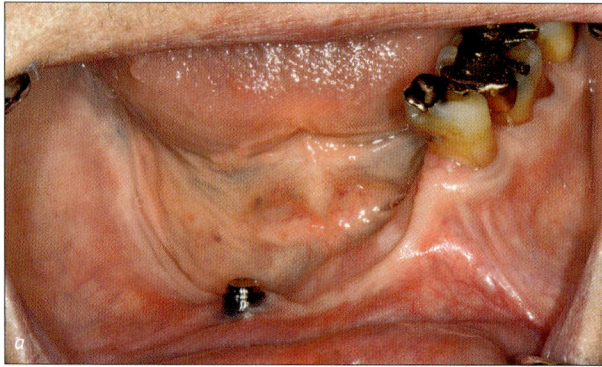

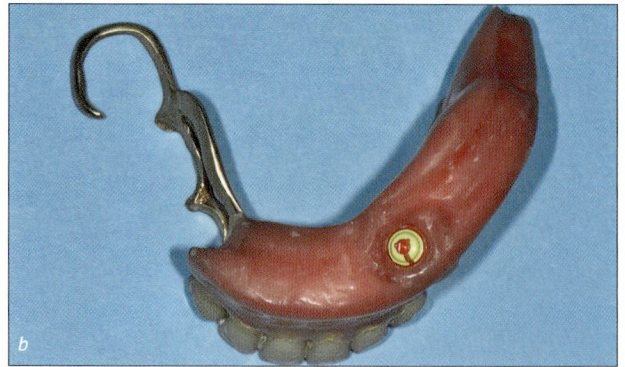

Figs 16a-b   Denture kinetics can be improved greatly even with one single implant if the residual abutment teeth are located only on one side of the arch.

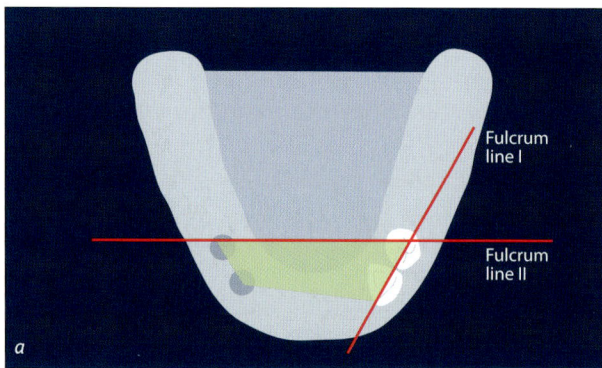

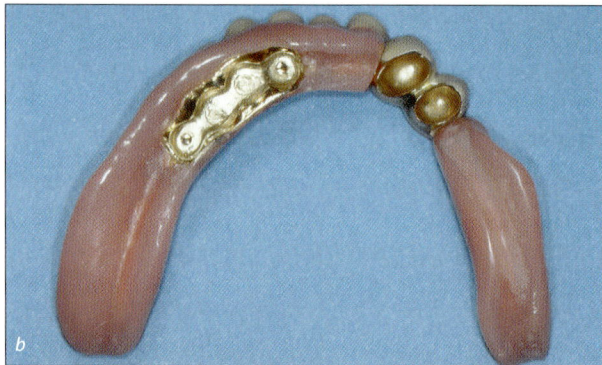

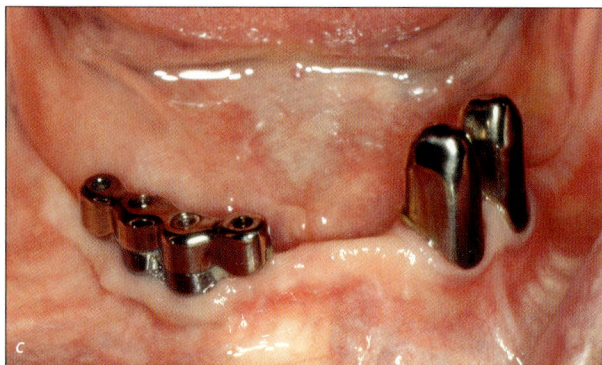

Figs 17a-c   In a severely depleted dentition, implants can serve as additional abutments and substantially improve denture kinetics. In this example, the linear unilateral fulcrum line was replaced by a bilateral one, and a supporting area was created.

Improving denture retention with implants

In elderly patients, denture retention is a critical issue. Partial denture retention is rarely perceived by old patients as being too low; a retention that is felt to be too strong precludes autonomous denture insertion and removal of the prosthesis for cleaning purposes. Even a small number of natural abutment teeth can provide sufficient retention for a partial denture, especially if these are distributed bilaterally. Adding retention to a partial removable dental prosthesis by means of implants may therefore be most useful in cases where only few abutment teeth are left or these are unfavorably distributed. The selection of the attachment system is critical, as the retentive forces of all available natural and implant abutments is cumulative. An eight-year retrospective study evaluated distal extension RDPs with retention but no support from distal implants (Bortolini and coworkers 2011). The study found a significant increase in patient satisfaction in a cohort of 29 consecutive patients with unilateral or bilateral distal edentulism.

The severely depleted dentition

The greatest improvement of denture kinetics through implants can be expected in partial dentures supplementing a severely depleted residual dentition. If the remaining abutment teeth are unfavorably distributed, implants may significantly improve denture stability and masticatory efficiency (Figs 16a-b), as conventional clasps rarely perform well when the abutment teeth are located unilaterally. Implants may effectively improve such partial dentures by creating an area of support and denture retention. Implants can also be combined with telescopic crowns on natural teeth (Figs 17a-c).

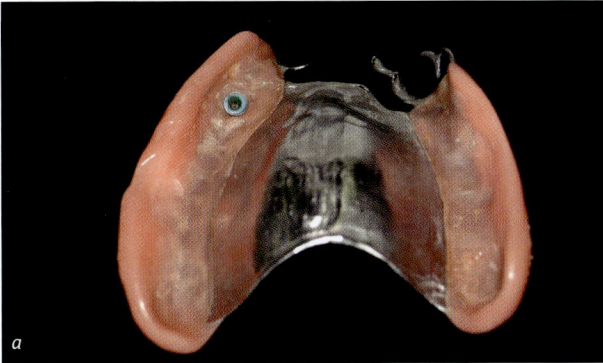

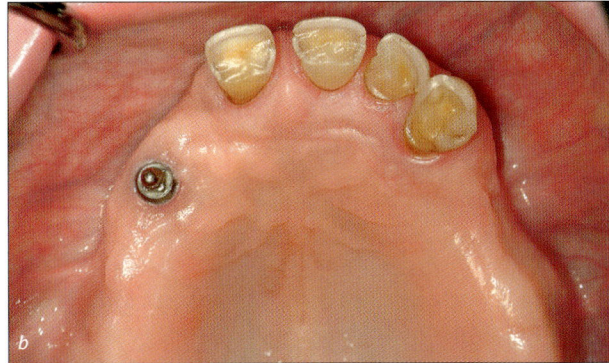

Figs 18a-b The implant replaced the visible clasp on the central incisor, whose shape was unfavorable for providing retention. This treatment provided a pleasing and esthetic outcome at moderate biological and financial cost.

Esthetic considerations

Besides the mechanical advantages, the use of implants in RDP design may help avoid visible clasps. An improved appearance may promote the patient's self-confidence and well-being in a social context. Additionally, when placed at least one premolar width distally of the adjacent natural abutment tooth, such an implant may serve as direct rest seat and further improve denture kinetics (Figs 18a-b). In the case shown in Figures 19a-c, the clasps of the lower RDP were not only highly visible but also rather ineffective, as the morphology of the lower lateral incisors did not provide much undercut. The existing denture was not renewed for economic reasons. After implant placement, the clasps were removed and the Locator housings were placed indirectly.

Choosing attachments

When combining natural teeth and implant abutments, it seems intuitive that retentive and frictional mechanisms should not be combined. However, clinical experience confirms that ball attachments or Locators can be combined with telescopic crowns or milled bars, as long as the two types of abutments are not immediately adjacent. This is of particular relevance if a natural tooth with a telescopic crown has to be extracted. In this case, the natural tooth can be replaced by an implant with a ball attachment, while the female part can by polymerized into the remaining secondary part of the telescopic crown.

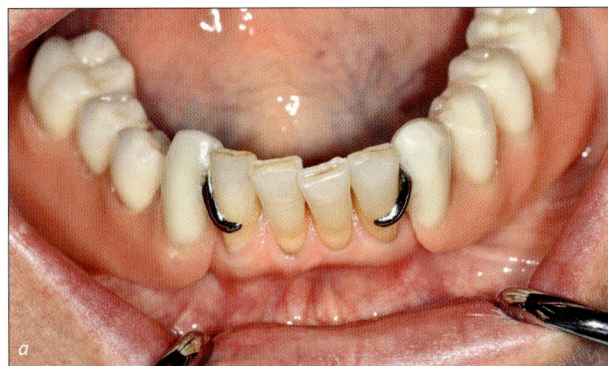

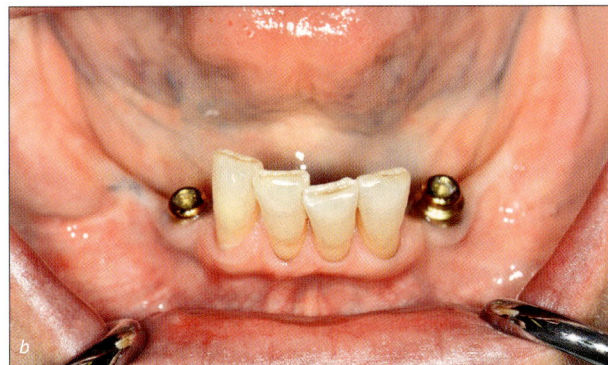

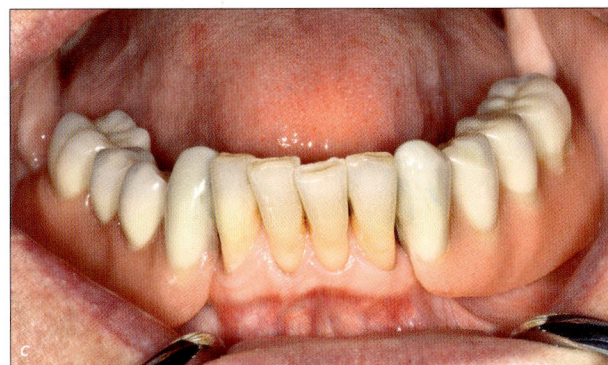

Figs 19a-c The lateral incisors were not suitable as abutment teeth. Implants were placed in both canine regions and replaced the ineffective and unesthetic clasps on the lateral incisors. The RPD was not renewed.

Preventive aspects

Any removable partial cast-chromium framework denture is the "natural enemy" of periodontal health. RDPs must therefore be designed to stay clear of the gingival tissues wherever possible. Large connectors should be located at a minimum distance of 5 mm from the gingival margin. RDPs also present a caries risk as they cover large enamel surfaces (Budtz-Jørgensen and Isidor 1990). RDPs should therefore receive a "bikini design," covering as little as possible of the natural tooth structures. Access for saliva will assist in keeping the tooth and the periodontal tissues healthy; it may even help remineralize incipient demineralized spots.

Clasps and their reciprocating arms, rest seats, and connectors create voids and change the natural "self-cleaning" tooth morphology, fostering the adhesion of biofilm. Consequently, implants may not only provide better RDP stability and retention, but may also play a major role in the prevention of caries and periodontal disease by reducing the need for such elements. No natural tooth substance will be sacrificed for preparing rest seats; no metal will cover the enamel. Hence, the prognosis of the abutment teeth may be enhanced if the residual natural dentition is not relegated to the task of assuring denture retention and support.

8 Implant-supported Overdentures for the Edentulous Patient

F. Müller

Although the percentage of completely edentulous patients in the working population is in steep decline, there is still a significant rate of edentulism in the elderly population, whether living independently or institutionalized.

Of all the indications for dental implants, edentulous patients probably show the most favorable ratio between effort/cost and benefit in terms of oral functional and psychosocial improvements. Tooth loss and removable prostheses are often associated with aging, morbidity, and finally death. Removable prostheses may present a handicap in a social context, especially when denture retention is limited to the effect of suction, muscular control, and occlusion. Edentulous persons in their third age who still live an independent and active social life will therefore often opt for fixed implant-supported restorations.

However, medical or anatomical risk factors may limit these options, and financial issues may play a role as well. In a study of edentulous patients who had worn both fixed and removable implant-supported prostheses for a period of two months each in random order, half the patients preferred to keep the removable reconstruction, while the other half opted for the fixed prosthesis (Feine and coworkers 1994).

In this study, removable prostheses were associated with easier cleansability and esthetic advantages. Indeed, replacing teeth with a removable prosthesis presents esthetic benefits, as anterior bone lost from the alveolar ridges can easily be replaced by the denture flange, which also allows the restoration of the former lip support of the patient. For fourth-age patients losing their autonomy and receiving help for the activities of daily living at home, or who live in an institution, a removable implant-supported prosthesis seems more favorable, as caretakers rarely have the time or the skills to clean fixed "high-tech" reconstructions adequately. Removable implant-supported prostheses also provide a greater degree of flexibility in denture design and retention mechanism, which is very helpful in case of a future functional decline and reduced neuroplasticity.

Number and position of implants in mandibular implant-supported overdentures

Even a careful and systematic evaluation of the literature in the field does not permit the recommendation of an ideal number of implants for mandibular implant-supported overdentures (Klemetti 2008). A carefully conducted longitudinal RCT by Meijer and his group investigated treatment concepts using bar-supported mandibular overdentures in edentulous patients (Meijer and coworkers 2009). Sixty patients of similar age were randomized into two groups. After receiving two or four implants, they were followed for 10 years. No difference was found in radiological and clinical parameters, patient satisfaction, or maintenance needs. However, an analysis of posterior bone loss indicated significantly more pronounced atrophy when only two implants had been placed (de Jong and coworkers 2010). As this seemed independent of any peri-implant bone loss, it may be related to the settling of the posterior denture saddle under occlusal load.

A similar pattern of posterior bone atrophy was confirmed in a retrospective study from Bern on overdenture wearers with two interforaminal implants, where posterior bone resorption increased with the distance from the fulcrum line (Kremer and coworkers 2014). In third-age edentulous patients, where masticatory-muscle atrophy is not yet clinically relevant, or in patients with a strong antagonistic dentition, it therefore seems preferable to create a larger supporting area by placing four implants in the canine and second premolar regions. Distal cantilever extensions are advisable to enlarge the supporting area even further, but often the denture height is not sufficient to accommodate the corresponding superstructure. Frequent fractures of these extensions may be avoided using recent CAD/CAM technologies for milled titanium bars (Katsoulis and coworkers 2015).

The higher occlusal loads made possible by implant-supported overdentures might also affect maxillary ridge atrophy. In two- or four-implant mandibular overdentures, maxillary anterior bone resorption was significantly higher over a 10-year period, than in a control group with complete denture-wearers (Tymstra and coworkers 2011). Therefore, when implants are placed in the mandible, it seems advisable to closely monitor the dentures for any need of relining in order to avoid anteriorization of the occlusion (Kreisler and coworker 2003).

In four-implant mandibular overdentures, implants should be limited to the interforaminal area. Although this provides a limited supporting area, the favorable amount of available bone as well as easier avoidance of the mandibular nerve appear to be a major advantage of this concept. Furthermore, the mandible is a flexible bone that deforms under masticatory load and during wide mouth opening, especially in the brachyfacial morphotype (Law and coworkers 2012; Prasad and coworkers 2013).

Experiences from the era of full-arch one-piece fixed dental prostheses has shown that some patients suffer from a "locked-in" feeling from large-span splinted reconstructions. Nowadays, segmenting fixed reconstructions is an acknowledged paradigm in restorative dentistry.

Although further research is needed on the clinical impact of mandibular flexure, placing the implants for a mandibular overdenture in the interforaminal area seems to be a sensible approach, given that a large supporting area can still be achieved by means of distal cantilevers. For this concept, the distribution of the four implants should ideally be in positions 5—3—3—5. However, depending to the shape of the alveolar ridge, the available bone, and the location of the mandibular foramen, a 4—2—2—4 constellation may become necessary (Figs 1a-b).

Basic principle: The distribution of four interforaminal implants should assure the distalmost position mesial of the mental foramen, and the lateralmost anterior position.

Such a distribution would optimize the supporting area, stay clear of the mandibular nerve, and avoid bulky superstructures where a natural denture morphology is important from a functional point of view. Care should be taken not to place the implants too close to each other, as this might lead to increased peri-implant bone resorption (Fig 1c).

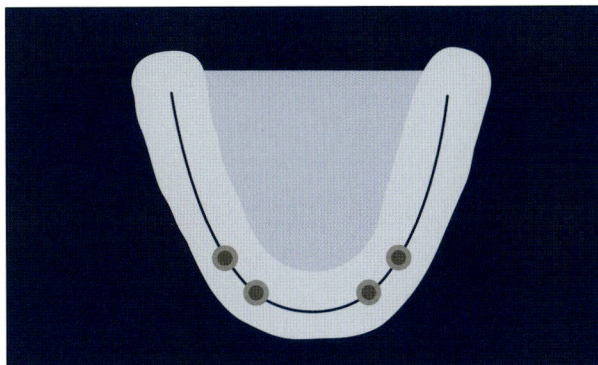

Fig 1a A mandibular four-implant overdenture should place the distal implants as distally as possible, yet still mesial to the mental foramen, and the anterior implants as laterally as possible. This concept stays clear of the alveolar nerve and avoids bulky superstructures in the sensitive anterior area. The ideal constellation is. 5—3—3—5.

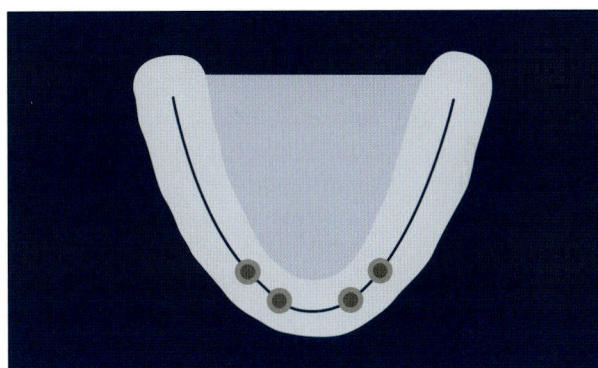

Fig 1b   The ideal constellation in Fig 1a could be modified to 4—2—2—4 if the shape of the ridge is rather "pointy" than "rounded."

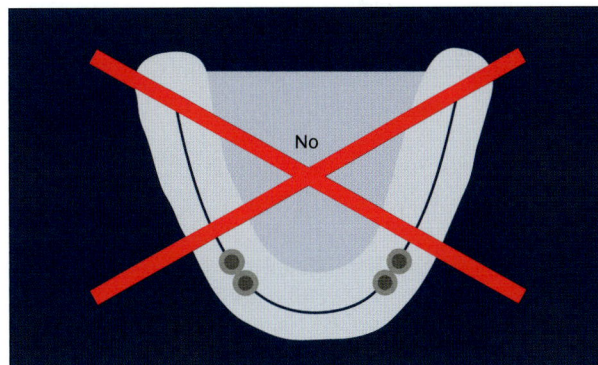

Fig 1c   Under no circumstances should the implants be placed too close to each other.

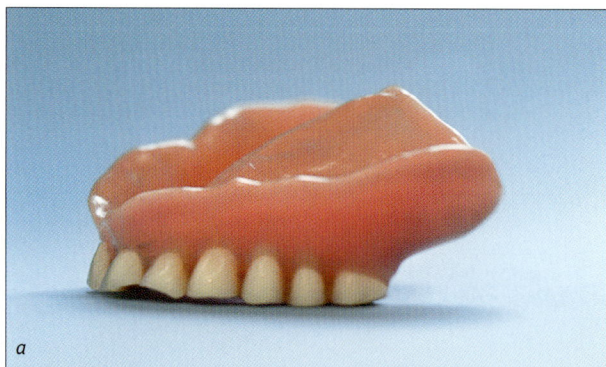

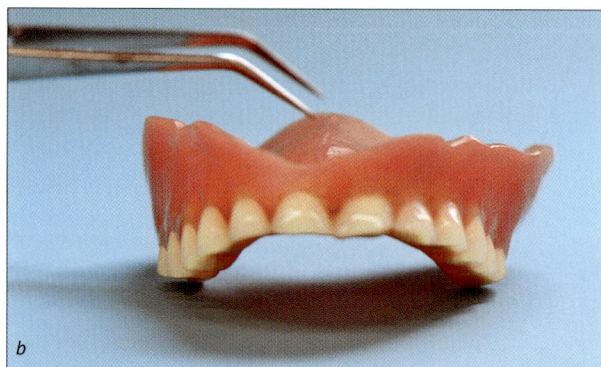

Figs 2a-b   Buccal (a) and frontal (b) view of a distally inclined occlusal plane in patient with Kelly's syndrome caused by a lower residual dentition.

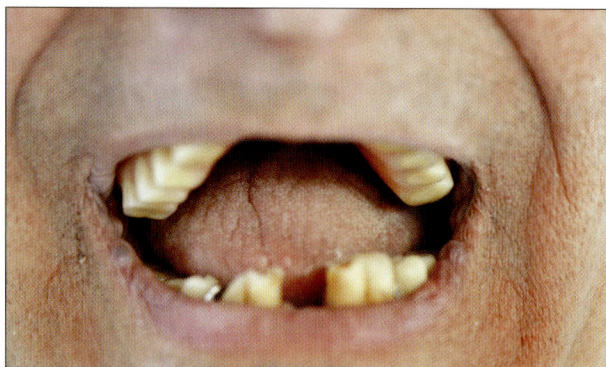

Fig 2c   Kelly's syndrome with barely visible upper incisors.

Three implants have also been proposed as support for a mandibular denture, but this concept only makes sense if the anterior alveolar ridge is shaped in a pronounced curve, so that using the canine position for the most anterolateral support would result in a cantilevered position of the lower incisors. In this case, an additional anterior abutment could be useful as indirect retainer. In this configuration, it is recommended not to add a retentive attachment, as—equivalent to the partial-RDP design—this is likely to fatigue and finally fracture when the distal cantilever is loaded during chewing. Splinting the implants by means of a bar could be an alternative concept.

The two-implant overdenture with linear support will always create a rotational axis, which leads to a distal compression of the tissues when the free end saddle of the denture is loaded during mastication. Correspondingly, accelerated posterior bone resorption may occur (de Jong and coworkers 2010; Kremer and coworkers 2014). Care should be taken to avoid excessive anterior occlusal contact, as the increased load on the maxillary anterior ridge risks creating Kelly's (combination) syndrome with flabby ridges and a distally inclined occlusal plane (Figs 2a-c).

As mentioned before, frequent remounting and possibly relining of the denture are required to avoid this phenomenon. As for the position of the implants for a two-implant overdenture, the canine region would again be preferable for mechanical and morphological reasons. Only in a strongly curvilinear anterior ridge should implants be placed in the area of the lateral incisor, to avoid rocking of the denture on the fulcrum line (Figs 3a-b).

Given the limited resources of the public health systems, the question arises as to whether one single implant in the mandibular midline might be sufficient to satisfy the needs of the edentulous patient. Indeed, one randomized controlled trial with edentulous participants supplied with either one or two mandibular implants for an overdenture showed a significant increase in patient satisfaction in both groups (Walton and coworkers 2009). Surprisingly, at the 12-month follow-up, 5 of the 42 patients in the one-implant group had already shifted from the positive half of the visual analog scale to the negative half (Walton and coworkers 2002). However, the difference in satisfaction between the one-implant and two-implant overdentures groups was not significant until the 5-year follow-up (Bryant and coworkers 2015). Implant survival seems excellent with this treatment

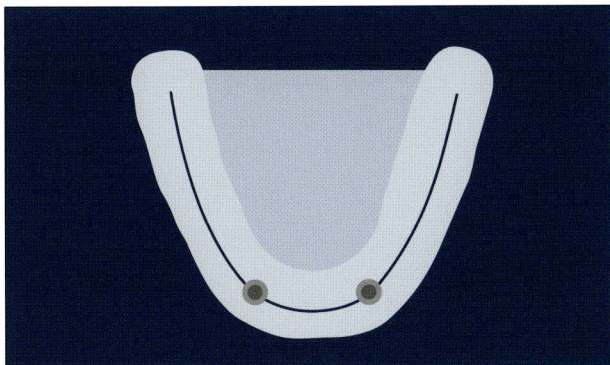

Fig 3a   If minimally invasive treatment is required, the two-implant overdenture is the first choice. Implants should be placed in the farthest anterior and lateral position. Depending on the shape of the ridge, this will most often be the canine region. Implants placed too far distally may cause a rocking movement of the overdenture shortly after insertion.

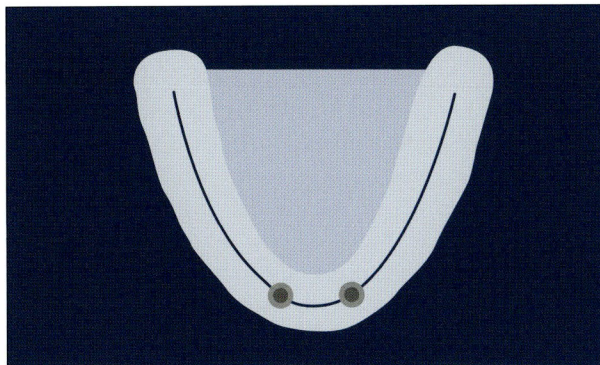

Fig 3b   Implant positions may vary depending on the shape of the ridge.

concept although long-term observations are still scarce (AlSabeeha and coworkers 2009; Bryant and coworkers 2015; Passia and coworkers 2014). Frequent denture fractures have been reported in some studies (Bryant and coworkers 2015; Passia and coworkers 2014), while others did not confirm this (Kronstrom and coworkers 2014). In a systematic review with a meta-analysis, it was confirmed that current evidence does not favor one or two implants in terms of implant survival (Srinivasan and coworkers 2016). The midline suture of the mandible often presents a lingual canal containing blood vessels and nerves, which requires consideration during implant placement (Oettle and coworkers 2015).

Finally, none of the published or ongoing studies on single-implant overdentures investigates the degree of posterior bone resorption. Even a minor premature contact in a complete denture will lead to denture rotation on the ridge during the last few micrometers before maximum intercuspation. The additional degree of freedom in a single implant overdenture would probably not preclude this movement. This kind of microrotation may accelerate resorption of the lateral parts of the alveolar ridge. Implant survival and peri-implant bone loss are important, but not the only success criteria for clinical decisions. Before recommending a single-implant concept, further research including patient-centered outcome measures, prosthodontic parameters, and functional aspects would be needed.

Number and position of implants in maxillary implant-supported overdentures

The mucosa covering the hard palate has a considerably greater resilience than that covering the mandibular alveolar ridge. The placement of only two implants to support a maxillary implant-supported overdenture must be approached with caution, as the overdenture might begin

rocking on the inevitable fulcrum line soon after delivery. Although early short-term experience with maxillary two-implant overdentures indicated patient satisfaction, prosthodontic and functional outcome measures are still missing (Zembic and Wismeijer 2014b). As a rule, a minimum of four implants is therefore recommended, with or without palatal coverage, with the anterior implants placed in the canine region and the posterior implants as close as possible to the chewing center. If the distal implants cannot be placed in the chewing center due to a lack of bone, the implant may instead be inserted immediately anteriorly to the maxillary sinus, as the functional benefit in terms of overdenture stability would not justify an intervention such as a sinus lift in a geriatric patient (Fig 4).

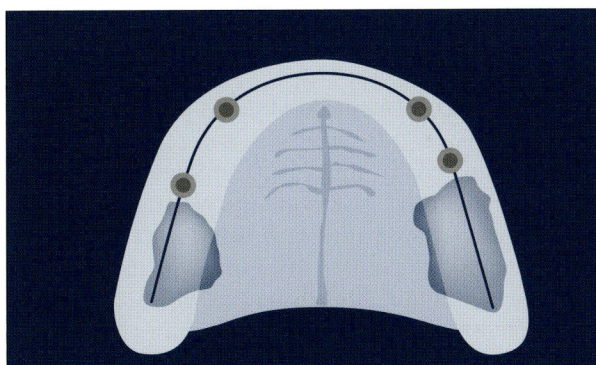

Fig 4   For a maxillary implant-supported overdenture, implants are ideally placed in the canine region and in the area of the chewing center (left side). Where the floor of the sinus precludes such position (right side), a more anterior position could be adopted instead (left side).

In younger patients, the mechanical advantage of a larger supporting area may outweigh the risks of such an intervention, and the clinical decision largely depends on the anatomical situation and the patient's functional state. The four-implant concept keeps the phonetic zone clear of bulky superstructures and encourages a more natural morphology of the palatal coverage, which in turn provides greater comfort and more natural speech. A shallow 0.5-mm-deep post-dam helps avoid food impaction under the prosthesis if a horseshoe-shaped palatal plate is used. The transition from the palatal coverage to the natural hard palate should be part of the cast chromium framework. Unlike a posterior palatal band for a partial denture, which is conveniently located in Donder's space, this transition is situated in a zone of the palate where the tongue is in constant contact, making it particularly important to assure a smooth transition from the artificial to the natural palate.

Some authors recommend placing implants in the maxillary tuberosities, as this provides the maximum possible supporting area. Unlike the mandible, the maxillary alveolar ridge does not flex during mastication, but the tuberosities should still not be considered the most favorable implant sites for other reasons. Firstly, access for clinical procedures such as connection of abutments or impression copings may be difficult, as elderly patients cannot easily be inclined backwards during treatment. Furthermore, there is a high prevalence of dysphagia amongst elderly persons. Dental instruments such as screwdrivers can be secured with dental floss, but small screws or abutments cannot (Deliberador and coworkers 2011), and there is a risk of aspiration. Finally, in the unlikely event of implant loss, the patient may be left with a poorer volume of tuberosity, creating a difficult situation for conventional denture retention.

The fourth-age patient

With age, there is less need for a large supporting area for an implant-supported overdenture, as the maximum bite force diminishes along with age-related muscle atrophy (sarcopenia) (Newton and coworkers 1993). Consequently, very old and fragile patients are less likely to present accelerated posterior bone resorption or the development of Kelly's syndrome, as described previously for a two-implant mandibular overdenture (Kremer and coworkers 2014). Given their fragile constitution, a two-implant overdenture according to the McGill and York consensus statements seems the first choice (Feine and coworkers 2002; Thomason and coworkers 2009). The advantages of a two-implant overdenture—rather than a four-implant overdenture—for geriatric patients include a minimally invasive intervention, reasonable

cost, and, most importantly, the possibility of the patient autonomously managing the overdenture. An overly retentive denture may cause panic if the patient cannot manage to place or remove the denture, which may cause profound distrust and disrupt their confidence in the dentist.

In fourth-age patients, it is also preferable for the occlusion, the vertical dimension, the shape of the denture body, and the dental arch to be changed as little as possible. This facilitates adaptation to the new prosthesis and avoids unnecessary challenges to the patient's neuroplasticity. Converting an existing complete denture into an implant-supported overdenture is an adequate therapy for fourth age patients, as long as the existing denture is reasonably functional and well tolerated. The low number of clinical treatment sessions required for such an intervention facilitates logistics in terms of patient attendance and meets the needs of the patient's increasingly fragile constitution. Conversion of a complete denture to an implant-supported overdenture could be done on the same day as abutment connection when no cast chromium framework is planned. In a dental arch in a suboptimal position, it may become necessary to add provisional autopolymerizing resin at chairside to provide sufficient support for the impression coping (Fig 5a).

As this is just a temporary support for the impression material, polishing could be performed later, together with the reline, in the dental laboratory. After creating sufficient space for the implant components and checking that there is no contact between the impression copings and the denture, for example by means of boxing wax or silicone, adhesive can be added to the denture base and a reline impression is taken (Figs 5b-d). Once the preferred retention insert has been chosen, the denture can be returned to the patient the same day (Figs 5e-i).

Patients will recognize the features of familiar prostheses to which they are already well adapted yet still appreciate the increased denture retention. Another way to avoid adaptation problems is to use a duplication technique. By copying the existing denture, features such as RC, OVD, and occlusal plane, as well as the position of the dental arch, can be incorporated into the new prosthesis. It is particularly important not to change the available tongue space, even if the posterior teeth of the existing denture are not mounted ideally. A lingual position of the dental arch may result in painful injury from accidental bites, as geriatric patients are less able to adjust their habitual movement patterns than younger patients.

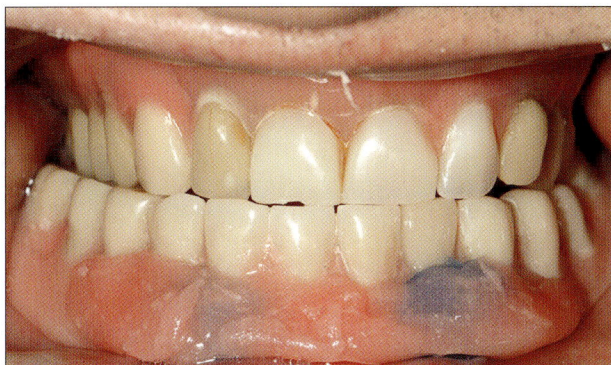

Fig 5a Conversion of an existing, suboptimal mandibular complete denture to an implant-supported overdenture. If the implants are placed "outside" the dental arch, the denture body needs to be provisionally extended with autopolymerizing resin to provide support for the relining material.

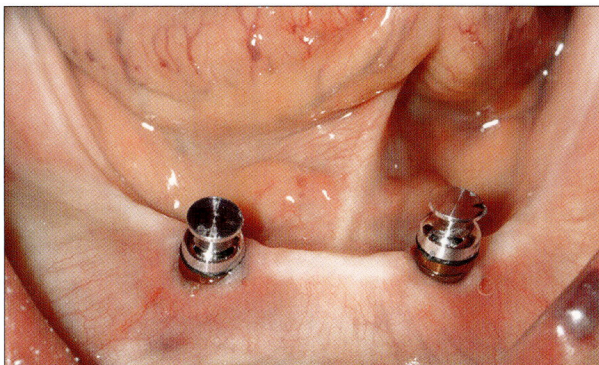

Fig 5b The impression copings are placed on the Locator abutments; it is also possible to use the female part of the Locator directly for the reline impression.

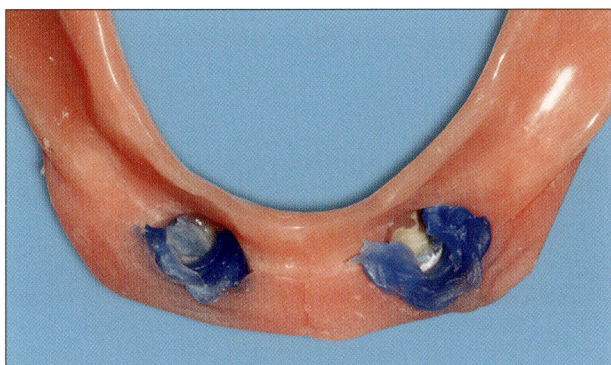

Fig 5c Boxing wax or a wash silicone impression to check if the denture base touches the impression copings.

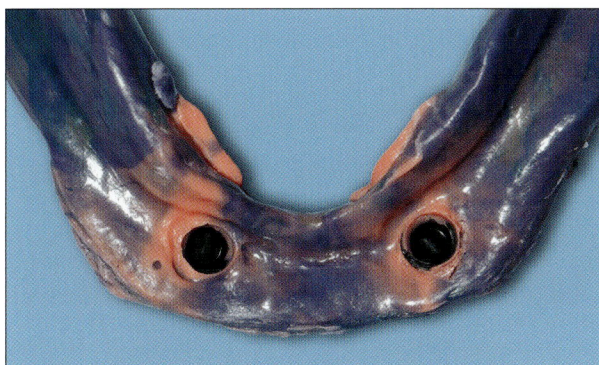

Fig 5d A reline impression with impression copings is taken.

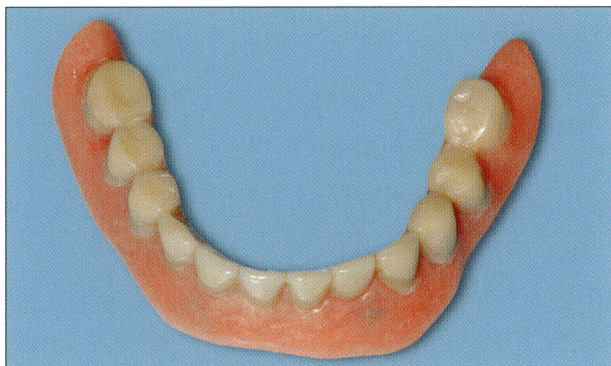

Fig 5e The vestibular denture flange needed to be slightly prolonged to accommodate the female part of the Locator attachment.

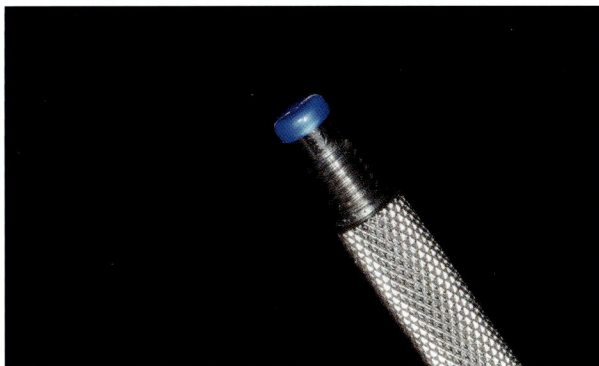

Fig 5f The blue insert is chosen in situations where "medium"-strength retention is required.

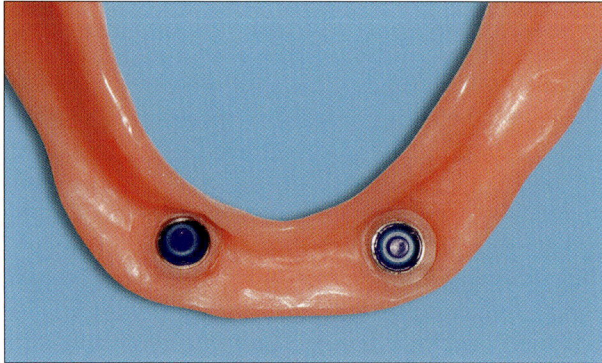

Fig 5g   The denture base with the female parts of the Locator attachments

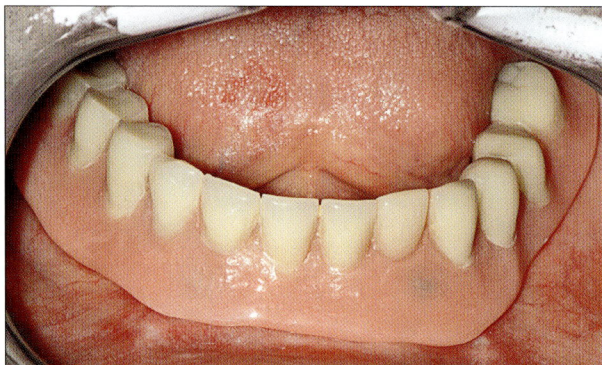

Fig 5h   Within one day, the patient had his well-adapted, yet suboptimal denture returned as a two-implant supported overdenture. The vestibular denture flange had to be slightly extended, as incisors were mounted rather lingual on the denture.

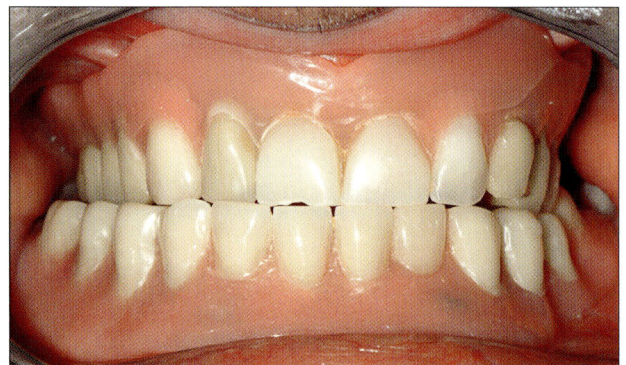

Fig 5i   OVD and RC are not changed and the patient "recognizes" his old, familiar denture.

However, copy techniques and the use of existing dentures are not widely used in dentistry. One explanation may be that the resulting prostheses are not pleasing to the dentists' eyes and may offend their professional pride in terms of appearance and function. However, in geriatric dentistry it is crucial to consider the patient's function and well-being as the first priority. The smile of a happy geriatric patient "recognizing" a prosthesis compensates for the missed opportunity to deliver a state-of-the-art denture design. The patient is the one wearing the denture—not the dentist!

Impressions for two-implant overdentures
Distal settling of a two-implant overdenture often creates a void between the denture base and the alveolar ridge in the anterior part of the denture, sometimes even shortly after delivery. This initial settling of the denture is physiological, as the denture-bearing tissues adapt to the posterior pressure under the denture saddles. Denture settling is a phenomenon well known in complete dentures, where a remount in the articulator is usually performed 10 to 14 days after insertion to correct the resulting occlusal discrepancies. In two-implant

overdentures, this settling process is even more visible, as it occurs only in localized areas supported by the mucosa rather than the implants.

An anterior void under the denture where no such settling occurs due to implant support may lead to the accumulation of food debris, which may be disturbing to the patient. An efficient way of avoiding anterior voids during the settling period is to simulate this process during impression-taking by forcing a slight compression of the denture-bearing mucosa. For this technique, the impression tray is prepared in contact with the denture-bearing tissues and an anterior dome of 3 to 4 layers of wax for the implant components. In the first step, the borders of the tray are adjusted and functional border molding is executed with a thermoplastic impression compound (e.g., Impression Compound, red sticks; Kerr, Orange, CA, USA) while the patient is performing functional movements. In a second step, a partial impression is taken of the edentulous mucosa using zinc oxide paste without exerting pressure and in the absence of functional movements (Fig 6a).

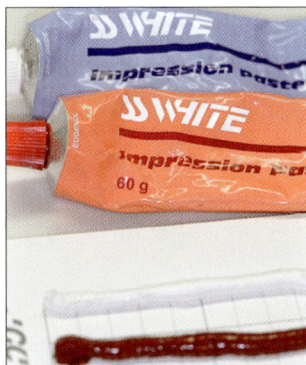

Fig 6a ZnO pastes are used for the impression of the edentulous mucosa (e.g., Zinc Oxide & Eugenol Impression Paste; SS White, Lakewood, NJ, USA).

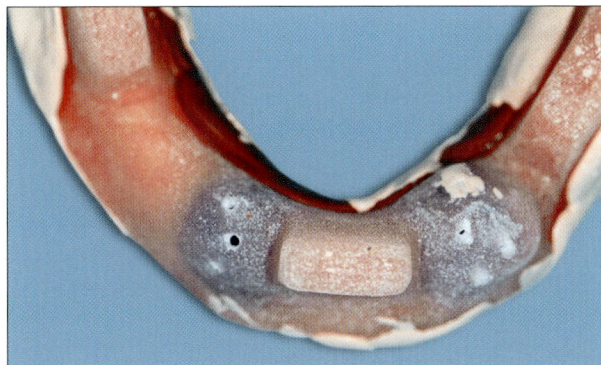

Fig 6b Sprue holes are added to the impression tray in the area of the domes.

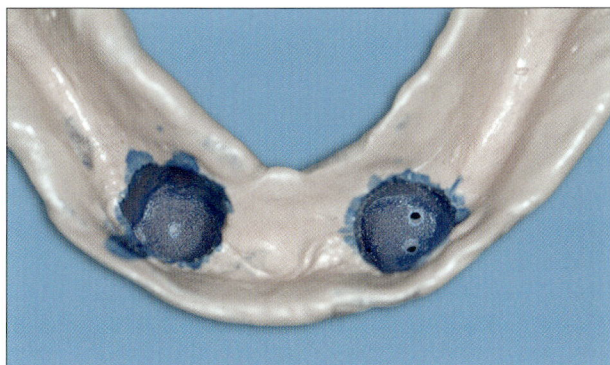

Fig 6c The domes are coated from inside with a silicone or polyether adhesive.

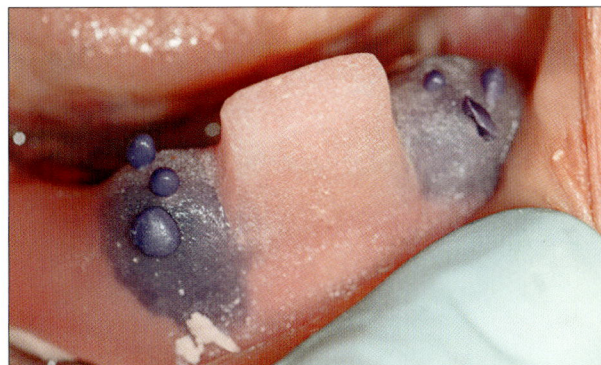

Fig 6d Silicone or polyether materials to add the remaining implant areas to the impression.

This first partial impression captures the edentulous mucosa in an unloaded state, with a tight inner seal. Care should be taken that no parts of the impression tray show through the initial impression, as these zones are likely to create painful sore spots once the denture is processed and inserted. In a third step, sprue holes are created in the impression tray in the area of the domes (Fig 6b) and the latter are coated from the inside with a silicone or polyether adhesive (Fig 6c). Then silicone or polyether materials are used to add the remaining implant areas to the impression (Fig 6d). This third part of the impression is performed under moderate pressure, anticipating the settling of the denture into the denture-bearing tissues. Careful inspection of the impression is necessary to verify a smooth transition of the silicone/polyether material to the zinc oxide paste (Fig 6e). A thin layer may be found on the zinc oxide paste; it can either be left on or peeled off before pouring the impression for the master cast.

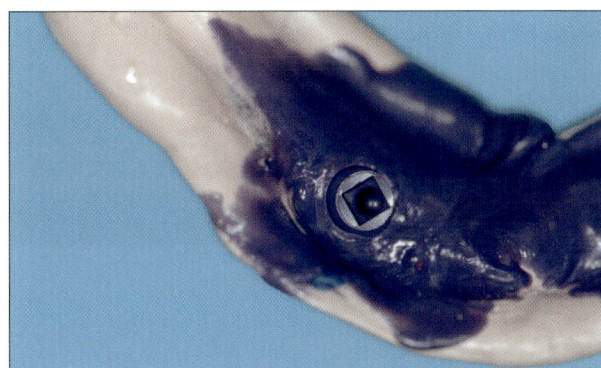

Fig 6e Careful inspection of the impression to verify a smooth transition of the silicone/polyether material to the ZnO pastes.

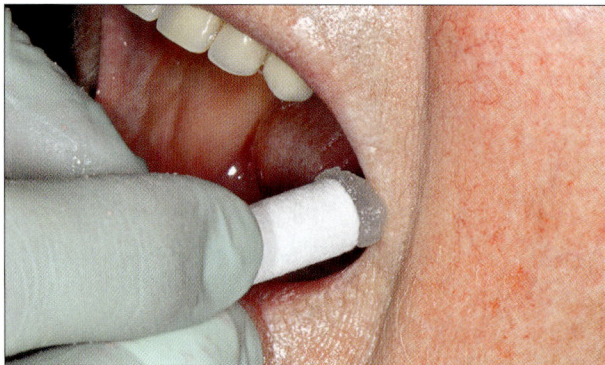

Fig 7a

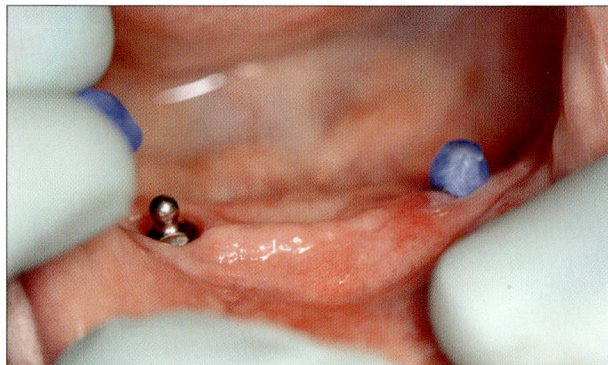

Fig 7b

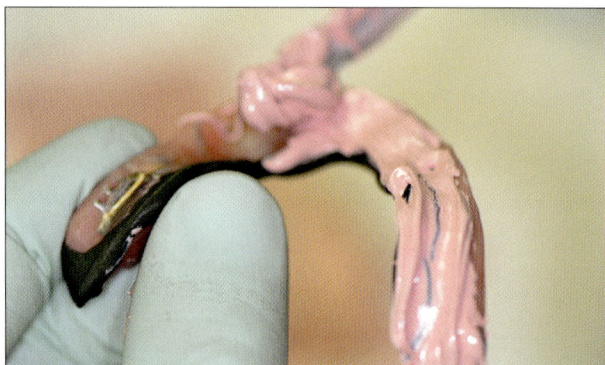

Fig 7c

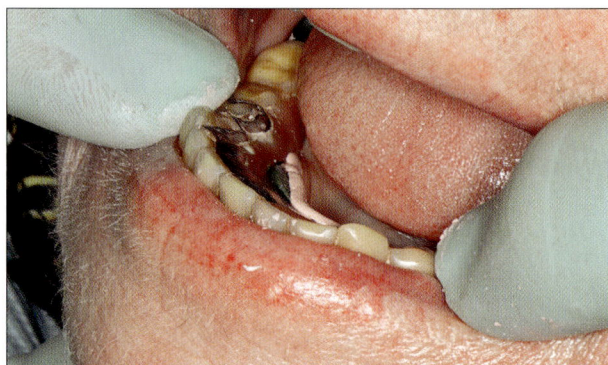

Fig 7d

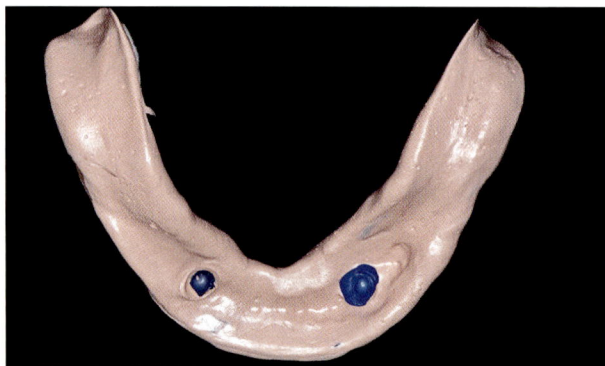

Fig 7e

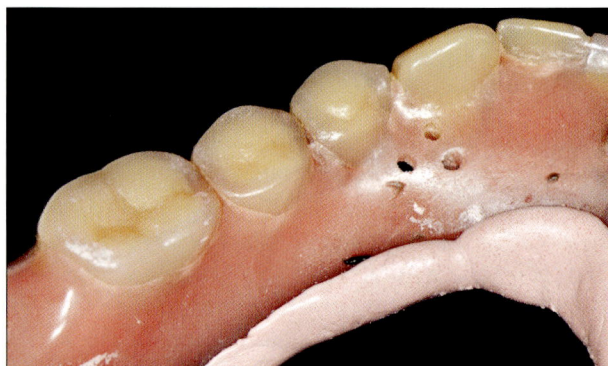

Fig 7f

Figs 7a-f   After border molding while the patient is performing functional movements, a static impression without pressure is taken of the edentulous parts.

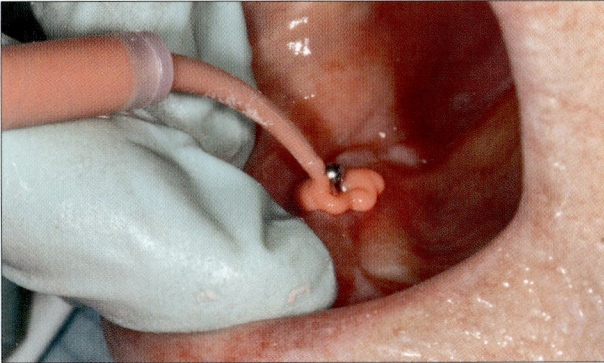

Fig 7g

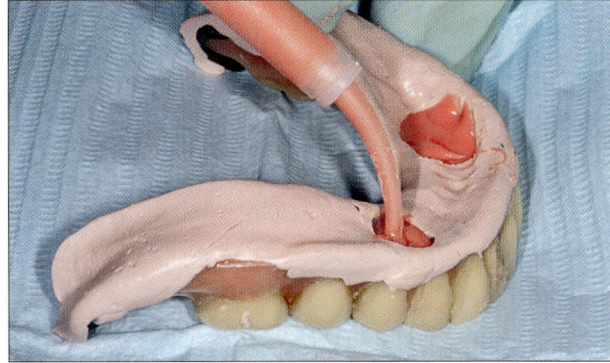

Fig 7h

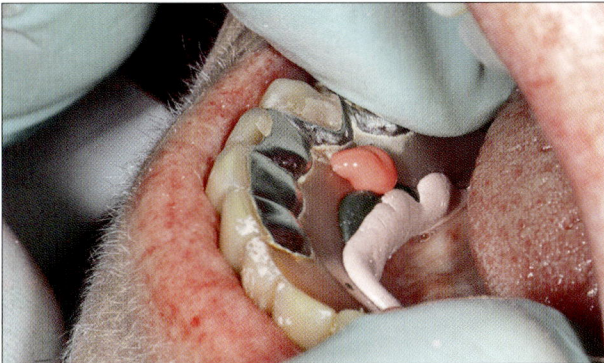

Fig 7i

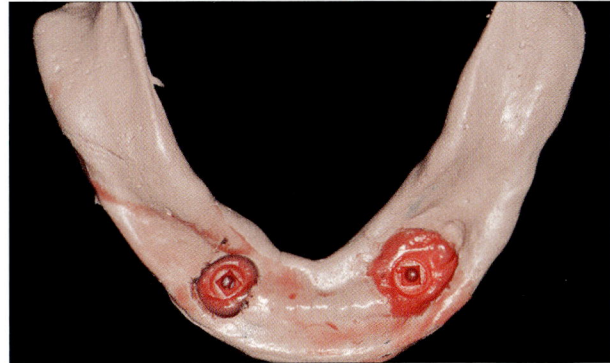

Fig 7j

Figs 7g-j   The implants are added to the impression by means of polyether material as moderate pressure, imitating the denture setting, is applied to the impression tray.

The question arises as to why such compression cannot be achieved in a one-step impression technique. The answer is that applying moderate pressure to a single-step silicone/polyether impression would result in multiple zones where the impression tray shows through. These pressure peaks will compromise denture comfort once the prosthesis is polymerized and inserted. With the two-step impression technique, the pressure will be more evenly distributed without causing discomfort. The same technique can be used for a reline (Figs 7a-j).

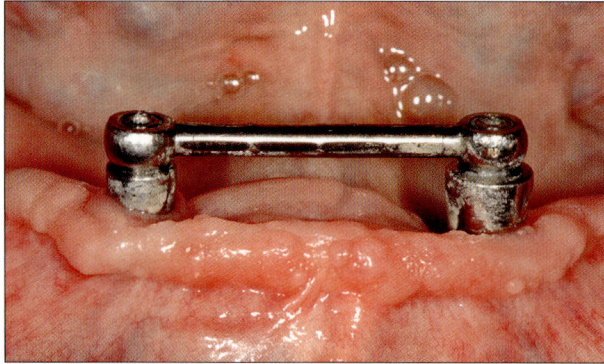

Fig 8   A two-implant bar provides very good retention for the overdenture, but may be difficult to clean for an elderly patient (courtesy of Martin Schimmel, Bern, Switzerland).

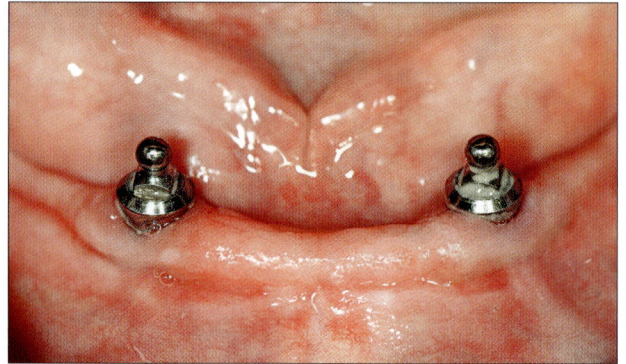

Fig 9   A two-implant overdenture with unsplinted attachments can be considered the "standard" type of mandibular overdenture for very old and fragile patients

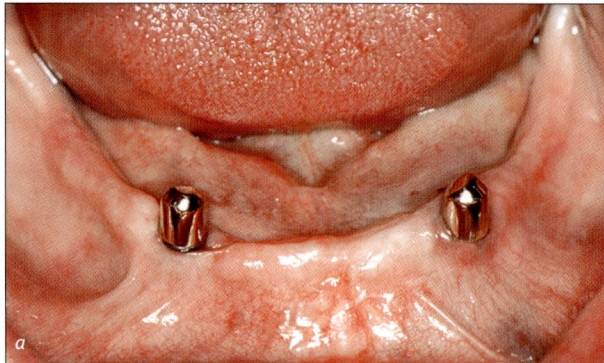

Figs 10a-b   Telescopic crowns are a suitable geriatric attachment system that provides retention via friction on parallel surfaces. The system provides maximum flexibility and requires very little maintenance (courtesy of Siegfried Heckmann, Erlangen, Germany).

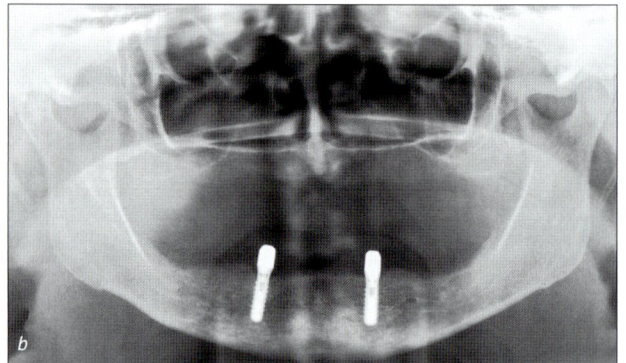

Attachment systems

An endless range of attachment systems is available in the market, and it would exceed the scope of this chapter to describe them all. The following section will therefore focus on commonly used attachment systems, even if the more recent ones are not well documented in the literature. The basic requirements of an attachment system for a geriatric overdenture are:

Attachment design and mechanical features

• Low volume to avoid bulky superstructures.
• Wear resistance to avoid maintenance and replacement.
• Possibility to compensate for axial divergences between implants.
• Smooth shape, to avoid injury when the denture is not worn (e.g., during the night).

Clinical requirements

• Adjustable retentive force (increase or decrease).
• Possibility of chairside repair and placement of the female part.

• Ease of handling and cleaning, even by a geriatric patient with reduced vision and dexterity.
• Low maintenance.
• Easy attachment removal, for a "back-off" strategy in the event of a functional decline.

Again, the literature does not conclusively recommend one ideal attachment system for the implant-supported overdenture. However, a recent review on attachment systems summarized the advantages and inconveniences of some commonly used systems (Andreiotelli and coworkers 2010). Whereas bar attachments require substantial vertical space and have high initial manufacturing costs, they provide good retention and require little maintenance (Fig 8). In contrast, ball attachments have a lower volume but require more adjustments due to increased wear (Fig 9). Only very few studies have been published on telescopic crowns and milled bars for implant-supported overdentures. Despite their high cost, they seem to satisfy the patient and require very little maintenance (Heckmann and coworkers 2004; Visser and coworkers 2009) (Figs 10a-b). Magnets, however, seem to provide the lowest retentive force (Andreiotelli and coworkers 2010; Fig 11).

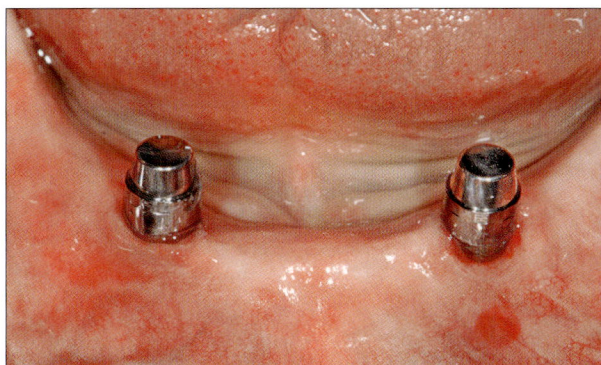

Fig 11 Magnets are attachments with low denture retention and particularly suited for patients with a weak hand force or requiring palliative care (courtesy of Martin Schimmel, Bern, Switzerland).

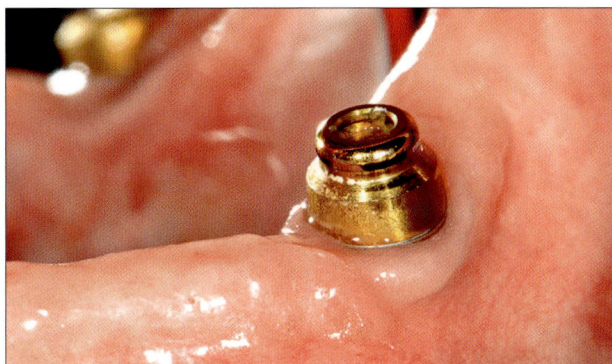

Fig 12a Locator attachments are widely used for a large range of indications.

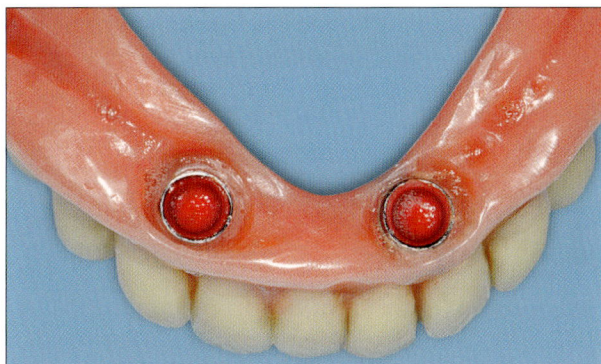

Fig 12b Locator attachments provide three degrees of retention from inserts with or without a central pin, respectively.

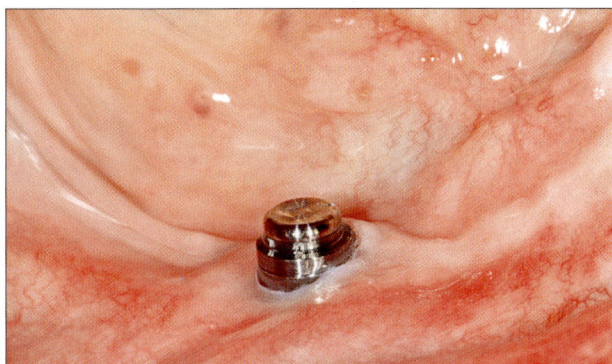

Fig 13a The CM LOC has the same volume and shape as the Locator, but no central hole that could trap food debris.

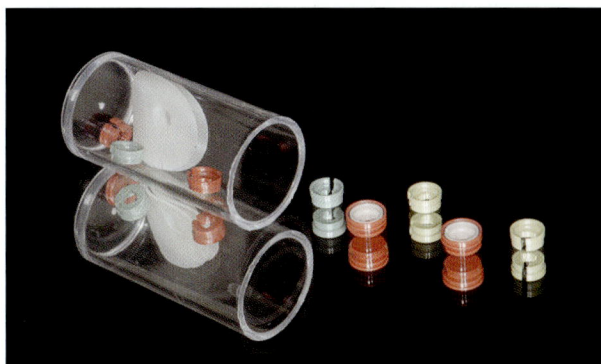

Fig 13b Female parts of the CM LOC.

Little long-term evidence exists on the use of Locator attachments (Zest Anchors, Escondido, CA, USA). In-vitro experiments indicate a high variability of the retentive force and an earlier loss of retention than with ball attachments or bars (Kobayashi and coworkers 2014; Figs 12a-b). The range of available attachment systems was recently complemented by the CM LOC (Cendres+Métaux, Biel, Switzerland), a titanium attachment with dimensions and shape similar to the Locator, but without the central hole (Fig 13a). In a newer version, the CM LOC Flex, the axis of the attachment can be aligned on a dome and subsequently fixed with resin cement. The female part consists either of a PAEK (polyaryl-etherketone) polymer (Pekkton; Cendres+Métaux) insert, which comes in four different retention strengths, from extra-low to strong, or a gold alloy (Fig 13b). The female part of the latter allows adjustment of the retentive force in two steps by turning the insert in its housing with a special instrument.

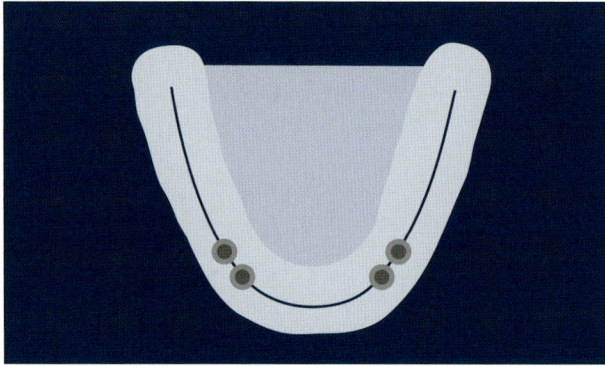

Fig 14a   For a four-implant overdenture, unsplinted attachment systems include the Locator, CM LOCs, or telescopic crowns, whereas ball attachments are little suited for this indication.

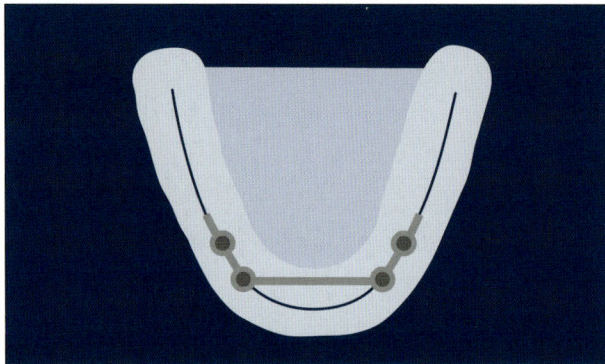

Fig 14b   Four-implant overdentures can also be used with prefabricated or milled straight bars with or without extensions.

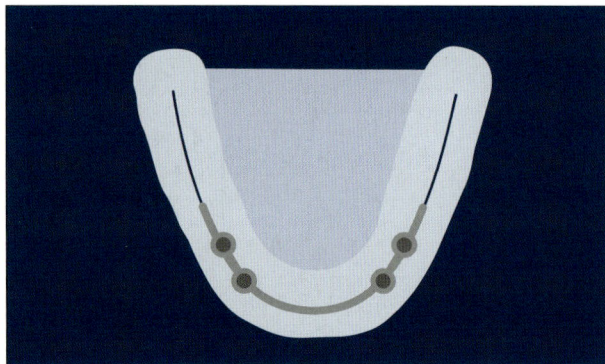

Fig 14c   Four-implant overdentures also allow for the use of individually milled bars that follow the contours of the alveolar mucosa.

With a larger area of support, a four-implant overdenture does not have a rotational axis and therefore allows a larger choice of splinted or unsplinted attachment systems (Figs 14a-c).

Telescopic crowns, Locator attachments, or CM LOCs are only some of the numerous possibilities amongst the unsplinted attachment systems. Ball attachments are less suitable for four-implant overdentures. Bars come with many different cross-sections, mostly round or ovoid, or parallel-shaped, the latter providing friction via intimate contact of the parallel surfaces of the bar and the corresponding female part. Milled bars may also follow the alveolar mucosa to maximize the parallel surface area without increasing the height.

As with the two-implant overdenture, there are splinted and unsplinted attachment systems (Figs 15a-c).

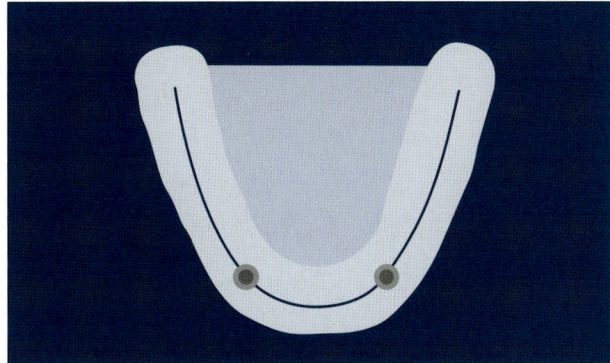

Fig 15a   For a two-implant overdenture, unsplinted attachment systems can be used.

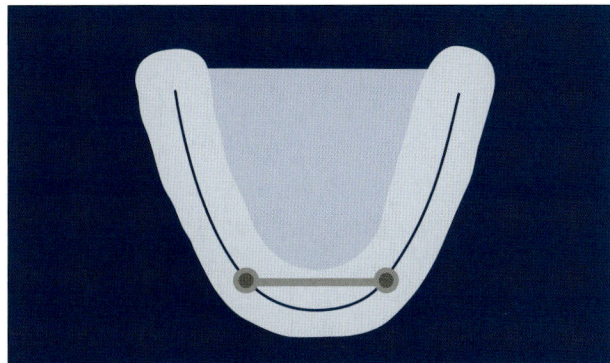

Fig 15b   For a two-implant overdenture, splinted attachments can be also used. Prefabricated Dolder bars in various shapes are available and can be used without cantilever extensions.

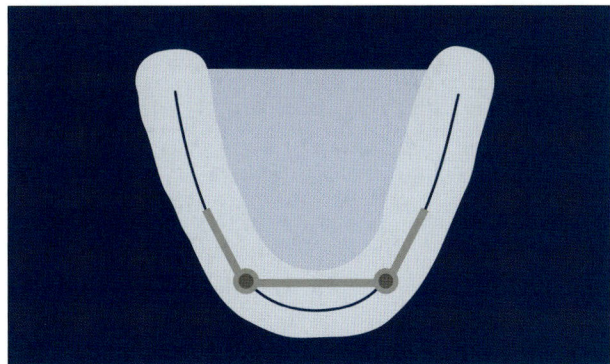

Fig 15c   Prefabricated Dolder bars with cantilever extensions can be used as well. This concept features a larger supporting area and, consequently, no rotational axis.

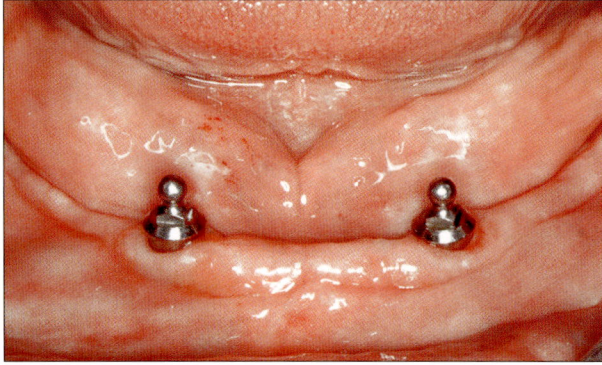

Fig 16   Ball attachments are robust, reliable, and inexpensive attachments for a two-implant overdenture and fairly forgiving if not cleaned perfectly; patients appreciate the distinct "click" when the denture is placed.

For geriatric patients, ball attachments have to be considered the basic attachment of implant dentistry. They are robust, reliable, and inexpensive (Fig 16).

They require little space, come with a huge choice of female parts, and have a very favorable cost-benefit ratio. Worldwide, they are the most commonly used attachment system for overdentures. Ball attachments provide a distinct "click" sound when the denture is seated, which is often perceived as reassuring. Patients used to a clicking retention mechanism will be profoundly disturbed if the click is missing, even if the denture is still retentive. Although ball attachments require regular maintenance, any repairs during these visits can be performed chairside and are generally associated with low cost. Service kits are available to deal with a loss of retention (Figs 17a-b).

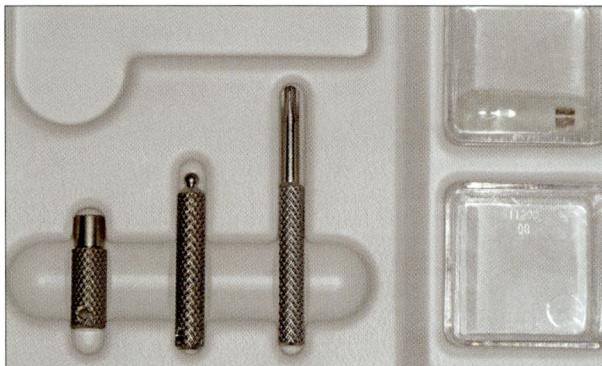

Fig 17a   A repair set (Cendres+Métaux, Biel, Switzerland) exists to facilitate the management of retention loss overdentures with ball attachments. An original ball attachment is used to check whether the attachment or the female part is worn.

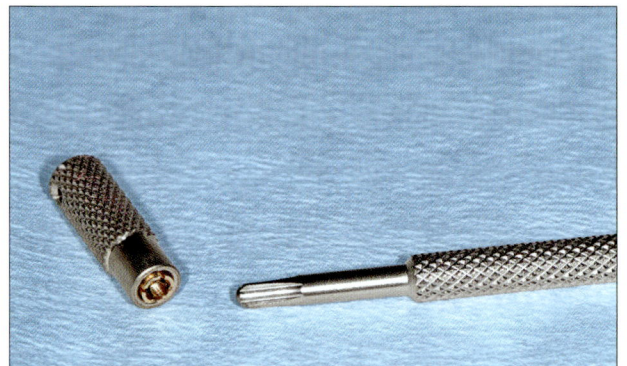

Fig 17b   The lamella insert of the Dalbo Plus attachment can be activated or replaced with a screwdriver.

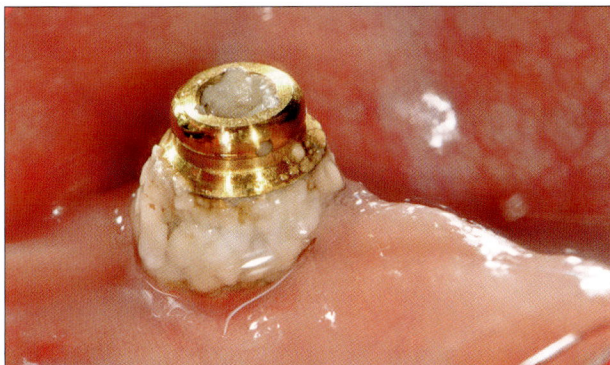

Fig 18a   The central hole of a Locator is difficult to clean and may trap food debris.

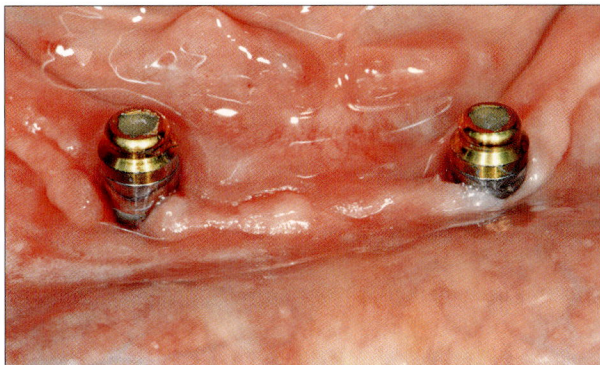

Fig 18b   A temporary filling avoids food trapping, but limits the choice of inserts to those without the central pin.

First, such kits contain a gauge with an original ball attachment, which can be used to establish whether it is the female part in the removable denture or the ball attachment itself that is worn. Secondly, there is a special screwdriver in the set, to turn the insert of the Dalbo Plus female part clockwise (Cendres+Métaux, Biel, Switzerland) in order to regain retention. Each one-eighth of a turn represents 125 g of added retention. If this is not sufficient to regain satisfactory retention, the lamella insert of the Dalbo Plus can be exchanged for a "soft-tuning" or "tuning" insert, which can be activated several times with the screwdriver.

Although adjustments and repairs for two-implant-overdentures with unsplinted attachments are frequent, these must not necessarily be seen as negative. The little turn of the female part to reactivate the retention takes only a minute or two, and the visit can be used to screen for oral carcinomas or other lesions, which are still frequent in old age (Ryan Camilon and coworkers 2014). At the same time, we can get an impression of patients' well-being and cognitive performance, and refer them for further examination if necessary.

For fourth-age geriatric patients, most attachment systems other than the ball attachment and the magnet will be too retentive and too difficult to clean. Especially the lingual side of a bar is often covered with substantial biofilm and calculus. As for the Locator attachments, the central hole may present issues, as it may fill with food debris and interfere with denture insertion. The prophylactic placement of a temporary composite filling can prevent this, but this limits the choice of inserts to those without the central pin (Figs 18a-b).

Short and reduced-diameter implants

Progress in implant surfaces, materials, and shapes has introduced a trend towards short and narrow implants. This minimally invasive treatment approach is very suitable for geriatric dentistry, because the surgical intervention presents one of the major barriers for accepting implant therapy in elderly adults, so simplification of the surgery may put the benefits of this therapy within reach of more patients. Furthermore, these novel implants extend the indication spectrum; even patients with anatomically challenging situations may benefit from the option of an implant treatment.

Short and narrow implants may also help avoid accessory interventions such as bone grafting; the operation will be shorter and less traumatic. Titanium-zirconium alloys (Roxolid; Straumann, Basel, Switzerland) alloys are an example of newly developed materials with enhanced mechanical properties. In a recent center study with eight European centers, the safety of 3.3-mm Roxolid implants and Locator attachments was confirmed for the edentulous mandible (Müller and coworkers 2015). Other small-diameter implants suitable for the edentulous mandible in geriatric patients are mini-implants, manufactured as one-piece or two-piece implants. Two-piece implants with a diameter of 2.5 mm have been documented in a prospective study on mandibular two-implant overdentures to provide a satisfactory survival rate of 95.5% after 6 years (Morneburg and Pröschel 2008). One-piece mini-implants are less well documented, and long-term survival data from prospective studies are still missing (Bidra and Almas 2013).

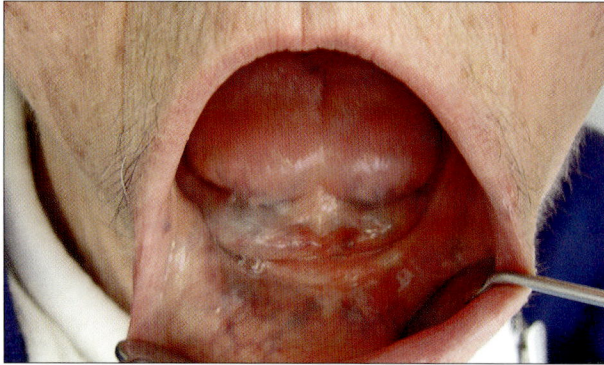

Fig 19a   Where alveolar ridge atrophy causes a vertical pressure of the denture base on the mental nerve, support from an implant may alleviate "electric" pain from the bolus.

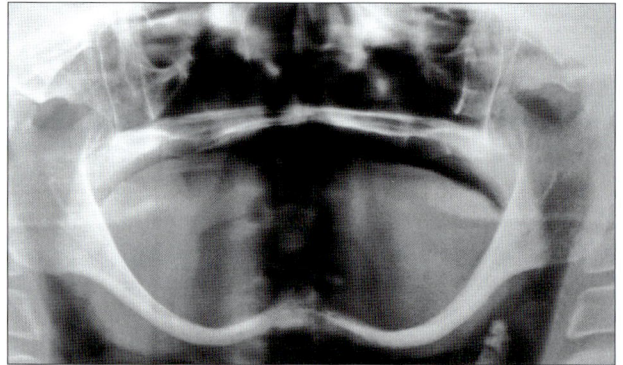

Fig 19b   Panoramic radiograph of the patient showing the atrophic ridge.

One-piece mini-implants do not provide prosthetic support, as the female part is not seated on the ball attachment of the implant. They solely provide retention, by means of a rubber O-ring placed in the female part. Their function is profoundly different from all other implant systems. Third-age patients appreciate such mini-implants, as they are designed for flapless placement and are relatively inexpensive. In fourth-age patients with largely atrophied ridges, these mini-implants may often be too long. With functional decline and reduced dexterity, the handling of the denture may also become difficult, as the heads of the implants are very small and the denture has to be placed with great precision. Removing a one-piece mini-implant when it is no longer useful can best be performed by simply cutting off the fragile head of the implant with a diamond bur. However, this approach may be difficult in a domiciliary setting.

In addition to reduced-diameter implants, short implants may be particularly suitable for elderly patients with severely atrophied mandibular ridges (Figs 19a-b).

These clinical situations present a problem in terms of denture retention and exposure of the mental foramen on top of the alveolar ridge. Loading a denture that exerts pressure on the mental nerve may cause significant pain and severe discomfort to the patient. Here, interforaminal implants may provide support for the denture base along with relief for the mental nerve. In these patients, implants are placed in the mandibular basal bone rather than in the (lost) alveolar ridge. The width of these implants is therefore not a limiting factor, and standard-diameter implants or even wide-platform implants may be used.

9 Surgical Considerations in the Aging Patient

S. Barter

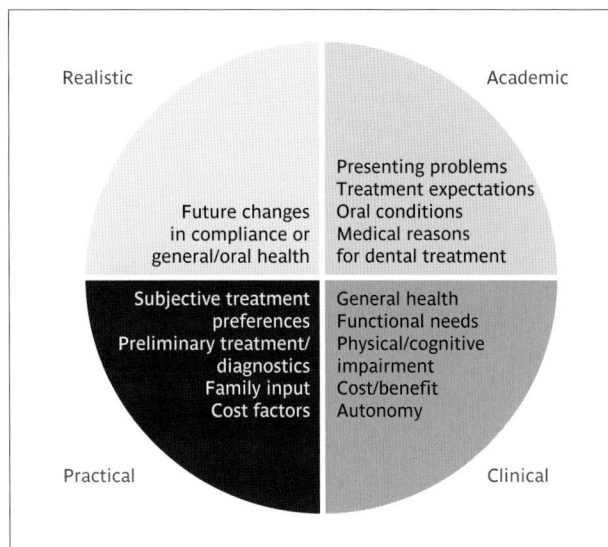

Fig 1 Treatment planning in the elderly patient (adapted from Bergendal and coworkers 2008).

The previous chapters of this Treatment Guide have shown that implant therapy can be successful in elderly patients and that it can provide measurable improvements in terms of their subjective and objective quality of life. Such improvements include functional benefits, perhaps most importantly the maintenance of adequate nutrition through better chewing comfort and efficiency, as well as the positive impact on esthetics and self-esteem. However, many factors must be considered when treating or managing elderly patients who are to be provided with or who already have implants. All treatment modalities have advantages and disadvantages; the surgical aspects of treatment require special consideration. It has been suggested that treatment planning for the geriatric patient can be seen as a sequence of four steps (Bergendal and coworkers 2008; Fig 1):

- The "academic" (ideal) treatment plan.
- The "clinical" treatment plan, relating to the general health, cognitive ability, and autonomy of patients in handling and caring for their dental restorations.
- The "practical" treatment plan, governed by subjective treatment expectations and the willingness to undergo specific procedures, as well as by financial and family constraints.
- The "modified" but realistic treatment plan that allows for adaptation due to changes in compliance or general/oral health that may occur as the patient ages.

The ideal—strategic—implant positions may be in regions that are affected by bone resorption. This implies a careful consideration of the required positions of the prosthetic tooth or teeth, the required implant positions, and the availability of bone in that region for implant placement—a process known as restoration-driven treatment planning. While this may lead to the conclusion that the ideal plan is not practical, perhaps due to the need for adjunctive surgery such as bone grafting, the same approach must be used for the modified implant treatment plan. It is no longer acceptable to merely place implants in the available bone volume and decide later how best to use them. The resulting prosthesis will often be inadequate in terms of function, phonetics, access for maintenance, and appearance. In the elderly patient with reduced capacity for adaptation and less ability to perform the necessary (perhaps complex) oral hygiene procedures, it may cause further difficulty, handicap, or disease.

The intended restorative outcome must allow for the individual patients' resilience and manual dexterity, their degree of autonomy, and their need for caregiver assistance. However, technical and biological complications are an almost inevitable consequence of all dental restorations; it is just a matter of time-to-failure. In the old person, the management of such complications needs to be anticipated and made a "designed-in" feature of the restoration. This will be discussed further in Chapter 12.

As surgeons, our first duty is to "do no harm"; surgery in itself is harmful, and the success of surgery has to be measured in terms of avoiding iatrogenic damage, adequate healing without avoidable disability, and achieving the planned outcomes.

The aim of this chapter is therefore to consider some surgical issues of particular importance in elderly patients. It is of course impossible to cover every eventuality; successful surgery is dependent on multiple site- and patient-specific factors, and a thorough and complete preoperative assessment and planning of all related factors is required in each individual.

Age-related changes in bone morphology and structure

With improving overall oral health, it can no longer be assumed that elderly patients will be edentulous; many adults retain a significant number of teeth throughout their lives, and implant therapy may be required for tooth replacement limited to single or multiple individual teeth, or small bridges. Neither can it be assumed that the elective edentulization of an aging individual to replace teeth with implants, as a "better or safer" option, is a valid treatment. Implants are not a tooth replacement; they are merely an option for the replacement of missing teeth (Donos and coworkers 2012). The maintenance of natural teeth should always be the primary choice where possible, in order to preserve proprioceptive feedback and simpler, less costly treatment.

However, many elderly patients will present with complete edentulism, with a previously heavily restored and failing dentition, or simply with individual failing teeth. When the remaining natural teeth are beyond further conventional restorative treatment, the replacement of teeth with fixed or removable implant supported prostheses, rather than conventional partial or complete dentures, may avoid the need for an old person to adapt to a radically different situation. As described in Chapter 5, the capacity of the elderly to adapt to such changes is reduced.

Histological changes

In the classical concept by Lekholm and Zarb (1985), there are four subtypes of bone quality (Fig 2).

Several other classifications of bone quality have since been suggested, but there is no universally accepted standard method.

However, bone quality depends on more than the relative density of bone in terms of the cortical and cancellous compartments. Bone quality in orthopedic medicine is a combination of factors that make bone fracture-resistant, such as the quality of the collagen content, mineral crystal size, the degree of vascularity and cellular vitality, accumulated microscopic damage, and the rate of turnover. All these can vary in elderly patients, especially given the prevalence of polymorbidity and polypharmacy prevalent in this age group, as discussed in earlier chapters.

These factors also have a potential impact on successful implant osseointegration; dense bone is not always stronger, and low bone density is not always related to osteoporosis. However, it has been shown that at any level of bone density (T score), aged bone is weaker and more liable to fracture than young bone (Hui and coworkers 1988). "Poor bone quality" has been associated

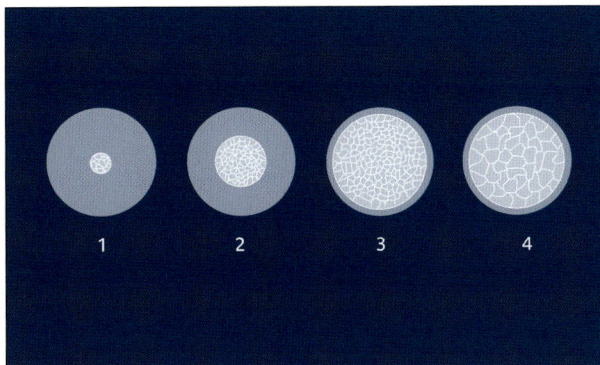

Fig 2 Grading system for bone-quality assessment (Lekholm and Zarb 1985).

with a higher implant failure rate (Goiato and coworkers 2014; Alsaadi and coworkers 2007). However, the presence of osteoporosis does not appear to be related to higher rates of implant failure (Bornstein and coworkers 2009; Slagter and coworkers 2008). Higher rates of implant failure have in fact been reported in dense mandibular bone, where perhaps the reduced trabeculation results in lower vascularity and decreased oxygen tension in the bone, with a consequent effect on bone healing and osseointegration. Bone with reduced oxygen tension and decreased numbers of vital osteocytes has been associated with a higher risk of osseointegration failure (Van Steenberghe and coworkers 2003). However, there are publications that show little difference in the survival of implants placed in "poor-quality" or "good-quality" bone, particularly when using implants with a microroughened surface (Stanford 2010).

Overheating of the bone due to poor surgical technique, inadequate irrigation, or the use of blunted rotary instruments can all contribute to bony necrosis at the osteotomy site. The concept of compression necrosis of bone has been described in the orthopedic field, with excessive insertion torques beyond the physiologic capacity of the bone causing plastic deformation, micro-fractures, and vascular ischemia (Winwood and coworkers 2006). It has been suggested that similar mechanisms may occur with implant placement, with concomitant resorption and loosening of the implant (Bashutski and coworkers 2009; Haider and coworkers 1991).

The highly atrophic mandible will often be primarily composed of cortical bone with little cancellous space, and the risk of thermal injury or excessive insertion torque is consequently greater, as is the risk of mandibular fracture (Chrcanovic and Custódio 2009), which is further discussed below. For a comprehensive overview of age-related changes in the histology and physiology of the bone, see Boskey and Coleman (2010). The impact of histological age-related changes in bone on the success of osseointegration of implants in the elderly is unclear. One could theorize that histological and anatomical changes, such as age-related deterioration of the inferior alveolar artery in the edentulous mandible, present a risk of poor bony healing (Bradley 1975; Bradley 1981). However, multiple studies have not shown any tendency to increased failure rates of implants with age (de Baat 2000; Op Heij 2003).

The many factors involved in the treatment of any one individual site or patient make meaningful assessment difficult. They include systemic and local site factors, but surgical technique and operator experience are often the most significant. Carefully performed surgery in a patient with appropriate disease control should result in a successful outcome, but as ever, surgery does not come with any guarantees, and patients or their representatives have to be appraised of this when considering implant treatment.

Morphological changes and surgical considerations

Bone resorption following tooth loss has long been a challenge for surgeons and prosthodontists in terms of obtaining satisfactory denture stability. It has a critical influence on the placement of implants in appropriate positions. Bone loss in the alveolar process following tooth loss is part of normal wound healing (Araújo and Lindhe 2005; Cardaropoli and coworkers 2003). The rate and degree of bone loss differs between patients and between sites within the same patient. This is further complicated by ongoing bone remodeling and resorption in the denture-bearing areas (Tallgren 1972). The long-term edentulous site or jaw may present with severely resorbed bone at the desired site of implant placement, particularly in long-term complete-denture wearers or in patients who lost some teeth at an earlier age but managed well with fewer functioning teeth or fixed or removable partial dentures.

The loss of one or more supporting teeth for the prosthesis may preclude successful rehabilitation without implants. However, anatomical changes in the edentu-

lous ridge bring special considerations in terms of implant placement. Following tooth loss, the alveolar ridge resorbs in an apicolingual direction (Lekholm and Zarb 1985; Cawood and Howell 1988). Important anatomical structures become more superficial, and the relative distance between the original (and therefore necessary) tooth positions changes.

Another claimed benefit of implant placement is the prevention of ongoing bone resorption. It has been suggested that implants may play a role in preventing progressive bone loss by stimulating the bone under load in a more favorable way than with complete dentures, preventing disuse atrophy. However, many studies also show implants as a potential cause of bone loss, due to crestal bone stress or peri-implant disease. Like any therapy, implants have a potentially favorable and a possibly harmful effect.

The immediate placement of implants into extraction sockets to prevent alveolar-bone remodeling has been suggested (Werbitt and Goldberg 1992). However, other authors consider this theory to be unsupported by conclusive evidence, and opinions remain divided (O'Neill and Yeung 2011; Schropp and Isidor 2008).

Mandible. In the mandible, the reduction in bone height results in muscular attachments becoming more superficial. The genial tubercles and mylohyoid ridge are less deeply positioned in the floor of the mouth. This results in a shallower lingual vestibulum and in muscle activity being more likely to cause denture displacement. The bony prominences may also cause painful pressure points below a denture.

Loss of bone height also results in the inferior alveolar nerve (IAN) becoming relatively more superficial. This will reduce the height of available bone for the placement of implants with an adequate safety margin without risk of damage to the IAN. Such damage can present a significant disability in any individual, not just "numbness or tingling."

There can be variations in the anatomy of the mandibular canal, including a posterior intraosseous division giving rise to a bifid canal, multiple branches (Carter and Keen 1971), or the presence of multiple mental foramina (Naitoh and coworkers 2009). The need for accurate and appropriate imaging in the resorbed mandible combined with a careful clinical examination cannot be overstated; the handicap produced by irreversibly altered sensation and neuropathic pain can be considerable, with reduced quality of life and psychological impact (Lam and coworkers 2003).

With progressive mandibular resorption, the mental foramina may eventually become situated on the crest of the ridge. In severe resorption, the main trunk of the IAN can become dehiscent and lie in a groove in the crest of the ridge for some distance. In either case, compression of the nerve by a denture base may cause pain. The advantage in terms of improved comfort of an implant-supported prosthesis can be dramatic for the patient. However, considerable care will be required in the placement of incisions and reflection of flaps to avoid nerve damage.

Peripheral nerve damage can be classified into neurapraxia, axonotmesis, or neurotmesis (Seddon 1942). Neurapraxia is the least severe form of injury and produces, according to Seddon, transient paresthesia or anesthesia with no conduction across the region of injury, but intact conduction in the proximal and distal segments. Recovery usually occurs within hours, days, or weeks, depending on severity.

Axonotmesis is a loss of axonal and myelin sheath continuity but with preservation of the connective-tissue framework (the epi- and perineurium). It results in conduction deficits distal to the site of injury, due to further degeneration of distal neural tissue, known as Wallerian degeneration. Axonal regeneration may occur, producing a degree of recovery.

Neurotmesis is a transection or disruption of the entire nerve fiber and may be partial or complete. Wallerian degeneration occurs and the sensory deficit is severe, with no spontaneous repair.

Nerve damage may produce a sensation of tingling (paresthesia), numbness (anesthesia), or reduced function (hypoesthesia), altered sensation (dysesthesia), the sensation of pain from a stimulus that would not normally result in pain (allodynia), or an abnormal increase in sensitivity (hyperesthesia).

Nerve damage can occur even without penetration of the canal; neurapraxia may arise from compression of the roof of the mandibular canal by the tip of an implant. It can also arise from the administration of an inferior alveolar block anesthetic.

The classical signs of nerve injury described by Seddon may be modified by the fact that the inferior alveolar nerve is contained within a bony canal. Edema within the confines of the canal may result in additional nerve compression and compromised vascular supply to the neural tissue. Bleeding into canal may have the same effect; in addition, hemoglobin is neurotoxic (Regan and Rogers 2003). Pain not responding to simple painkillers such as ibuprofen or acetaminophen may be neuropathic in origin and require special management (Renton and Yilmaz 2012).

The submandibular and submental spaces also become more superficial with progressive mandibular atrophy. In a radiological study, lingual concavities with a depth of 6 mm were reported in 2.4% of assessed cases (Quirynen and coworkers 2003). There is a greater risk of perforation of the lingual cortical plate causing damage to the vessels in the floor of the mouth, with a risk of hemorrhage.

Cross-sectional imaging studies have demonstrated that the sublingual and submental arteries may not only pass close to the lingual cortical plate in the mandibular midline but that branches of these arteries may enter accessory foramina along the lingual cortex (Hofschneider and coworkers 1999). Numerous studies have reported the formation of sublingual hematomas related to implant surgery, possibly even several hours after treatment (Dubois and coworkers 2010; Isaacson 2004). In some cases, this bleeding may be severe and cause an acute airway obstruction (Niamtu 2001). Although very rare, this is potentially more likely with implant placement in the mandibular first premolar position, a common site of implant placement for overdentures (Givol and coworkers 2000; Kalpidis and Setayesh 2004).

It is of course important to consider the risk of mandibular fracture when implant surgery is performed in the atrophic mandible. Fractures may occur during or after implant placement (Goodacre and coworkers 1999) and may result in further complications after fracture repair. The incidence reported is variable, but is commonly quoted at around 0.2% (Rothman and coworkers 1995). Peri-implant bone loss associated with implants in an atrophic mandible appears to be an important risk factor for mandibular fracture; it has been suggested that implants be removed before 50% of the peri-implant bone are lost. However, the same authors also wisely highlight the risk of mandibular fracture during the removal of an implant, should this become necessary (Raghoebar and coworkers 2000).

Given that the removal of bone to place implants will inevitably weaken the structural integrity of the mandible, preserving an adequate bone volume and not violating the buccal and lingual cortical plates—and in particular the inferior border—is vital. Cross-sectional imaging of the atrophic mandible is recommended to assess the degree of hard-tissue reduction required to remove prominences and achieve a flat bed for implant placement. In addition, the greater the number or length of implants placed, the higher the risk of fracture. A stress fracture of the edentulous mandible should be considered as part of the differential diagno-

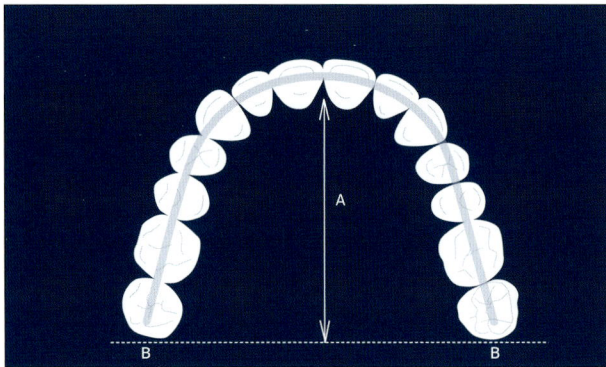

Fig 3a   The required arch form is determined by the "neutral zone" between the lips and tongue, providing the correct occlusion, phonetics, and extraoral soft-tissue support.
A = Anteroposterior arch length
B = Posterior extent of dental arch

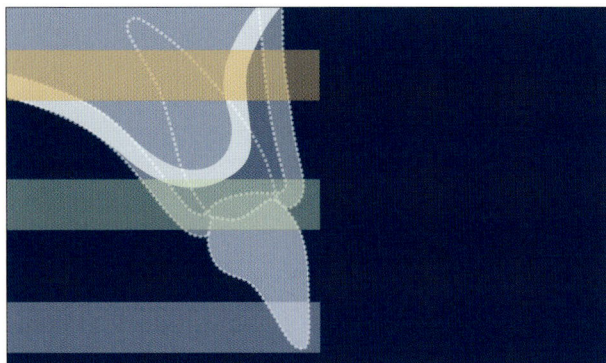

Fig 3b   The occlusal/incisal tip position (blue) has to remain constant; soft tissue (green) and alveolar crest (orange) resorb in an apicolingual direction, away from the required tooth position.

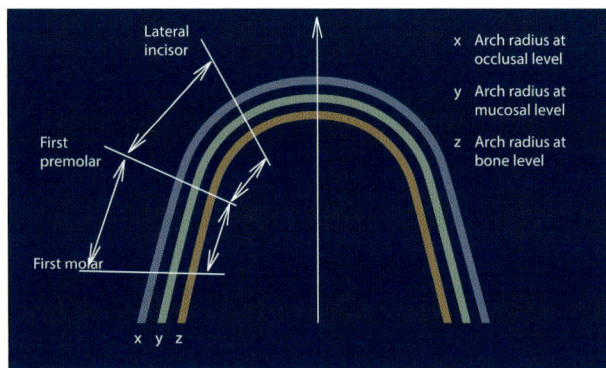

Fig 3c   Consider a reconstruction needing 6 implants in the first molar, first premolar and lateral incisor positions: tooth position and screw access holes are needed at position x, occlusal level. As the degree of ridge resorption increases, the radius of the available bony ridge decreases. This is more pronounced in the anterior maxilla.
x = Desired tooth position (normal arch radius)
y = Moderately resorbed ridge
z = Severely resorbed ridge

sis of persistent pain associated with implants (Rothman and coworkers 1995).

It has been suggested that proper informed consent for implant placement in the atrophic mandible should include warnings related to this infrequently reported but significant risk (Soehardi and coworkers 2010). Many authors have observed that there is an age-related degeneration in the vascular supply to the mandible from the inferior alveolar artery (IAA) (Bradley 1975) and that this may be linked to mandibular alveolar atrophy (Eiseman and coworkers 2005). However, there is a considerable collateral supply from vessels in the adjacent muscles (masseter, mentalis, and medial pterygoid) that penetrate the periosteum and from the vessels in the floor of the mouth (sublingual, submental, and mylohyoid arteries). The degeneration of the vascular supply from the IAA has been linked to localized alveolitis ("dry socket") (Chiapasco and coworkers 1993), poor socket infill, and poor outcomes of guided bone regeneration (Ersanli and coworkers 2004) as well as to a higher incidence of osteoradionecrosis of the posterior mandible (Bras and coworkers 1990). Careful flap design and management is necessary to preserve this blood supply in elderly patients where the central mandibular blood vessels may be less efficient.

Maxilla. The pattern of bone resorption in the maxilla generally also runs in an apicolingual direction, as described by the various classifications for the resorbed jaw (Lekholm and Zarb 1985). Reduction in maxillary height as a consequence of bone resorption also results in changes in the geometry of the arch and the relationship between implant and tooth position that can cause issues in the surgical planning of a full-arch reconstruction, whether with an overdenture or a fixed reconstruction. The radius of the dental arch at the occlusal level will need to remain relatively constant to ensure that the prosthesis is in the "neutral zone," providing adequate extraoral soft-tissue support while not impinging on the tongue space. However, the bony ridge will resorb in an apicolingual direction, and in doing so will become reduced in radius. This requires placing the implants at a more proclined angle; if the implants are on a narrower radius, they may be placed too close to one another. The difference in radius change is more pronounced in the anterior maxilla (Figs 3a-c).

The progressive resorption of the maxilla also results in the remaining bony crest approaching the air spaces of the maxillary antra and the nasal cavity. This will frequently preclude implant placement without augmentation.

Augmentation in the posterior maxilla can be achieved with subantral augmentation using the "sinus lift" procedure, which is safe and predictable in the hands of a skilled and experienced surgeon. However, the question is whether patients can tolerate the procedure and are willing to accept both the risks and the extra time required, as the graft must mature before implants can be placed. That some biomaterials may offer as reliable a grafting outcome as autogenous bone, previously considered the gold standard, removes the need for harvesting bone and avoids the associated morbidity (Kim and coworkers 2009; Handschel and coworkers 2009). The risk of hemorrhage in a sinus lift will need to be appropriately considered in aged patients, particularly those more at risk for medical reasons (as discussed in Chapter 5). The incidence of sinusitis following grafting is largely related to perforation of the Schneiderian membrane and escape of graft materials into the sinus, which causes inflammation and may cause a loss of patency of the ostium (van den Bergh and coworkers 2000; Doud Galli and coworkers 2001). Sinus lifts of course do not replace the lost alveolar bone; they provide a volume of bone to facilitate the placement of implants, but the positions of these implants will not necessarily be closely related to the positions of the missing teeth. Some authors have observed that implant placement in the correct position for a fixed reconstruction also requires lateral augmentation. Bone grafting will not always be practical here: reconstruction of the vertical component of bone loss will not be simple, and in elderly patients, the complexity of the surgery required will rarely be desirable or justifiable.

Other authors suggest that a "simplified" approach to sinus augmentation is offered by placing graft material into a subantral space created via the implant osteotomy: the osteotome technique, first described by Summers (1998) and further modified in many different ways. However, it is the opinion of this author that this technique is ineffective for several reasons and, given the associated risks, is largely obsolete for the following reasons:

- The evidence base surrounding the osteotome technique has a significant degree of heterogeneity; drawing meaningful conclusions is difficult (Tan and coworkers 2008).
- Many of the studies showing success rates comparable to the survival rates for short implant placement in the posterior maxilla employed the osteotome technique where the residual bone height would have allowed the use of short implants without grafting; further, sometimes no graft was placed due to a suspected perforation—and the implant outcome was the same. There is no impact on the health of the sinus when penetrated by a fixed object (Brånemark and coworkers 1984; Stamberger 1991); while there may be no advantage in terms of implant penetration beyond the floor of the antrum, there is no harm, either.
- It is known that displacement of graft particles into the sinus can result in acute or chronic sinusitis (Wiltfang and coworkers 2000); membrane perforations cannot be detected reliably using this procedure, and the rate of membrane perforations increases with reduced residual alveolar height (Ardekian and coworkers 2006).
- It is known that significant remodeling of the graft placed in this manner occurs and that the bone gain is limited to small amounts on the walls of the implant, with little bone at the apex (Brägger and coworkers 2004; Leblebicioglu and coworkers 2005).
- The primary determinant of implant success is the height of the remaining residual ridge (Toffler 2004).
- It is further known that such bone is unlikely to add significantly to biomechanical load transfer; this load is primarily borne in the posterior maxilla, by the cortical plates, and then dissipated to the palatal and zygomatic bones (Yacoub and coworkers 2002; Gross and coworkers 2001a; Gross and Nissan 2001b). Unless the packing of graft matter into the sinus is complete to the walls of the antral space, small amounts of additional bone are relatively useless (Tepper and coworkers 2002).

As there appears to be more variability in implant survival in the grafted sinus than in the unaugmented posterior maxilla (Graziani and coworkers 2004), the use of shorter implants, where possible, may be the preferred option to reduce surgical morbidity in elderly patients with sufficient residual alveolar height.

Given the lack of a clear advantage of the osteotome technique, the additional risks associated with the technique can be considered more significant than the potential limited advantage. The risk of implant displacement into the sinus becomes greater as the residual alveolar height diminishes (Chiapasco and coworkers 2009); displacement can still occur after many years in function (Iida and coworkers 2000; Ueda and Kaneda 1992).

There have been several reports of benign paroxysmal positional vertigo (BPPV) with the osteotome technique, attributed to the dislodgement of otoliths in the semicircular canals caused by the malleting employed in this procedure (Chiarella and coworkers 2008). This can be a significant disability in patients of any age, but in elderly patients with a decline in balance and proprioception, BPPV could result in a considerable change in their quality of life. The incidence may well be underreported, as the symptoms often do not manifest for days or weeks afterwards and may not be associated with the procedure (Vernamonte and coworkers 2011; Kim and coworkers 2010; Peñarrocha-Diago and coworkers 2008; Di Girolamo and coworkers 2005; Kaplan and coworkers 2003).

Attempting to simplify surgery and avoid sinus lifts by placing implants only in the anterior maxilla, where sufficient bone volume remains, may increase the risk of implant failure. A good anteroposterior spread of implants is needed (Lambert and coworkers 2009). Consequently, some clinicians advocate protocols utilizing a combination of longer, angled implants to avoid the need for sinus elevation. The stated rationale that this "simplifies" the procedure is questionable, as the protocol often requires a significant vertical reduction in height to provide the necessary space for prosthetic components. The extensive flap elevation and bone removal required do not appear less invasive than the sinus lift procedure. Furthermore, in the event of implant failure or complications, the bone removal required for the procedure may leave a situation that is impossible to restore even with a conventional complete denture, leaving the patient with significant disability and disfigurement.

The use of other sites in the maxilla for implant placement with special protocols, such as the zygomatic or pterygomaxillary region, requires complex surgery and difficult prosthetic procedures. There is again an increased risk of morbidity, and peri-implant mucosal inflammation is often a problem because of restricted access (Aparicio and coworkers 2006). Such procedures are unlikely to be suitable in the elderly patient.

Given that it is not possible, even with considerable augmentation, to reconstruct significantly resorbed sites to their full pre-disease contour, fixed implant rehabilitations may require the missing tissue to be made up for in the prosthesis itself. Full-arch fixed prostheses in resorbed jaws commonly require flanges or volumes of pink-colored material to provide the necessary extraoral tissue support or the desired esthetic appearance of the teeth, or to prevent air escape from affecting phonetics. This will increase the difficulty of effective plaque control and increase the risk of peri-implant disease and bone or implant loss.

Strategies for simplifying surgical procedures in elderly patients

Any complication may assume greater significance in the elderly patient as a result of its impact on patients' quality of life and on the practicality of the treatment required to treat those complications. The importance of planning for implant placement relative to the intended prosthesis is well documented. In addition, we must plan for maintenance, replacement of prostheses, adaptation of prostheses to future implant loss, or possible changes in the type or design of prosthesis as patients becomes less able to care for or manage the reconstruction. In short, we have to plan for the contingency of reverting a potentially problematic situation to one than can continue to benefit the patient—or at least not cause inconvenience or disability. From a surgical viewpoint, such strategic planning will include implants in key positions and a choice of surgical approach that is the least invasive but still offers a predictable outcome with the lowest risk. To a certain extent, this will also depend on operator experience.

The loss of the vertical component of alveolar ridge height may result in proximity of the IAN or maxillary air spaces at the desired implant location, as described above. Vertical ridge augmentation is challenging and shows considerable variation in clinical outcome, with limited data available (Rocchietta and coworkers 2008). Like all augmentation procedures, there is increased morbidity and a greater risk of complications. In situations of limited bone height in the maxilla or mandible, the use of shorter implants can be considered a reasonable treatment option.

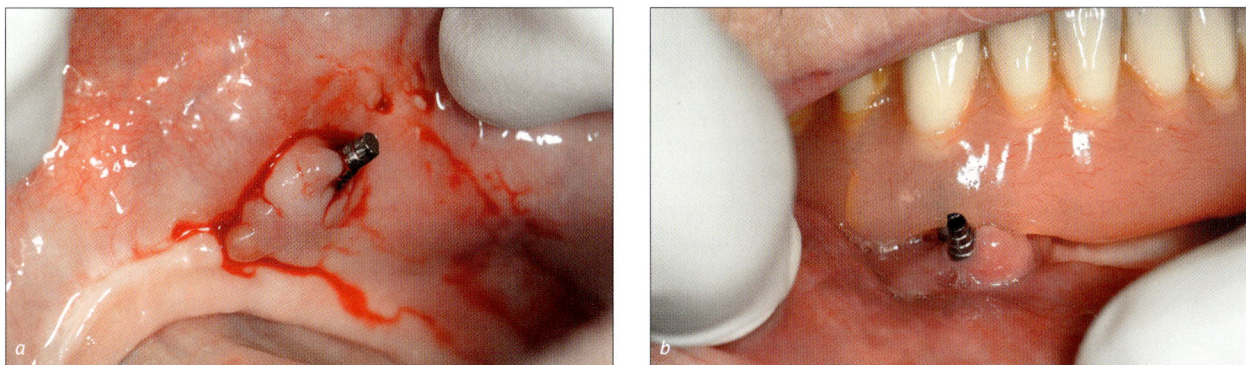

Fig 4a-b   One-piece mini-implant has fractured the buccal plate and is displaced into the vestibular tissue.

Short implants appear to perform just as well as longer implants in bone of similar density (Renouard and Nisand 2006). Even shorter implants (4 mm) have been used with some success, although the dense cortex of mandibular bone appears to be affected more by implant diameter and stress peaks than implant length (Slotte and coworkers 2012). It has been suggested that the reverse may be true in the maxilla (Baggi and coworkers 2008). As the most coronal 2 to 3 mm of the implant transfers most of the functional load to bone (Pierrisnard and coworkers 2003), and given the higher incidence of lower bone density and the lack of cortical plate in the posterior maxilla, this may present a case for considering appropriate sinus augmentation, depending on patient suitability in terms of risk-to-benefit and cost-to-benefit ratios. The same consideration may be applied to lateral ridge augmentation in situations of reduced alveolar width. While perhaps more predictable in outcome than vertical augmentation, there is still increased cost, morbidity, and risk.

The use of reduced-diameter implants may to some extent offer an alternative solution in narrow edentulous ridges. However, we have to consider the load-bearing capacity of the implant and of the narrow bony ridge. The risk of fracture increases as implant diameter reduces, even with one-piece implants with integrated abutments made of titanium alloys such as Ti-Al-V (Allum and coworkers 2008), and these materials have been demonstrated to be less biocompatible than commercially pure titanium in cell cultures and animal experiments (Han and coworkers 1998). The clinical significance in implants for human use remains a topic of critical discussion, but other more biocompatible alloys of titanium-zirconium

used in implants 3.3 mm in diameter have been successful for fixed and removable prostheses (Barter and coworkers 2012; Chiapasco and coworkers 2012; Al-Nawas and coworkers 2012), if only in relatively short-term studies. The use of implants less than 3 mm in diameter is not well documented, being largely related to their use in the edentulous arch and in single tooth non-loadbearing sites, with few data on success rates (Klein and coworkers 2014). It is also reported that stress values in crestal cortical bone increase as implant diameter decreases, increasing the risk of peri-implant crestal bone resorption (Baggi and coworkers 2008; Ding and coworkers 2009). In an already resorbed jaw, the effect could be significant. Age-related reduction in cortical bone thickness and elasticity occur in the jaws as in other bones and in particular seem to affect the mandible (Sarajlic and coworkers 2009). When the cortical plate is thin or there is peri-implant bone loss, it is possible for the implant to break through the buccal plate under load (Figs 4a-b)

Finally, solid implants with integrated abutments, typical of some mini-implant designs, may present problems as they are less adaptable to changes in patient compliance. A patient suffering from cognitive decline may be intolerant of a previously successful implant overdenture and refuse or be unable to wear it. Conventional two-piece implant designs may allow for the relatively simple removal of the abutment, which may otherwise cause trauma to the intraoral tissues, resulting in pain and a reduced ability or inclination to eat. This is not possible with a one-piece implant design, and removing or modifying the implant in such a patient may not be so simple. This will be discussed further in Chapter 11.

Flapless surgery has been advocated as simplifying the placement of implants. Avoiding periosteal stripping with flap elevation undoubtedly reduces postoperative morbidity, but "blind" implant placement carries a risk of inaccurate placement, inadequate bone thickness around the implant, perforation of the cortical plate, or violation of adjacent anatomical structures. Computer-guided surgical templates are not a new technique, and flapless placement with such templates has been shown to reduce postoperative morbidity.

However, the accuracy of placement has been questioned in systematic reviews of the published literature. Computer-guided surgery is a promising development that may facilitate less invasive surgery, reduce surgical risk, and improve access to implant treatment for medically compromised patients. However, as with all new techniques, it is important to understand the considerable technical details and inherent limitations (Tahmaseb and coworkers 2014).

General surgical considerations in the older patient
The reduced physiological reserves of the elderly patient and their declining capacity to tolerate stress have been discussed in Chapter 5 on medical considerations. The elderly patient may be less able to cope well with long and difficult procedures, and this will need to be taken into account when deciding on what treatment option is best suited to the patient. The skill and experience of the operator will largely determine how quickly a surgical procedure can be completed safely and accurately, and referral to a specialist surgeon may be advisable in many cases.

Treatment under local anesthetics is generally preferred in geriatric patients, where physiologic changes affect drug absorption, metabolism, and excretion. The only local anesthetic that has been extensively investigated in elderly patients is lidocaine (Oertel and coworkers 1999). However, amide local anesthetics such as lidocaine are primarily metabolized by the liver, and there is an age-related decrease in this capacity. Furthermore, patients with decreased hepatic blood flow (e.g. congestive heart failure) or reduced liver function may metabolize local anesthetics at a significantly slower rate, resulting in increased plasma drug levels and a greater risk of toxicity (Malamed 1997). The metabolites of lidocaine are also potentially toxic, with a potential impact on patients with impaired renal function.

However, articaine, while an amide local anesthetic, is primarily metabolized in the bloodstream and has a significantly shorter half-life than lidocaine. The metabolites are non-toxic. There were no significant differences in plasma concentrations and the half-life of articaine between young and old healthy individuals (Oertel 1999). It should be remembered that articaine is highly bound to serum proteins, and this binding capacity does change in the elderly patient, particular in the chronically ill who may have low serum albumin levels.

The time that the operation may take will need to be considered within the constraints of the amount of local anesthetic required—prolongation of the procedure as a result of reduced capacity of the patient, with "topping up" of local anesthetic, may give rise to insidious overdose in the elderly patient. As discussed in Chapter 5 on medical considerations, the incidence of complications with local anesthetic solutions is greater in debilitated elderly patients, particularly in polymorbid individuals where interactions may occur with prescribed medications. Further advice can be found in Chapter 5.

Patient age, as well as the duration and complexity of the surgical procedure, have been linked to the degree of postoperative morbidity experienced with third-molar surgery (Jerjes and coworkers 2010; Bello and coworkers 2011). It seems reasonable to expect that similar effects may be observed with more protracted and complex procedures related to implant surgery.

There are other considerations related to complex or lengthy procedures in elderly patients. Certain conditions such as arthritis or gastric reflux may result in an inability to remain comfortable in the chair for long appointments and can contribute to stress during the procedure—both for the patient and the operator—threatening the successful completion of the treatment. Other conditions such as diabetes, dementia, and osteoarthritis may affect the scheduling of the treatment during the day. Arthritic changes in the spine may make optimal positioning of the patient in the chair impossible, with a consequent impact on access, lighting, and visibility of the operative site. These may contribute both to the time taken to complete the procedure and to the stress on both patient and operator. Even the practicality of certain imaging techniques may be affected: it may not be possible to position a patient with kyphosis correctly for a CBCT or panoramic investigation. For example, a patient with Parkinson's disease may not be able to remain still during the exposure.

All of these factors will have to be considered in treatment planning and appointment scheduling; more and shorter procedures may be advisable. However, the overall appointment time at each visit may need to be proportionally longer so as not to rush the patient, which may cause them additional stress. More time may be needed for the patient to rest occasionally; sarcopenia and masticatory-muscle fatigue may affect the ability of patients to keep their mouths open for long periods without a tremor of the jaw. Anxiety regarding the nature of the treatment may also be a significant stressor. Oral and inhalational sedation can normally be safely tolerated in elderly individuals, and intravenous sedation may be considered—with adjustments for increased benzodiazepine sensitivity in older patients. However, some techniques may not be suitable for medically compromised elderly patients in an outpatient environment, and a general anesthetic in an inpatient setting may be more appropriate, despite the increased risks associated with age and some medical conditions.

Swift, calm, smooth, and comfortable delivery of the operative treatment by a skilled and experienced practitioner is of course essential. However, treatment is nothing without care; the pastoral care element and consideration for the different needs of each individual elderly patient are of equal importance. This continues into the postoperative phase, throughout treatment and into ongoing maintenance care.

Postoperative period and healing

The provision of postoperative instructions in a clear and understandable fashion is important in all patients. Hearing difficulty, anxiety, or memory or cognitive impairment may all result in a lack of proper understanding of important aspects of postoperative home care and could adversely affect the treatment outcome. Giving verbal postoperative instructions may not be adequate for any patient, especially at the time of surgery. Written postoperative instructions should be provided in large enough print; instructions provided a week or two before the procedure can also be very helpful. This allows the patient and any family member or caregiver the opportunity not only to ask relevant questions in good time, but also to make any necessary preparations, particularly with regard to maintaining adequate food and fluid intake.

The elderly patient may take longer to recover in the period immediately after completion of even relatively simple procedures; muscular stiffness, orthostatic hypotension, and fatigue can all increase the risk of falls, and so they should be permitted adequate time before leaving the dental chair to accommodate and be escorted/supported on discharge as required.

While there appears to be no general increase in the risk of infection in patients over 65 years of age, this age group in general has a higher incidence of conditions or prescription medications that that may predispose them to infections, or present a risk of adverse drug events (ADEs) with prescribed postoperative antibiotics. As discussed in Chapter 5, infections in the elderly patient may tend to begin earlier, develop more quickly, and be more difficult to resolve, so prompt action is required.

Adequate postoperative pain control is of course essential. Pain has many components in addition to the sensory mechanisms, including emotional and behavioral elements. The experience of pain is influenced by biological, psychological, and cultural factors. The basic principle of pain control is the preemptive administration of analgesics, which may help prevent the potentiation of noxious stimuli (Scully 2014).

Some of the many factors influencing analgesic use in the elderly patient have been discussed in Chapter 5. NSAIDs should be used with caution, especially in patients with gastric problems or renal disease and in those taking ACE inhibitors or beta-blockers for hypertension, or anticoagulants. Centrally acting painkillers such as opioids carry a higher risk of confusion, drowsiness, or falls in elderly patients. Older patients are more at risk of poor compliance with medication regimes, especially new additions to extensive drug regimes. Written instructions should always be given along with careful oral explanations, particularly in relation to the timing of medication and whether the drug should be taken as prescribed, or as required. Small drug labels or manufacturers' instruction sheets may be impossible to read for visually impaired patients and it is useful to have information sheets that can be printed at varying font sizes for commonly used medications.

Many authors have observed age-dependent differences in wound healing. The response to injury can be divided into four main phases: hemostasis, inflammation, proliferation, and tissue remodeling or resolution (Gosain and DiPietro 2004). As discussed, the inflammatory response decreases with age (Swift and coworkers 2001), and this will affect healing, as will the age-related reduction in cellular migration and proliferation. Changes in collagen structures with age will have an effect on remodeling. However, it appears that while healing may be delayed in older adults, the overall process and results are not otherwise affected (Guo and DiPietro 2010). Most of the studies on wound healing in elderly patients relate to skin healing. It is clear that there are histomorphological changes in the skin with aging; there are reductions in collagen and elastin volume and quality, vascularity, and the production of granulation tissue. Some of these changes are due to extrinsic factors such as solar UV light exposure (Thomas 2001), which will of course not apply to intraoral wounds, making this environment a potentially better predictor of the impact of age on wound healing. However, there are few studies relating to this, and where they exist, the effect of polymorbidity and polypharmacy factors in the elderly is frequently not assessed. Medical factors affecting tissue perfusion and oxygenation such as cardiovascular disease, COPD, and smoking are all implicated in impaired wound healing, as are conditions such as diabetes and medications such as corticosteroids. Wound closure in older individuals was clearly delayed even when eliminating potential age-related factors, indicating that aging does slow mucosal wound healing, and the typical finding of a greater impact in males was reversed, with a greater incidence of delay in females. It was hypothesized that wound healing might be modulated by different mechanisms, depending on tissue type (Engeland and coworkers 2006).

Bone healing is also slower in old age. It has been postulated that this is related to decreased levels of the cyclooxygenase 2 (COX 2) enzyme, which plays an essential role in bone repair (Naik and coworkers 2009).

While many studies indicate that increasing age has little effect on osseointegration in otherwise healthy individuals, no comparable studies exist relating to guided bone regeneration in the elderly patient. Animal studies have indicated a delayed bone-healing response in guided tissue regeneration models; given the previously discussed changes in bone healing with age, this would appear to be relevant to the older patient.

Fortunately, serious complications associated with dental implant placement are uncommon. However, the risk of complications may increase with the complexity of the procedure and with multiple patient related risk factors. Proper surgical training should be acquired before attempting such procedures. Complications will inevitably occur despite our best efforts to prevent adverse events. It is therefore important to assess the risks not only in terms of prevention, but also in terms of what treatment may arise should such a risk actually occur. Above all, accurate placement in carefully planned positions to achieve the equally carefully planned prosthetic outcome is mandatory; the practicality of retrieving an unfavorable outcome by means of revision surgery is difficult in all patients and may be impossible in an elderly individual.

10 Oral Hygiene in Geriatric Implant Patients

F. Müller

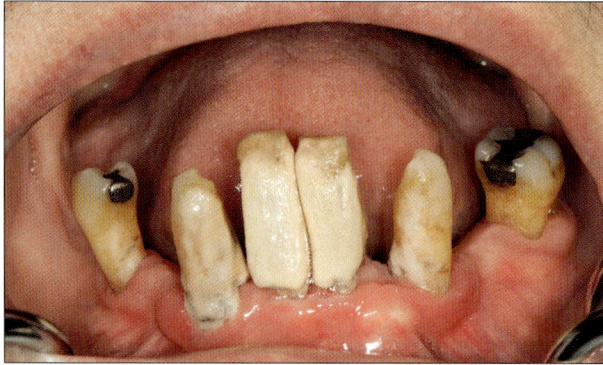

Fig 1   Oral hygiene is not always a priority in old age. Reduced vision, tactile sensitivity, and manual dexterity render oral hygiene difficult.

Maintaining effective oral hygiene becomes increasingly difficult as manual dexterity deteriorates. It seems generally acknowledged that oral hygiene in elderly patients is poor (Fig 1), especially if they live in care homes or other institutional environments (Peltola and coworkers 2004). In frail elderly patients with reduced masticatory efficiency and poor coordination of the masticatory and facial muscles, retention of food debris is common; the "self-cleaning" effect that occurs with effective chewing and bolus formation is reduced. Accordingly, tongue coating with accompanying halitosis is a common finding in elderly adults.

Oral and general hygiene may no longer be a priority, as along with a withdrawal from the work environment and social life, the need for a "proper" appearance may be felt as less important. Priorities also change with degrading general health; it seems logical that an elderly person is more preoccupied with the more vital needs arising from chronic diseases and disabilities.

Implant-supported reconstructions of any type may impede the removal of biofilm. Implant-supported prostheses or partially dentulous jaws with prosthetic restorations are distinctly different in morphology from the natural dentition, which affects the self-cleaning effect during mastication.

Poor oral hygiene was found in 23 out of 35 edentulous long-term care residents with—mostly fixed—implant-supported dental prostheses. However, only 18 subjects displayed moderate to severe soft-tissue inflammation (Isaksson and coworkers 2009). While the objectives of effective oral hygiene remain the same in geriatric patients, methods and techniques have to be adapted to the individual's functional decline and handicap.

Peri-implantitis in old age

In younger patients, peri-implantitis seems likely to be associated with inadequate oral hygiene. However, little is known about the reaction of the periodontal tissues to bacterial load in geriatric patients, and even less about the reaction of their peri-implant tissues. In a split-mouth study involving 15 volunteers, experimental gingivitis was compared to experimental peri-implantitis caused by a 3-week period of undisturbed plaque accumulation (Salvi and coworkers 2012). During the experimental period, the implant sites developed more inflammation than the natural teeth ($p < 0.04$), although the natural teeth presented a higher plaque index ($p < 0.02$). However, these patients could hardly be described as geriatric, having an average age of 58.7 ± 10.9 years. Another study reported that the levels of *P. gingivalis, T. forsythia, F. nucleatum,* and *T. denticola* in the saliva of 89 "geriatric" patients were related to the severity of the periodontal disease, but again, the average age of the cohort was below 70 years (Shet and coworkers 2013).

It has also been demonstrated that the absence of preventive maintenance in patients with pre-existing peri-implant mucositis is associated with a higher incidence of peri-implantitis after 5 years (Costa and coworkers 2012). Immunosenescence generally increases the susceptibility to infection and impaired wound healing and elderly individuals do not respond as robustly to immune challenges as the young do.

A Swedish cross-sectional study screened 3,041 patients aged 65 years or older who had at least one dental implant and who were identified by a Swedish municipality as being eligible for subsidized care. In the final cohort of 26 participants, the authors reported less inflammation around the dental implants than around the corresponding natural teeth. Clinical experience often shows abundant plaque accumulation on implant abutments; removing the plaque then reveals healthy peri-implant tissues (Figs 3a-b), a finding confirmed in this study, where 38% of the patients had high plaque scores but no correlation was found between plaque scores or bleeding index (Olerud and coworkers 2012).

A different study found significantly more soft-tissue inflammation as well as cheek and lip biting in edentulous patients over 80 years of age who were provided with fixed dental implant prostheses, compared to a younger control group with similar prostheses ($p < 0.05$), although the implant survival rates were similar in both groups. Here it has to be borne in mind that cleaning fixed dental prostheses is extremely difficult for geriatric patients (Engfors and coworkers 2004; Fig 2).

Pending more and stronger evidence, it is recommended that the prevention and treatment of peri-implantitis in geriatric patients are approached with the same protocols as in younger adults but with appropriate allowance being made for age and setting.

General setting for oral hygiene

Oral hygiene must remain part of the routine of daily personal hygiene. Sufficient time should be planned for cleaning the teeth, mucosa and, if present, removable prostheses. Elderly persons unable to stand for long periods may appreciate a chair in front of the sink. Reading glasses or even a magnifying loupe should be used to enhance visibility (Fig 4). Good lighting is also helpful. Removable dentures may sometimes be slippery when covered with saliva, so filling the sink with water or a towel may prevent fractures if the denture is accidentally dropped during cleaning (Fig 5).

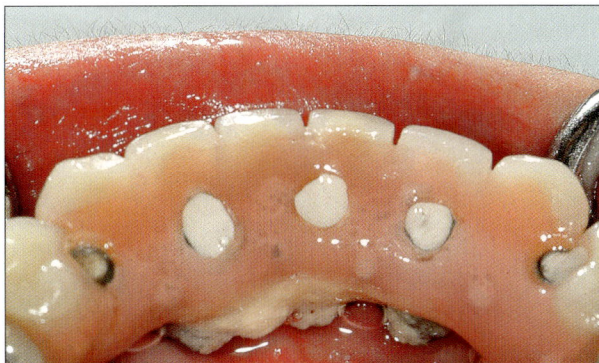

Fig 2   Fixed implant-supported dental prostheses are particularly difficult to clean for elderly patients with reduced dexterity and impaired vision.

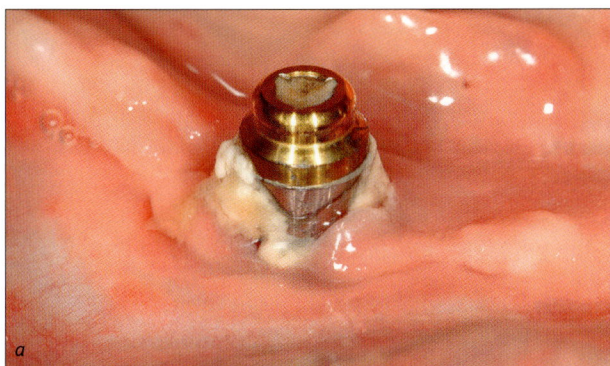

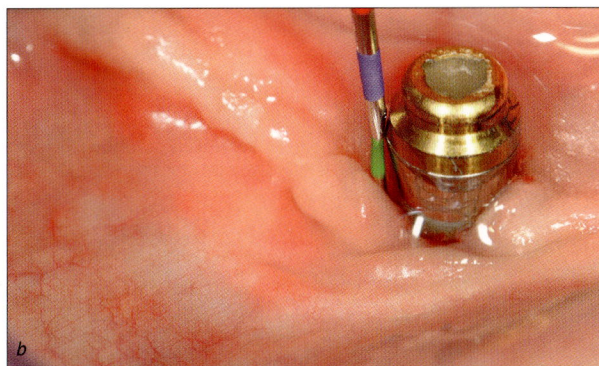

Figs 3a-b   The peri-implant tissues in elderly persons often show no signs of inflammation, despite abundant plaque. Locator attachments may fill with food debris, preventing the denture from being seated (a). A central filling with temporary composite material may prevent this, but it requires the use of inserts without a central pin (b).

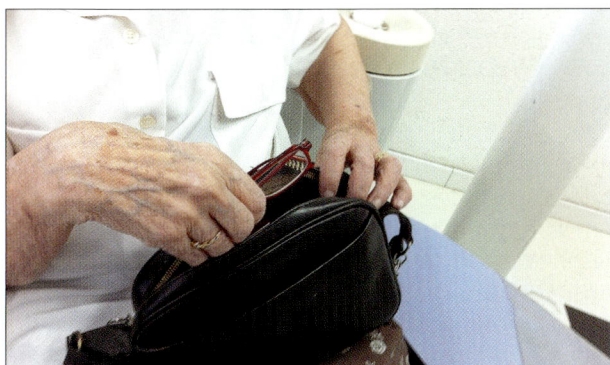

Fig 4   Most elderly patients require reading glasses for performing meticulous oral hygiene. Glasses may also be useful during the dental consultation when oral findings are shown and explained to the patient. Do not hesitate to ask patients if they use glasses, as they may be too shy to admit that they cannot see very well.

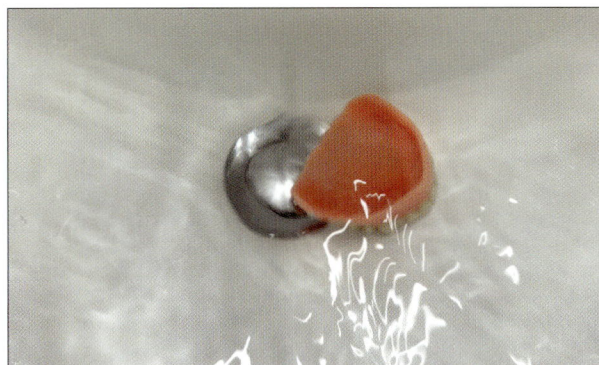

Fig 5   Filling the sink with water or a towel helps prevent denture fractures in case the denture is accidentally dropped.

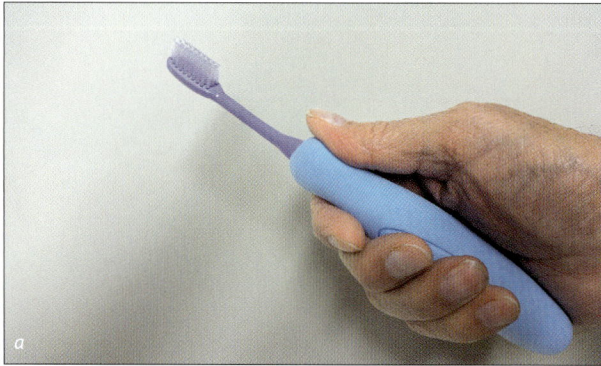

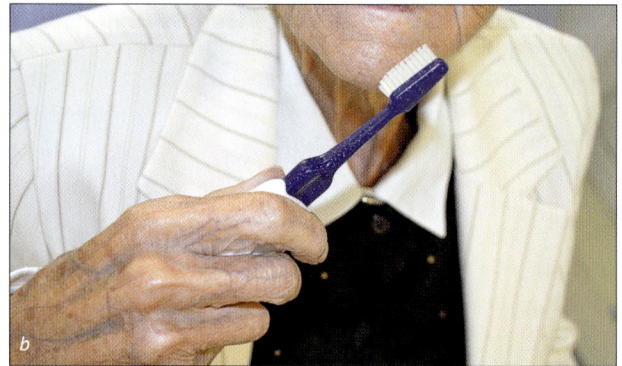

Figs 6a-b   Prefabricated thick handles facilitate "safe" and efficient handling of a toothbrush by geriatric patients. The plug-on handles are dishwasher-safe and can be re-used with a new toothbrush. (a) Inava System toothbrush (Cocooncenter, Châlons-en-Champagne, France). (b) Extra Grip (TePe, Malmö, Sweden).

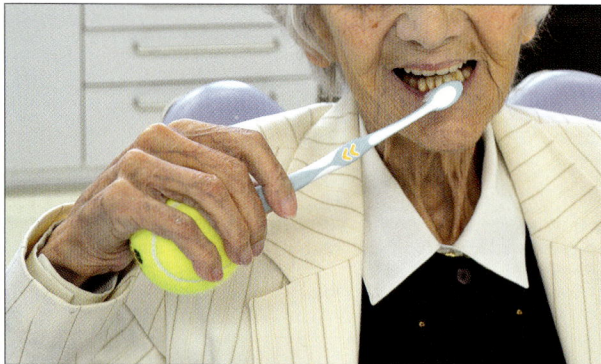

Fig 7   A tennis ball can also be used to adapt a toothbrush handle to an elderly person's reduced manual strength.

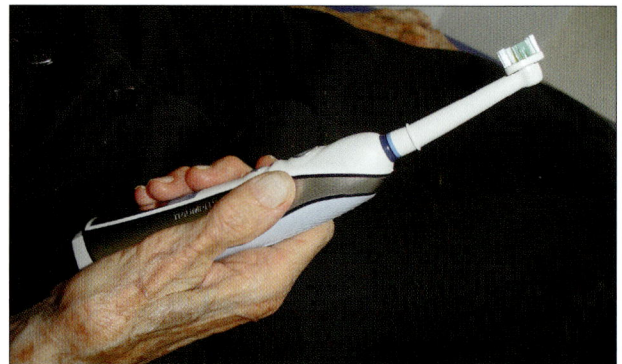

Fig 8   Power toothbrushes have a conveniently thick handle and offer good cleaning efficiency. However, they sometimes require substantial force and dexterity to switch on.

Choice of appropriate oral-hygiene tools

The altered perception and dexterity of geriatric patients requires individually selected and adapted oral hygiene tools to match the patient's intraoral status, visual acuity, and manual skills.

For example, in patients with osteoarthritis or sarcopenia, a larger-handled tool provides a more effective grip. With the growing elderly population, manufacturers are now providing prefabricated tooth and denture brushes with thicker handles. Plug-on handles are also available, which are dishwasher-safe and can be re-used (Figs 6a-b). A tennis ball or a bicycle handlebar grip may similarly be used to assist in holding a toothbrush firmly (Fig 7). For patients with severe osteoarthritis, handles can also be individually shaped using silicone impression putty, which can subsequently be converted to a more durable resin.

Most electric toothbrushes have a thick and easy-to-hold handle that contains the battery (Fig 8). Although their cleaning efficiency is excellent, their noise and vibration may not be appreciated by elderly persons, especially in the case of ultrasonic brushes. Furthermore, these brushes are sometimes difficult to turn on, especially if the power button is protected by a waterproof rubber layer. It would be preferable to have a model where the power can be turned on by pushing the brush on the table with both hands. Sometimes three-headed brushes are recommended that brush the lingual, vestibular, and occlusal surfaces at the same time. These brushes are efficient, but when a loss of periodontal attachment has resulted in lengthening of the clinical crowns, the lateral bristles risk not reaching the gingival margin due to the occlusal stop. Other than that, any toothbrush will do, provided it is used regularly and efficiently. Most geriatric patients prefer their reliable old friend—the traditional manual toothbrush.

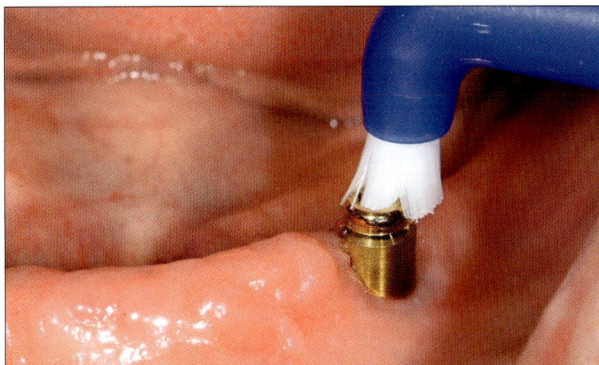

Fig 9   The central cavity of Locator attachments quickly accumulates bio-film and food debris. Special bristle brushes may help to keep them clean (TePe Implant Care; TePe Malmö, Sweden).

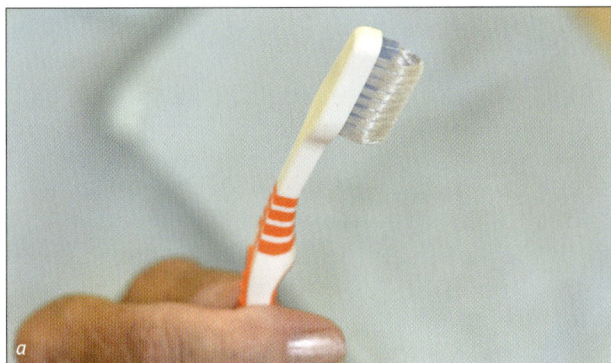

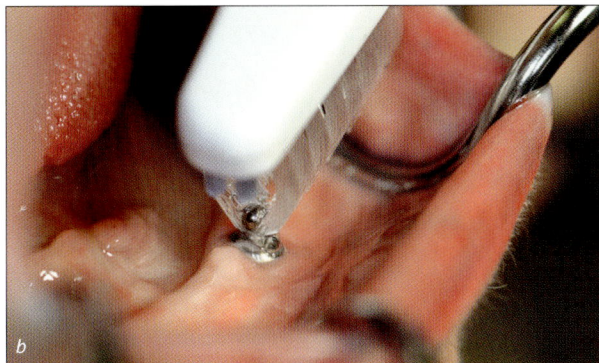

Figs 10a-b   For ball attachments, a special brush with bent bristles is available that facilitates cleaning the undercut of the ball. This brush may also be used for cleaning implant-supported bars (Access Oral Care; 3M ESPE, Seefeld, Germany).

Implant superstructure hygiene

Implant-supported prostheses sometimes present shapes that require special cleaning tools. Cleaning implant-supported restorations is therefore more complex than cleaning natural teeth. In the above-mentioned Swedish study, the 26 geriatric implant patients rated the ease of cleaning of their implants an average 5 on a scale from 0 to 10 (Olerud and coworkers 2012). Given that most patients tend to give rather positive answers in interviews, this score indicates at least some difficulties.

The Locator attachment, for example, has a cavity on the occlusal aspect to accommodate a central pin of the retention insert. This cavity quickly fills up with biofilm and food debris, which may ultimately preclude denture insertion. Special rigid bristle brushes may help keep these cavities clean (Fig 9). Alternatively, the cavity can be filled with a composite filling (Figs 3a-b). The latter should be provisional so that the abutment driver can still be used if required, and temporary composite materials such as those used for filling screw access canals have proved to be successful.

For ball attachments, a special brush with bent bristles is available that facilitates cleaning the undercut of the ball (Figs 10a-b). This brush can also be used with bars or all other low-profile attachments with undercuts. Bars are often less easy to clean on the lingual aspect and require special attention.

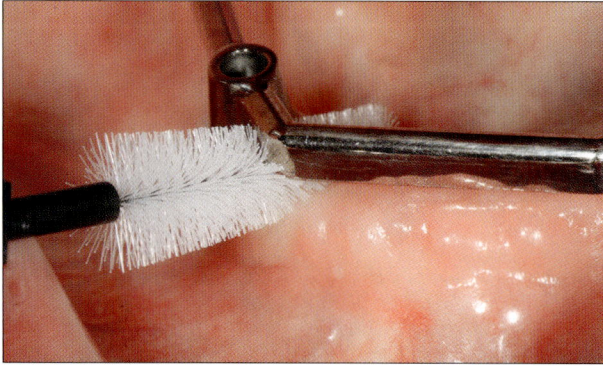

Fig 11   Interdental brushes, also available in larger sizes, are effective in cleaning the mesial and distal surfaces of the implant abutments, but fail to clean the lingual side (CPS soft implant; Curaden, Kriens, Switzerland).

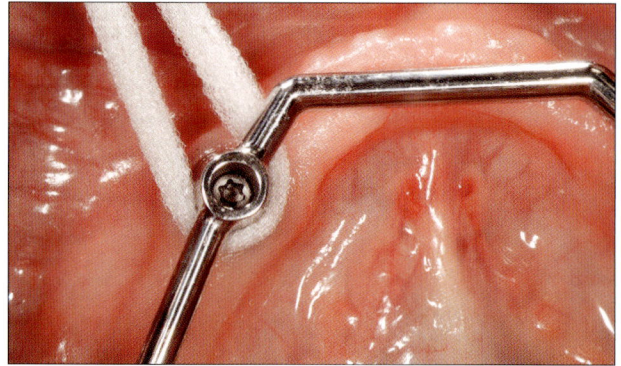

Fig 12   Dental floss may be effective in cleaning below the bar and around the abutments, including the lingual surface, when passed around the abutments.

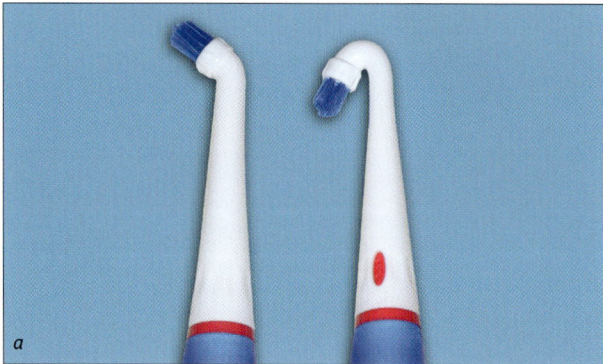

Figs 13a-b   Curved brushes with small heads may be an alternative for cleaning the lingual side of bars and for implant-supported fixed dental prostheses. (a) Reverse and Focus Tip Brush (Erskine Oral Care, Macksville, NSW, Australia). (b) TePe Implant Care (TePe, Malmö, Sweden).

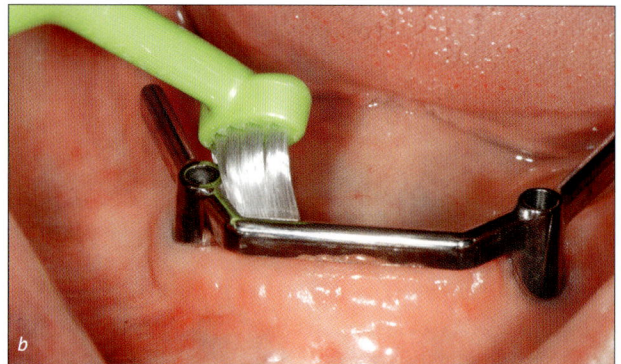

Interdental brushes are effective in cleaning the mesial and distal surfaces of the implant abutments, but despite being available in larger sizes, these fail to clean the lingual side (Fig 11). Dental floss may be effective in cleaning below the bar and around the abutments, including the lingual surface, when passed around the abutments (Fig 12), but may be difficult to thread in place for an elderly person with reduced dexterity or visual acuity. Bent small-headed brushes may be an alternative in cleaning the lingual side of bars and for implant-supported fixed prostheses (Fig 13a-b). The latter should also be unscrewed in the dental office for professional cleaning of the implants and the superstructure, at intervals adapted to the patient's own ability to keep the restoration clean. Again from a hygiene point of view, the most critical areas are located between the prosthesis and the mucosa of the alveolar ridge as on the lingual side of the implant abutments. Beyond the tools mentioned above, there is an exhaustive variety of oral-hygiene instruments designed for cleaning implant-supported prostheses, with new products appearing on the market almost every month.

Denture hygiene

It seems trivial but needs to be explicitly mentioned to a patient receiving an implant-supported removable prosthesis: the denture needs to be taken out for cleaning!

Patients also need to understand that not only the denture teeth need cleaning; the intaglio surface of the denture also requires a through brushing at least once a day. Special denture brushes are available that reach all regions of the denture base (Fig 14), even where small edentulous ridges render the cleaning of the denture's intaglio surface with a conventional toothbrush impossible.

Acrylic dentures can be cleaned exactly like household tableware; most patients understand that mechanical brushing is mandatory when it comes to doing the dishes and that the same principle applies to their dentures. No expensive fluoride toothpastes are required—cheap dishwashing liquid or hand soap will do. The latter has the added advantage to have a distinctly unpleasant taste, which may encourage better cleaning—if only to avoid the terrible taste.

Although the use of ultrasound baths or denture cleansers may help loosen stains or debris and perhaps provide a feeling of freshness in the mouth, they are not mandatory for keeping a denture clean. A recent Cochrane review on interventions for cleaning dentures in adults revealed that despite a lack of comparative studies, both mechanical and chemical cleaning seem superior to placebo (de Souza and coworkers 2009).

Occasional professional cleaning at the dental office or laboratory is useful if stains and deposits are not removed by the daily routines. Various methods are available, including cleaning in a vinegar-based cleansing bath with mechanical cleaning performed by swirling stainless-steel needles in a magnetic field (C2S, Lyon, France or Renfert, Hilzingen, Germany) (Figs 15a-c).

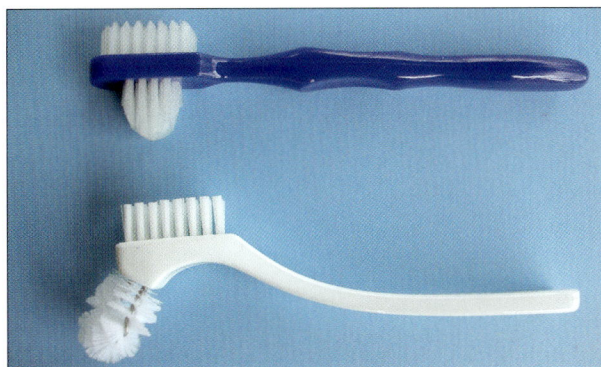

Fig 14   Denture brushes are large and rigid and have one side shaped to reach the narrow ridge parts of the denture base.

If professional cleaning is required too often, a layer of clear acrylic can be added to cover any surface details or retention niches and make the surface of the prosthesis smoother.

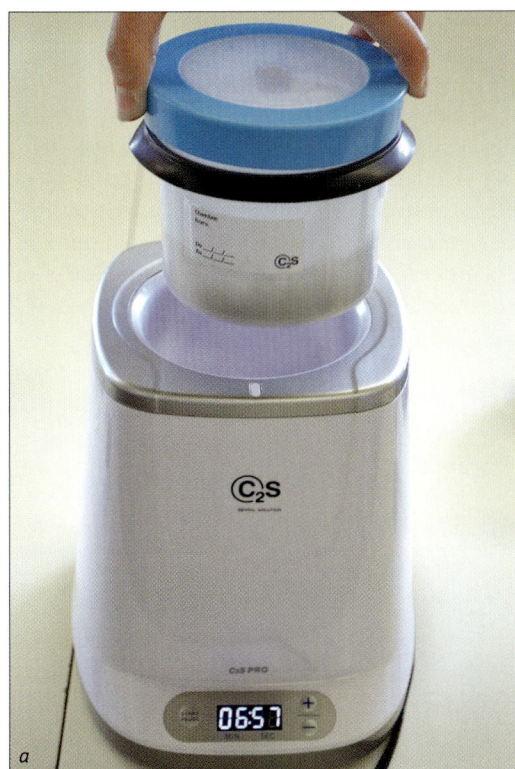

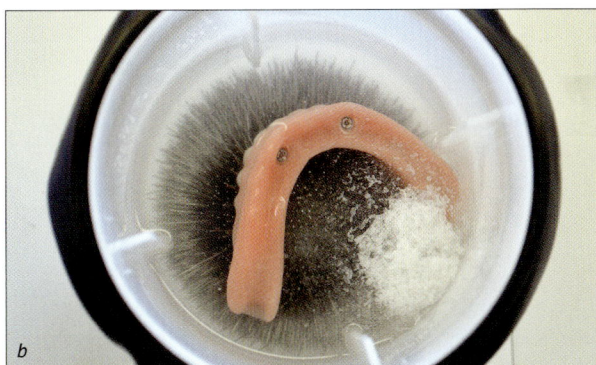

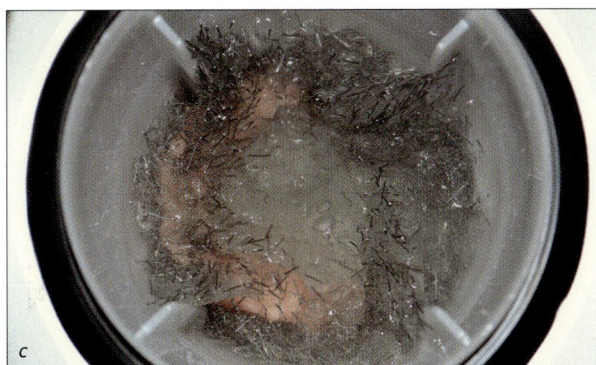

Figs 15a-c   In-office denture cleaning may be performed in a vinegar-based cleansing bath (C2S, Lyon, France).

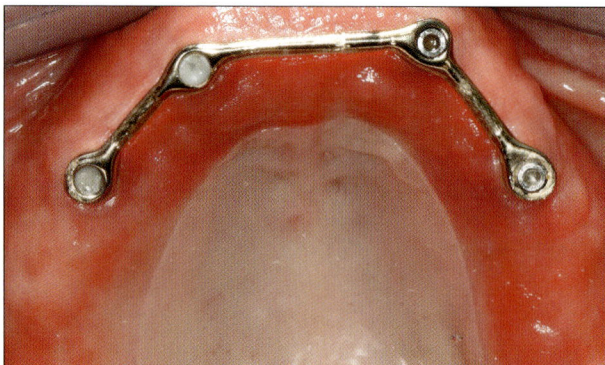

Fig 16   Biofilm may cause denture stomatitis.

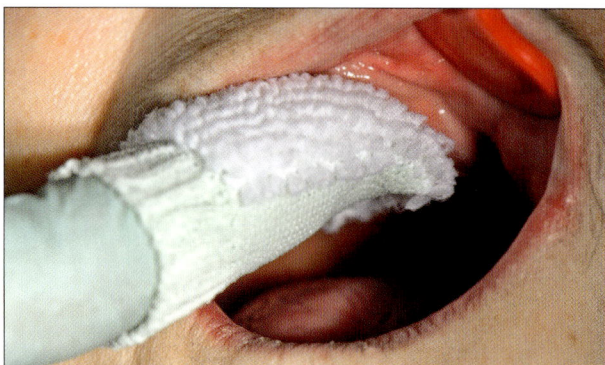

Fig 17   Microfiber glove to wipe down and massage the oral mucosa and edentulous ridges (Dr Hahn's Ibrush; Tootec, Tübingen, Germany).

Denture storage during the night

To wear or not to wear the denture at night—that is a question often heard from patients. Several aspects have to be considered. When anterior teeth are replaced and removing the denture is esthetically disfiguring, patients may prefer wearing their denture during the night for their self-esteem. They may also want to maintain their "prosthetic privacy" and keep their dental status a secret (Müller 2014). Meticulous hygiene is of even greater importance with nocturnal denture wearing, as the oral mucosa is never left uncovered for a prolonged period. Under these conditions, the oral mucosa presents the same changes as the skin under a wide finger ring. Additional mechanical load and prolonged biofilm exposure may cause denture stomatitis, which in its most common form is characterized by redness and swelling of the mucosa, corresponding to the shape of the denture base (Fig 16). Leaving the denture out during the night seems therefore preferable, if the patient is willing. A recent cohort study in 524 randomly selected seniors confirmed a 2.3-fold risk for developing aspiration pneumonia when a denture is worn during the night (Iinuma and coworkers 2015). Storing the denture overnight under dry conditions is recommended to challenge the survival of bacteria and fungi in the biofilm. The slight distortion of the prosthesis caused by dehydration in dry storage may be reversed by soaking the denture in clear water before inserting it the next morning.

Edentulous ridges and tongue

Although plaque adheres well to hard objects such as teeth and dentures in the mouth, a substantial bacterial load may also accumulate on the edentulous mucosa and on the tongue. As mentioned before, less vigorous chewing in elderly persons diminishes the self-cleaning effect during eating. Deposits on the tongue appear clinically as a yellowish or brownish tongue coating. The latter has even been identified as a risk factor for pneumonia in edentulous elderly patients (Abe and coworkers 2008).

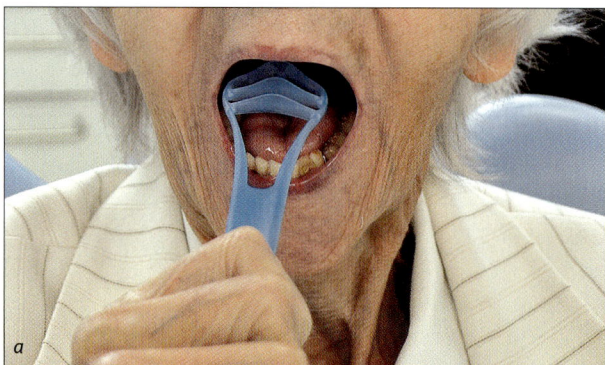

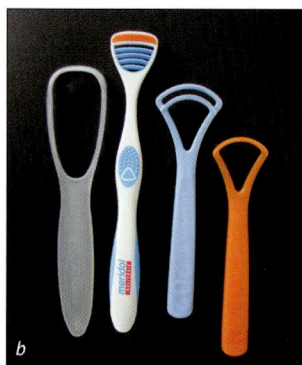

Figs 18a-b   Tongue scrapers exist in various forms and shapes.

Microfiber gloves are available to wipe and massage the oral mucosa and edentulous ridges (Fig 17). Although a toothbrush may also be used for gently massaging the tissues, some elderly patients, especially those with cognitive impairment, refuse to allow a toothbrush in their mouth. For these patients, the microfiber gloves are a more gentle way of scrubbing at least some of the biofilm off. These microfiber gloves also allow a vestibular wipe in special-care patients (or in children who refuse to open their mouth for more conventional oral hygiene).

Tongue scrapers exist in various forms and shapes (Figs 18a-b). Tongue scraping reduces the bacterial load in the oral cavity and helps reduce halitosis (Van der Sleen and coworkers 2010). An initial gagging reflex may be perceived as unpleasant, but this is often less marked in the evening.

Oral hygiene in an institutionalized setting
Along with the loss of autonomy, oral hygiene becomes more and more the responsibility of the caregiver staff. In geriatric nursing, maintaining the patient's autonomy is one of the priorities of care; consequently, patients are expected to perform oral hygiene themselves for as long as possible. Gradually, patients will first require supervision and motivation, then assistance. With further functional decline, the procedures have to be performed entirely by the nursing staff. Occupational therapy may help to maintain autonomy, especially in residents with a mild cognitive impairment (Bellomo and coworkers 2005). At this stage, implant-supported dentures may become problematic, as knowledge regarding such "high-tech" prostheses is scarce amongst caregivers. The threshold for not wearing a denture becomes lower as patients tend to become less demanding with age, frailty, and multimorbidity.

General recommendations for oral hygiene in patients with mild functional impairment include:

Mild dependency
- Supervise and motivate oral hygiene.
- Employ occupational therapy to maintain autonomy for as long as possible.
- Choose tools adapted to the individual functional capability of the patient.

Brushing technique for bedbound patients
- Sit the patient upright in bed (lower risk of aspiration).
- Hold a kidney dish under the chin.
- Place yourself behind the patient.

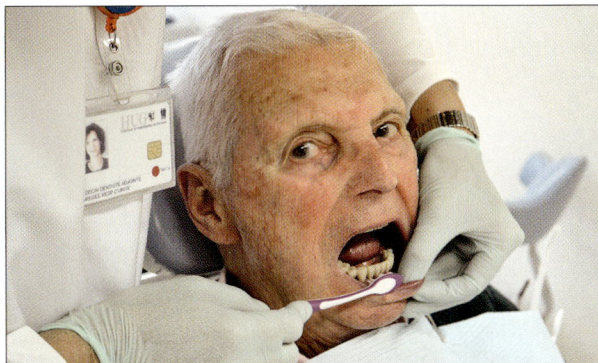

Fig 19 In bedbound patients, the caregiver should be behind the patient and keep the mouth open with the left hand. This allows the right hand to perform the usual cleaning movements.

- Support the patient's head with one hand.
- Brush teeth with the other hand using your "own" technique.
- Remove the denture twice a day for thorough cleaning and rinse after each meal.

Comforting measures
For patients who are unconscious, ventilated, or have problems spitting or swallowing, comforting measures may be indicated:

- Wipe oral cavity with gauze soaked with tea or rinsing solution.
- Apply ointment on the lips.
- Cool the mucosa with pineapple lozenges.
- If oral infections are present: wipe with 0.1% chlorhexidine.
- If xerostomia is present: use sprays of artificial saliva or humidifying gel on the tongue.
- If dentures are present: preferably leave them out and store them in a safe and dry place.
- Assure oral comfort by removing sharp edges from restorations or implant superstructures.

In a clinical setting, the proposed measures may be combined or modified according to the patient's individual oral status and health. If natural teeth are still present, the increased risk of coronal and root caries may require prevention by intense fluoridation with gels, varnishes, or toothpaste (Pretty and coworkers 2014; Srinivasan and coworkers 2014b). As xerostomia exacerbates the risk of caries and mucosal inflammation, symptomatic relief of xerostomia should be included in any preventive scheme for geriatric patients.

11 <u>The Ailing Patient</u>

F. Müller

Introduction

In the fourth stage of life, when dependency sets in and physical, mental, or social frailty dominate life, dental care and preventive needs become distinctly different (Pretty and coworkers 2014; Fig 1). Access to oral health care may be limited by multiple barriers such as poor mobility, unavailability of mobile dental services, or simply cost (Nitschke and coworkers 2005). Patients with a cognitive impairment may find it difficult to express a treatment need. Even in ailing patients who are able to explain their need for treatment, a striking modesty concerning their needs and expectations can often be noted (Vigild 1993), and they may understate the difficulties they are experiencing. Routine checkup visits are not mandatory for long-term care residents, and ailing patients maintain their right to self-determination concerning their health care, unless allocated a legal guardian. Access to dental services for ailing patients who receive domiciliary care is even more restricted, as it may be difficult obtain support from health professionals in organizing a visit at, or by, a dentist. Yet ailing patients should, as far as possible, expect to receive the same high-level comprehensive oral health care, whether living at home or a LTC facility.

Treatment planning for ailing patients

Treatment planning has to take into consideration the patient's physical and mental handicaps as well as the possibility of declining autonomy in managing fixed or removable prostheses and essential oral hygiene. As mentioned, the ailing patient might not be interested in long and invasive treatment procedures, such as implant placement or bone augmentation. Chronic diseases and the effects of their treatment may also limit the range of possible surgical interventions. A lack of saliva, perhaps

caused by polypharmacy, increases the risk of caries and renders the oral mucosa more delicate. Muscle coordination is likely to be impaired, and swallowing disorders can occur. Furthermore, psychological afflictions such as depression have a high prevalence in ailing and elderly patients, which may affect the prosthodontic treatment outcome and recall compliance. Treatment planning also has to take into account the patient's life expectancy and the cost/benefit ratio of the planned intervention.

Often the most limiting factor in treatment planning can be the patients' resistance or resilience to any dental intervention. For how long will they be able to sit in the dental chair? Can they open the mouth and remain still? What will my working conditions be in terms of visibility and accessibility, will patients be able to tolerate a supine position in the dental chair (Fig 2)? How will they react to an impression tray? Will they be frightened by radiographic apparatus? How can we manage bed-bound patients in a domiciliary setting? And lastly, will the patient be able and sufficiently compliant to follow simple instructions? All these issues need to be clarified before commencing a treatment that, once started, must be finished. Even with many years of clinical experience, this is one of the most difficult decisions in geriatric treatment planning. Some patients have a "day form"—they appear fit and compliant one day, while the next day they may be disoriented, fatigued, or absent-minded.

> It is essential to evaluate ailing patients' capability to undergo dental treatment in a preparatory treatment phase to avoid failure and premature abandonment of a restorative treatment.

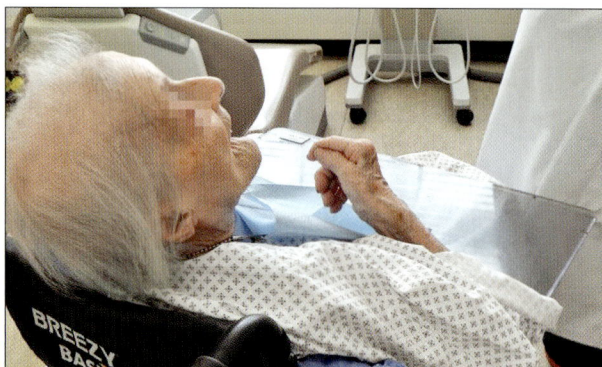

Fig 1   *In the fourth stage of life, dental needs become distinctly different.*

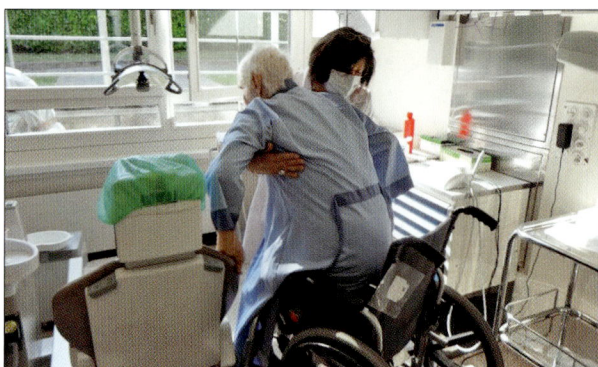

Fig 2   *Transferring the ailing patient to the dental chair may be difficult.*

Ailing is not a linear process, and general health may deteriorate at any time. The medical history must be updated regularly and the treatment plan adapted if necessary. However, the practicality of maintaining complex or even simple implant-supported restorations that were provided when the patient was more able physically and mentally should not be underestimated. Even simple treatments for minor technical complications may be very challenging; the meticulous procedures required for the treatment of peri-implant disease will often be so difficult as to be beyond consideration, and this should be anticipated in planning the treatment for elderly patients before they become too frail.

Ethical considerations

Ailing patients are considered a vulnerable patient group, and dentists, as part of the patient's social network, have a responsibility to detect and react to elder abuse. Elder abuse may be defined as violating a vulnerable older person's human and civil rights. Psychiatric illness and physical frailty, sensory impairment, social isolation, and physical dependency are important causes of vulnerability to abuse (Cooper and Livingston 2014). Maltreatment of elderly, very old, and dependent persons is more common than generally assumed, and violence against elders has a reported prevalence of up to 10%. Psychological maltreatment may comprise vilification, belittlement, infringement of rights, or ignorance of vulnerable seniors. In addition to physical violence, the withdrawal of food, clean clothes, or economic means are all forms of abuse. Dentists should be mindful of assessing whether or not any accompanying caregiver or guardian is trustworthy and whether they should be present during the consultation and decision-making process. Ailing patients' decisions for or against a suggested treatment should always be respected. The dentist's role is to provide the professional knowledge required for adequately informed consent, without influencing or manipulating the patients' decisions. Assessing the capacity to consent to treatment is not always easy; in case of doubt, a referral to a memory clinic for an in-depth examination may be indicated.

Our care for ailing elders should adopt a humanitarian and holistic approach (Fig 3), especially as medicine has become high-tech and machine-driven. Ailing, elderly patients may be intimidated, for example, by a 3D tomography unit, and the negative psychological impact on the treatment or the patient's trust in the dentist may outweigh most of the diagnostic value of such an intervention. Respect and recognition of the patient's values and lifetime achievements should feature in the doctor-patient relationship, as this will in turn engender the patient's trust in and respect for the dental professional. Shuman and Bebeau (1996) summarized some

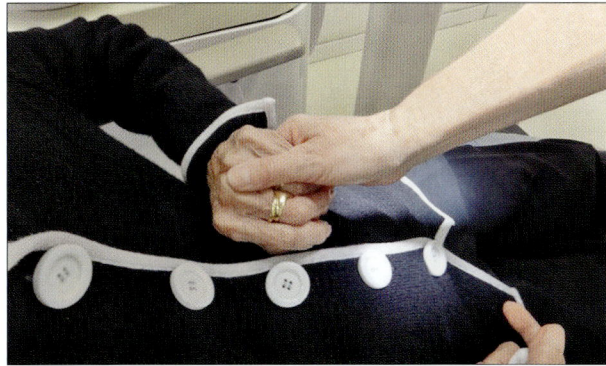

Fig 3   Caring for ailing elders should adopt a humanitarian and holistic approach.

basic ethical principles of the treatment of vulnerable elders as follows:

Autonomy	Right to self-determination
Non-maleficence	Duty to do no harm Duty to prevent harm to others Duty to remove harm from others
Beneficence	Obligation to do good for the benefit of others
Justice	Obligation to treat others fairly, not discriminate, distribute resources fairly
Truth-telling	Duty to tell the truth
Fidelity	Obligation to keep promises

Dentists would do well to remember the age-old maxim:

"Patients do not care how much you know, until they know how much you care."

Implants in the ailing patient

When considering implants in the treatment of ailing patients, two distinctly different scenarios have to be distinguished:

The first scenario is the placement of new implants, which is critical, given that the ailing patient may increasingly lose the capability to manage implant-supported prostheses and perform adequate oral hygiene. The widespread assumption that patients request "tight" and firmly fitting dentures does not apply to all elderly adults. Some patients openly admit that their oral comfort dominates their prosthodontic treatment choices. However, considering the abovementioned ethical aspects, it seems unreasonable to withhold the means of modern dentistry to an ailing patient if they request implants for a justified indication. Also, there are many different varieties of "ailing," and recommendations

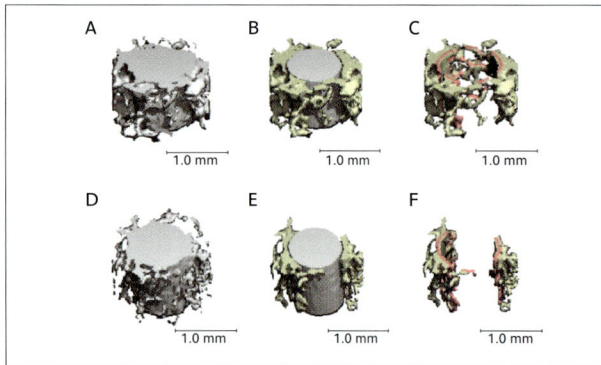

Fig 4   *Defective implant osseointegration under protein undernutrition in animal experiments (reprint with permission from Dayer and coworkers 2010).*

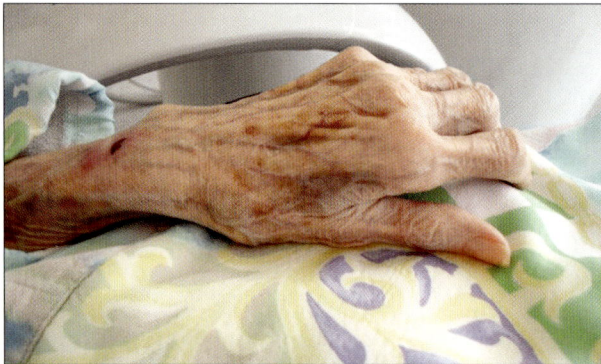

Fig 5   *Muscle weakness and reduced dexterity in frail elders may preclude the autonomous management of a sophisticated implant-supported prosthesis.*

therefore cannot be generalized. However, when opting for implants, the circumstances should be as close to ideal as possible. Animal experiments showed a lower rate of implant-to-bone contact if a low-protein diet was provided during osseointegration (Dayer and coworkers 2007; Fig 4). Food supplements should therefore be considered during the healing phase, particularly when masticatory performance is inevitably impaired.

The second scenario applies to functionally declining patients who had implants placed while they were still fit and the surgical intervention was no barrier. Ideally, these patients can benefit from their implants for the rest of their lives if maintenance of their implant-supported prosthesis is assured. There is a need for an active and strict follow-up program, with appropriately adapted recall intervals, so as not miss the point for "backing off" to a technically less sophisticated prosthodontic solution (Fig 5).

> Monitoring the use and handling of fixed and removable implant-supported prostheses in ailing patients seems mandatory. When functional decline and frailty preclude denture management, "backing off" to a less sophisticated and simplified restoration with or without the implants may become necessary.

In practical terms, this back-off strategy could imply the replacement of a fixed reconstruction by a removable prosthesis, which is easier to manage and clean for the patient or the caregiver. Great care should be taken to duplicate as many features as possible from an old fixed reconstruction to which the patient has become well adapted, to facilitate adaptation to the new prosthesis by avoiding unnecessary challenges to neuroplasticity.

Technically, in a few years' time, an existing fixed implant dental prosthesis might be scanned intraorally and an identical dental arch milled or 3D-printed as a removable prosthesis. Backing off could also mean the gradual simplification of the current overdenture attachment system. For example, bar, Locator, or CM LOC attachments seem more difficult to manage than ball or magnetic attachments.

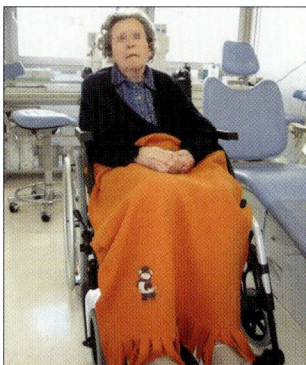

Fig 6a The edentulous patient had two interforaminal implants to support her mandibular overdenture.

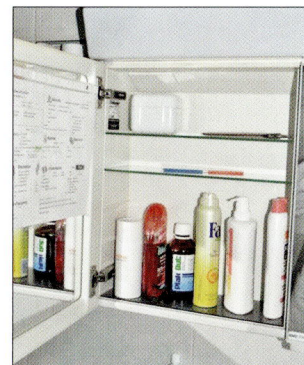

Fig 6b Her dentures had been stored in the bathroom cabinet for months as she became too weak to seat the denture with the famous "click."

Figures 6a-e depict a geriatric patient for whom the optimum time for a backing-off strategy was missed. Her dentures had been stored in the bathroom cabinet for months as she became too weak to seat the denture with the famous "click." The nursing staff accepted this situation as inevitable and the patient did not ask for a dental visit, although she was on a recall program and did have the contact details. At a first glance, when she opened her mouth, considerable food debris was seen, with just a glimpse of the heads of the two ball attachments. The peri-implant mucosa had grown over large parts of the implant, precluding denture insertion. The process of frailty had progressed rapidly, and transporting the patient to the dental office even for a minor excision of the gingiva was disproportionate, given her condition. It was decided to unscrew the ball attachments and replace them with healing caps. A localized reline with a tissue conditioner filled the female part of the ball attachments. The patient re-used her dentures during the days and for meals, although she relied on denture adhesives until she passed away around 2 years later.

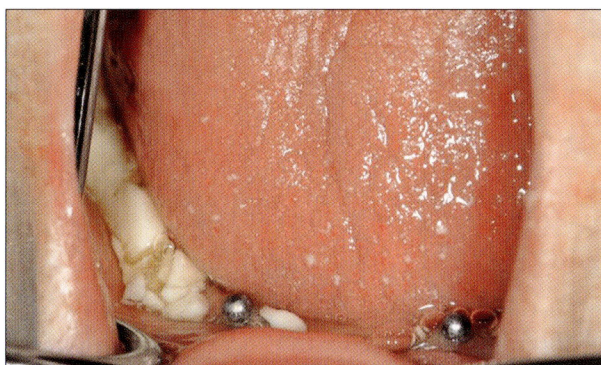

Fig 6c Large morsels of food debris; only the heads of the two ball attachments are visible.

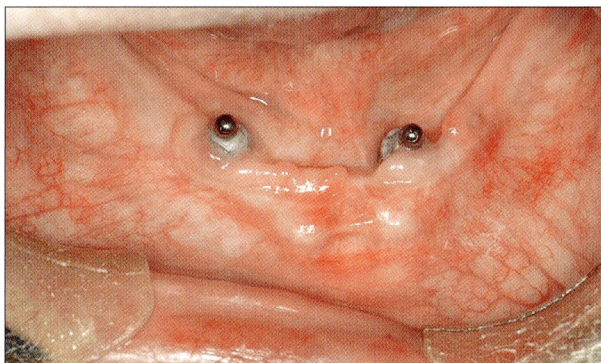

Fig 6d Peri-implant mucosa overgrowing the implants, precluding denture insertion.

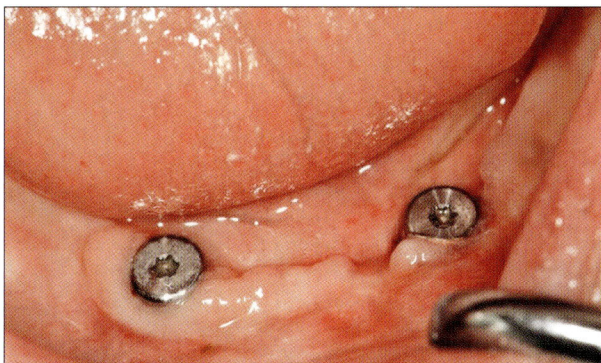

Fig 6e The back-off strategy meant unscrewing the ball attachments and replacing them with healing caps.

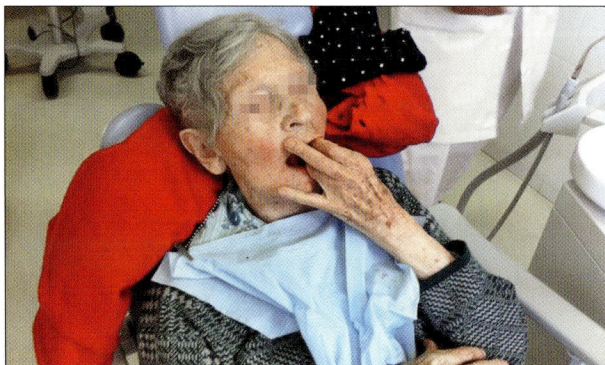

Fig 7   With progressing dementia, patients become less compliant for dental interventions. The extraction socket puzzles the patient, who explores the wound with her fingers.

Such a situation demonstrates the advantage of two-piece implant systems over one-piece "mini-implants" where it is impossible simply to unscrew the abutment. The sectioning of a one-piece implant to remove the intraoral part, causing soft-tissue trauma with potential concomitant infection and pain, would not be a simple back-off procedure. Furthermore, a high-speed rotary instrument to render the implant comfortable may not be available in a domiciliary setting, and the procedure could also be impossible in terms of patient compliance without recourse to sedation or general anesthesia, with the associated risks and serious implications for the patients' medical condition.

The cognitively impaired patient

The prevalence of cognitive impairments increases with age, with more than half of the population suffering from dementia at the age of 90 years or over (Graves and coworkers 1996). Several types of dementia exist, with Alzheimer's type being the most prevalent. Clinical symptoms vary greatly and include a progressive loss of memory accompanied by diminishing language skills, dyspraxia, impaired cognition, and a decline in executive functions, as well as a loss of social competence (American Psychiatric Association 1994). The disease progresses slowly but although treatment may alleviate the symptoms, a cure does not yet exist. Impaired motor coordination is one of the clinical symptoms; in the final stages of the disease, even chewing movements may become "de-programmed."

Persons with dementia generally have poorer oral health and fewer teeth than healthy controls (Syrjälä and coworkers 2012). Effective motor control of complete dentures is also affected. Weight gain seems to reduce the morbidity of the condition; hence, improving the chewing efficiency by prosthodontic means seems intuitively beneficial (Faxen-Irving and coworkers 2005; White 1998). In the final stages of the disease, dentures are rarely used, and implants may cause injury, infection, discomfort, and pain (Taji and coworkers 2005). Dental treatment becomes increasingly difficult when access to the mouth is violently refused by demented patients (Fig 7). Conscious sedation or even general anesthesia may become necessary. Existing implants should be "put to sleep" in good time by connecting gingiva-level healing caps. When necessary, adhesive pastes may be prescribed for denture use when necessary.

Palliative dentistry

Terminally ill patients for whom a cure is not possible will receive palliative care, which no longer focuses on curing the disease but aims to alleviate discomfort and pain. It is an approach that improves the quality of life of patients and their families, facing the problems associated with life-threatening illness, through the prevention and relief of suffering by treatment of pain and other problems, be they physical, psychosocial or spiritual (WHO 1990). Palliative dentistry deals with the specific oral symptoms patients experience from either their disease or its treatment that have a direct impact on their oral health related quality of life (Wiseman 2006). Most often, these are side effects of chemotherapy, which renders the oral mucosa sensitive to the point where this precludes denture wearing or adequate oral hygiene (Fig 8). Radiotherapy may additionally affect the salivary glands and cause xerostomia (Fig 9).

At the same time, the patient may need some unrelated dental treatment, for example the repair of a fractured filling or a denture reline. These conventional treatments also have to be planned in view of the patient's life expectancy and quality of life. A need for dental treatments in a palliative-care setting is not rare, and it would be desirable to have a dentist and a hygienist in each palliative care team (Fig 10). Most treatment demands for a dental visit are related to pain or denture maintenance, but esthetic repairs are also common (Schimmel and coworkers 2008).

When removable prostheses are not worn, implants may be problematic if they cause injury or infection. If this is the case, the dental treatment should be limited to the elimination of sharp and disturbing elements from the oral cavity, which in some cases means unscrewing the attachments and putting the implants to sleep. Local chlorhexidine gel and mouth rinses may help control infection and thus alleviate pain. In palliative dentistry, it is even more important to respond to the patient's requests, as this vulnerable group does not have many available options in terms of treatment.

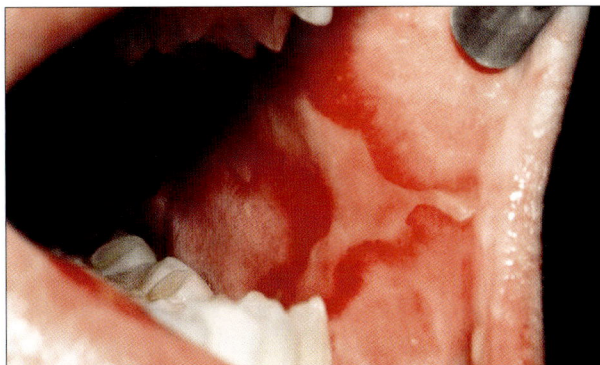

Fig 8   Radiotherapy renders the oral mucosa sensitive, and dental restorations or prostheses may cause pain and injury (after MacEntee and coworkers 2010).

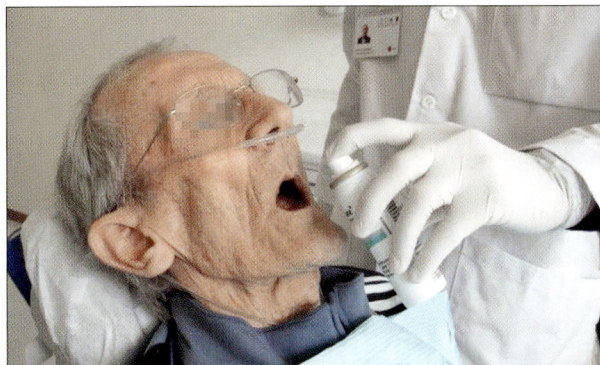

Fig 9   Artificial saliva alleviates the symptoms of hyposalivation.

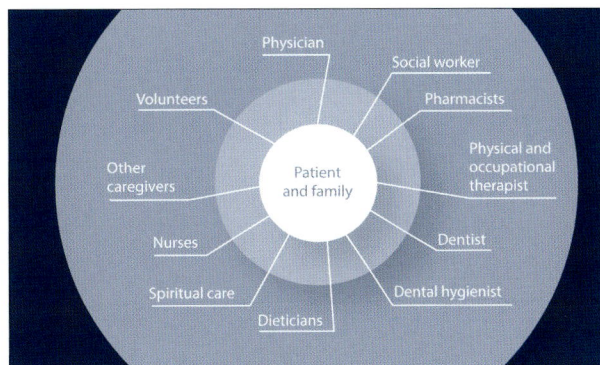

Fig 10   The patient- and family-centered care team should ideally comprise a dentist and a dental hygienist.

12 Management of Technical and Biological Complications

S. Barter

A great proportion of the literature relating to implants in the elderly patient focuses on the provision of implants and related prostheses. It is clear that chronological age alone is not a barrier to successful implant integration; the substantial benefits to oral health, function, and quality of life that can be provided are shown in other chapters of this book. However, we must consider not only the provision of such treatment, but also the inevitable ongoing maintenance requirements.

In elderly patients, planning a simple prosthesis designed for their current and likely future needs should be relatively predictable. However, as a result of an aging population, we will face an increasing number of patients who were provided with implant-borne prostheses at a time in their lives when they were younger, fitter, and more able. At the time of provision, it was relatively easy for them to seek and receive preventive or interceptive treatment for their implant-retained prostheses. The need for such treatment will not decline as the patient ages; in fact, it may be more necessary even as it becomes less practical.

Much as we would like to think our treatment will be perfect and that the prostheses we make will last forever, this is unlikely to be the case. Biological and technical complications will occur in many patients, and the risk is only likely to increase with the time the restoration has been in place. This may have implications on the oral health and well-being of the patient, can influence the possibility of continuing with an implant-retained prosthesis, and will inevitably bring further cost. Patients need to be advised of both the inevitability of the required maintenance and of the nature of the complications that may arise, not only from the surgical procedures involved but also in terms of technical complications with the prosthesis and the risk of peri-implant disease.

There are well-known criteria that are accepted as defining success, rather than the survival of an individual implant, but not all studies report the data necessary to determine whether these criteria were met. In general, studies looking at survival rates consider whether the prostheses under review have remained in service for the duration of the study. However, considerable numbers of "surviving" prostheses have suffered technical complications, whose prevalence may be greater than indicated in the literature due to underreporting—most studies report experiences in hospitals or specialist centers and may not reflect the wider primary-care situation.

The etiology of biological complications is patient-related and multifactorial: genetic susceptibility to periodon-

tal disease, medical factors such as diabetes, poor oral hygiene, etc. However, biological complications may also arise from iatrogenic factors such as poor surgical technique, poor prosthesis design, excess cement, or similar operator-related faults. It is one thing to reduce the risk of peri-implant disease by increasing patient compliance, but quite another to ensure that patients can actually manage what is required. For older patients with conditions that may preclude adequate compliance, their caregiver will need to be able to do what is necessary. Risk management begins with the planning of the most suitable prosthesis, not with its delivery.

Similar considerations apply to technical complications, which are largely related to prosthetic design and to the nature of the materials used. Recent systematic reviews suggest a minor improvement in our ability to avoid esthetic, and some technical, complications when comparing data in the last decade or so with older data, although the incidence of biological complications has remained relatively unchanged and the rate of all such complications is still high (Pjetursson and coworkers 2014).

The validity of such findings has to be considered against the weaknesses in the data and, therefore, the conclusions that we may draw. In general, most studies are uncontrolled, retrospective, and have low power in terms of the number of patients included. Many systematic reviews fail to assess the reliability of the included studies and may not detail any control group. When complications are reported, it is necessary to consider the level we use to measure success—it is not valid to use an individual implant as a success marker. If several implants in the same "favorable" patient are used as individual units for analysis, this may not result in valid statistics if, in that individual, it is the patient-related factors that have the greatest influence on the outcome (Chuang and coworkers 2002).

Studies reporting the rate and nature of complications may be interesting and valuable if they can be used to guide the clinician in choosing the best treatment plan for an individual patient. However, the patient is the one who will ultimately tell us whether they share our view of success. Patient-centered outcomes are equally important measurements and are not always reported.

When considering the success of our treatment overall, we need to consider different factors (Papaspyridakos and coworkers 2012a; Chung and coworkers 2009):

- Have we achieved the intended rehabilitation as planned and agreed with the patient?
- Have we satisfied the desired patient centered outcomes?

- Over time, is the rate of technical complications low and only requires simple intervention?
- Is hygienic maintenance achievable and maintains peri-implant tissue health?
- Is the longevity of the prosthesis adequate such that the original and on-going costs of treatment and maintenance produce good health economics?

There is little data on whether the rate of complications increases in the elderly patient. Studies indicate that osseointegration is unaffected by age alone. Is this relevant? Is the failure of an implant to integrate a greater problem than a significant peri-implant bone defect with soft-tissue inflammation and suppuration? Or, for that matter, healthy implants supporting an implant-retained overdenture that is now intolerable to a patient suffering from a neurodegenerative disease who refuses to wear the denture but suffers severe oral ulceration from the intraoral components? How easily will such conditions be treated in an elderly patient of increasing frailty?

Technical complications

- Implant fracture
- Abutment loosening/fracture
- Screw loosening or fracture
Fixed prosthesis
- Misfit
- Loss of screw hole seal
- Loss of cement
- Damage to veneering material
Removable prosthesis
- Wear or loss of retaining components
- Damage to or loss of prosthesis

Mechanical complications with implant-retained prostheses are common and almost inevitable as a result of functional wear. It is difficult to evaluate accurately the true incidence of technical complications. In one study, the authors observed that four large systematic reviews (Lulic and coworkers 2007; Pjetursson and coworkers 2007; Aglietta and coworkers 2009; Tan and coworkers 2004) provided data from less than 100 reconstructions on cumulative complications at five and ten years. Concluding their own study, they highlighted the fact that the literature alone cannot be used to choose between different treatment options for a particular patient (Brägger and coworkers 2011).

Implant fractures are rare (Fig 1a), but more commonly associated with reduced-diameter implants (Allum and coworkers 2008). However, a fractured retaining screw

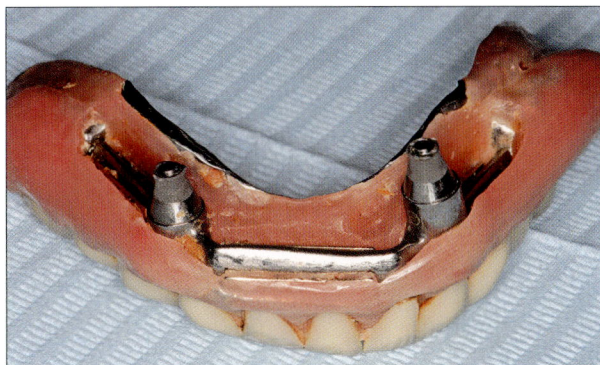

Fig 1a   A mandibular overdenture with reduced-diameter implants that have fractured as a consequence of poor prosthetic design.

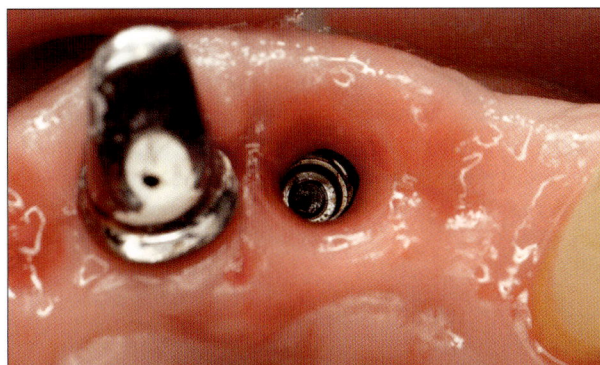

Fig 1b   A fractured abutment-retaining screw—difficult to retrieve in a patient with Parkinson's disease.

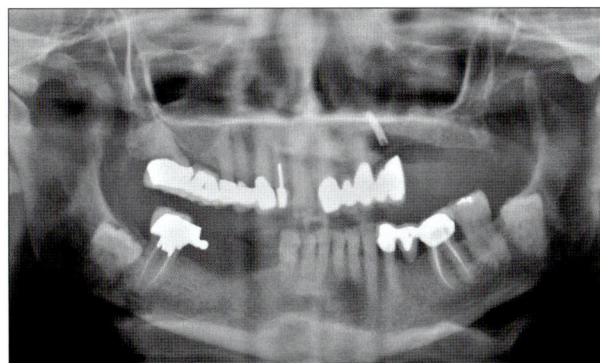

Fig 2   The fractured implant is impossible to retrieve and precludes further implant placement in this position.

inside an implant may be impossible to retrieve (Fig 1b), which not only renders the implant useless but also hinders the placement of a new implant in a suitable nearby location (Fig 2).

In fixed prostheses, problems with component fit are associated with biological problems such as mucosal inflammation and marginal bone loss due to bacterial accumulation, or increased wear and consequent risk of loosening or fracture of components (de Torres and coworkers 2011).

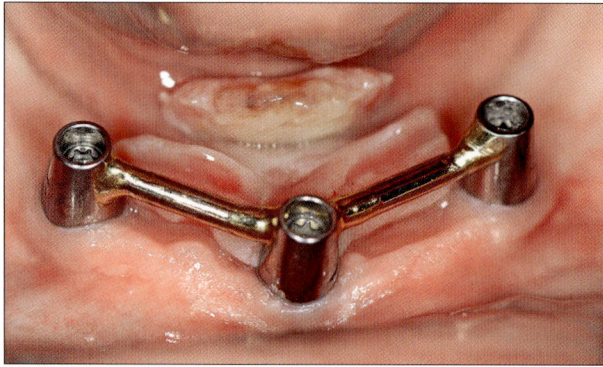

Fig 3   Hyperplasia and ulceration associated with an overdenture.

Biological complications

- Traumatic ulceration of soft tissues
- Soft-tissue hyperplasia/hypertrophy
- Mucosal recession
- Peri-implant disease
- Implant loss or removal
- Combination syndrome

A discrepancy of 150 μm may be acceptable (Jemt and Book 1996). However, discrepancies of up to 500 μm may be difficult to detect clinically, especially when the margins are subgingival. Periapical radiographs are recommended, but non-parallelism of the primary beam can cause misdiagnosis (Kan and coworkers 1999; Sharkey and coworkers 2011).

Technical complication rates for full-arch fixed implant prostheses have been estimated at 24.6% per 100 restoration-years; in more recognizable terms, two-thirds of prostheses in this study had suffered some form of complication at five years, and at ten years, this figure was over 90% (Papaspyridakos and coworkers 2012b). These numbers are consistent with other studies on the same topic.

Screw loosening remains one of the most frequently reported complications in implant-supported single crowns; in fixed and removable prostheses, the most common events appear to be fracture of the veneering materials or dentures, or loss of overdenture retention (Papaspyridakos and coworkers 2012b; Pjetursson and coworkers 2012; Bozini and coworkers 2011).

In overdenture patients, the most common complication is loss of retention, normally due to wear and tear of the retaining elements. As would be expected, this will be time-related, but it is also related to other factors such as the nature of the opposing dentition, prosthesis design, and parafunction (Payne and Solomons 2000). Overdentures often have a higher rate of complications in the immediate post-insertion period relating to comfort and have a need for more frequent maintenance, with associated costs (Zitzmann and coworkers 2005).

Age-related changes in the resilience of the oral mucosa are more commonly seen after the age of 70. Histological changes in mucosal structure and vascularity cause a loss of resilience, while increased susceptibility to mechanical and chemical trauma causes ulceration (Nedelman and Bernick 1978). The mucosa is more atrophic, and inflammatory changes last longer, even where clinical symptoms are less intense. Oral mucosal conditions are more prevalent in elderly populations and are more frequent in denture-wearers (Jainkittivong and coworkers 2002; Fig 3).

Mechanical irritation from ill-fitting dentures may cause hypertrophic conditions such as denture stomatitis, even when then prosthesis is implant-supported. Multiple risk factors may also be implicated, for example candidiasis and systemic factors such as diabetes. Hyperplasia of tissues under a bar or a fixed bridge may also occur due to inflammatory changes and may not only cause discomfort; access for effective oral hygiene may be more difficult, further worsening the condition (Figs 4 to 6).

The increased friability of the oral mucosa may lead to recession around implants, particularly in the presence of a thin tissue biotype. While some elderly patients may not be concerned about any degradation in the esthetic appearance, the exposure of the textured implant surface will lead to increased rates of plaque formation, again potentially worsening the peri-implant tissue health and leading to peri-implantitis.

The periodontitis-susceptible patient is at greater risk of peri-implant disease (Ong and coworkers 2008; Heitz-Mayfield 2008). While there are established protocols for the treatment of periodontal disease that are effective in preserving teeth, there are no accepted protocols that have been shown to be superior in treating peri-implant disease (Claffey and coworkers 2008).

It is consequently invalid to anticipate that long-term implant success in the periodontitis-susceptible patient can be achieved using the same principles of periodontal treatment, for established peri-implant disease.

Biological complications are possibly as underreported as technical complications; peri-implant tissue conditions are often reported in different ways or may not be reported at all in some studies (Berglundh and coworkers 2002). The reporting of peri-implant marginal bone loss by means of radiographic evaluation may not always be reliable. An accurate evaluation requires reproducibility of the exposure and positioning of the film/sensor. Panoramic imaging, used in many studies, is rarely valid as a technique for such evaluation; it is only possible to visualize the proximal bone levels, which gives limited information.

The relevance of detection and reporting of biological peri-implant conditions is illustrated in a study of mandibular fixed full arch reconstructions (Gallucci and coworkers 2009a). While most of the implants had survived after five years, peri-implant health parameters showed a statistically significant difference over this time, which was attributed to "oral hygiene being more challenging." When the peri-implant health parameters were considered, the true implant success rate was significantly worse. Oral hygiene may be difficult with greater amounts of "pink prosthetics," or, worse still, may be impossible when the prosthesis has a flange (Figs 7 and 8), perhaps to achieve adequate esthetics or to prevent escaping air from causing phonetic difficulties.

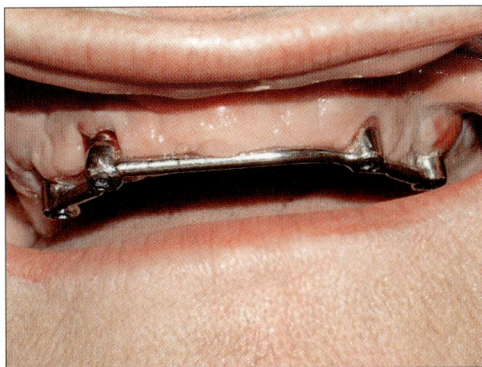

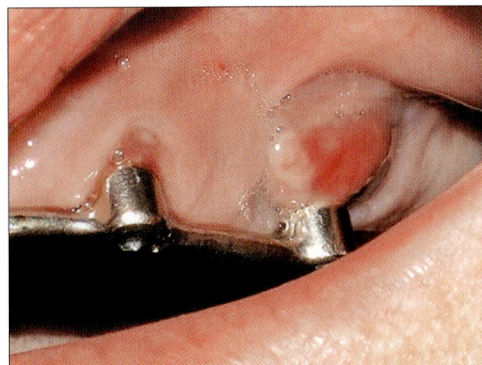

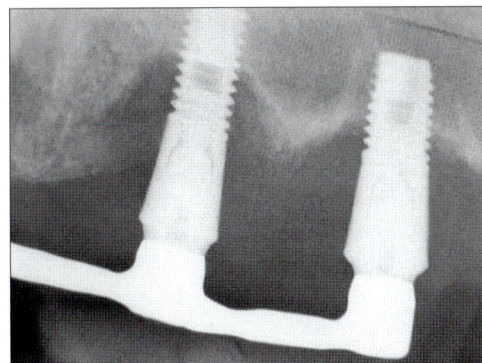

Figs 4 to 6   These images show soft-tissue hyperplasia under a maxillary bar; cleaning was difficult and therefore neglected, leading to advanced peri-implant bone loss.

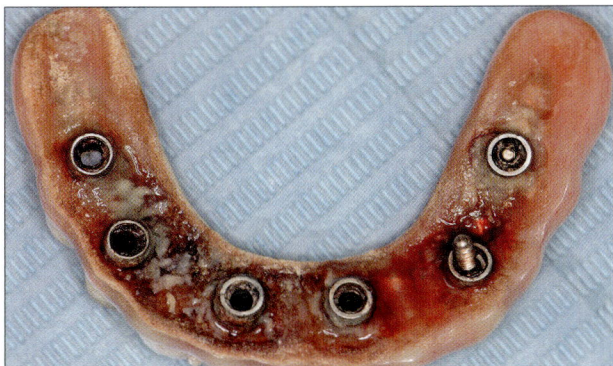

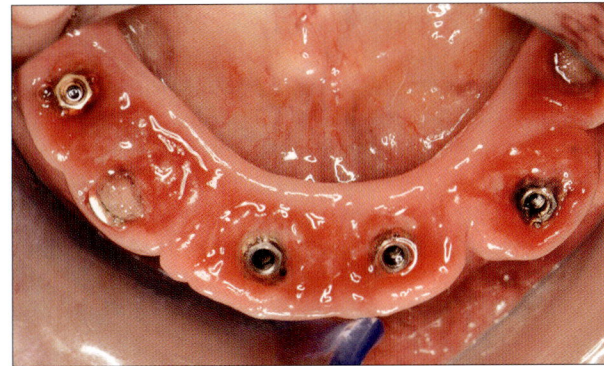

Figs 7 and 8   The design of this fixed reconstruction, with both upright and angled implants, made access for adequate oral hygiene impossible, leading to severe mucositis and peri-implant marginal bone loss.

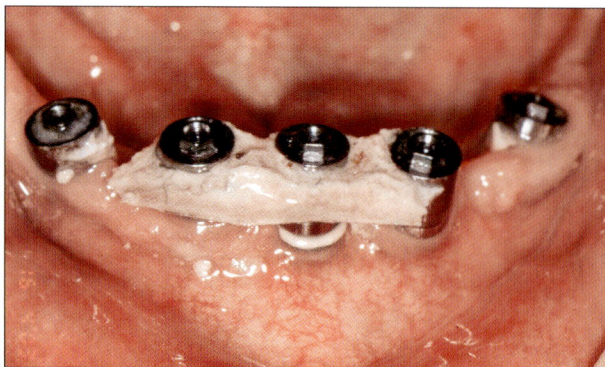

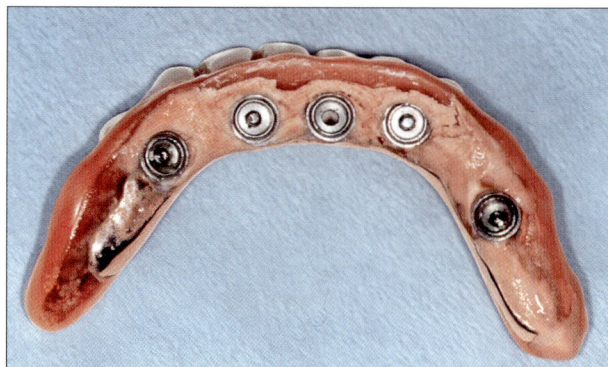

Figs 9 and 10   This prosthesis was ultimately retained by one screw (the others having been lost or fractured) and many years' worth of accumulated calculus. The patient's caregivers and relatives were completely unaware that the patient did not have natural lower teeth.

Peri-implant crestal bone loss exceeding 2 mm has been reported as a common biological complication in fixed prostheses, with an incidence of approximately 20% over five years and 40% over ten years. Peri-implant mucositis showed a similar increase over time, rising from approximately 10% at five years to 20% at ten years (Papaspyridakos and coworkers 2012b). A similar doubling of incidence was observed with soft-tissue hyperplasia, which will also make peri-implant cleaning more difficult.

Age-related changes in collagen turnover, immunosenescence, the effect of medications, the impact of a lifetime of smoking, medical conditions, and psychosocial factors including stress or depression are all examples of factors that may affect the control or progression of periodontal disease in elderly patients—factors that are not yet fully understood. To date, there are no studies investigating the relationship between advanced age and the progression of peri-implant disease.

Some studies have shown that plaque accumulation in the older patient is more rapid than in the younger individual (Brecx and coworkers 1985; Holm-Pedersen and coworkers 1980). Other studies have suggested that the composition of plaque may vary with age and that the role of different bacteria in plaque may change with advancing age. However, there is no evidence to suggest that there is any association between advancing age and peri-implant plaque composition in either healthy or diseased sites (Mombelli 1998). There are many other factors of potential greater significance in the progression of peri-implant disease, such as medical conditions

and most importantly the ability of the elderly patient to perform home care effectively. The cumulative increase in the microbial burden is likely to have an adverse effect on stagnation areas that are inaccessible for daily home care.

When it is more difficult for the patient to clean their prosthesis or access professional care, there may be a greater likelihood of peri-implant disease. In a small study examining fixed prostheses on implants, it was found that nearly 40% of implants described by patients as "difficult to clean" were affected by peri-implantitis (Schuldt Filho and coworkers 2014; Figs 9 and 10).

The treatment of peri-implant disease in a geriatric patient may become progressively less practical; even non-surgical therapy that does not require the removal of a fixed prosthesis can be difficult to provide and may be impossible in an institutional setting, or for a patient with neurodegenerative conditions. The progression of the disease may lead to more severe infection with a need for surgical intervention in a hospital setting, which is likely to be undesirable for all patients.

There are no studies investigating age-related differences in the outcome of regenerative surgery in either periodontal or peri-implant defects. However, given the variability in outcome of such procedures in the age groups commonly studied, the additional difficulty in performing these procedures and the potential reduced healing capacity associated with common medical conditions in the geriatric patient may render the consideration of this treatment unlikely.

The effect of multiple factors

There will always be multiple site- and patient-specific factors that influence the outcome of treatment with implants in terms of benefits and risks. Such factors may have complex interactions, which may not be immediately apparent to the unwary clinician who is planning treatment on a purely technical or mechanistic level.

For example, in a denture patient with xerostomia, the provision of an overdenture may provide significant help with the relief of mucosal irritation. However, if the xerostomia is a result of Sjögren's syndrome associated with rheumatoid arthritis (RA), there can be a higher incidence of peri-implant crestal bone loss in patients with connective-tissue diseases (CTD) such as scleroderma and RA, possibly as a result of reduced mucosal vascularization resulting in impaired bone nutrition. There may also be higher peri-implant bleeding indices attributed to the vascular immunological component (Kovács and coworkers 2000b; Mosca and coworkers 2009).

There could also be pharmacological implications, as patients may be taking corticosteroids or immunosuppressants, potentially requiring management of adrenal insufficiency and impaired healing. The same patient may be taking non-steroidal anti-inflammatory drugs and have a higher bleeding tendency.

Impaired manual dexterity may make the insertion and removal of the denture more difficult. Problems with the accurate placement or removal of the denture can also cause increased wear on the retentive elements of the denture, or increase the risk of fracture. Patients may not remove the denture as often as recommended for cleaning; oral hygiene may also be affected by impaired dexterity, and a specific plan with aids such as adaptation of toothbrush handles may be indicated.

Professional hygienic intervention may therefore be required more frequently, with increased cost and implications for the patient in terms of accessing the necessary care.

A further factor may be the effect of a well-retained implant-supported lower overdenture on a previously successful conventional complete upper denture. A moderately stable and retentive complete upper denture may not in itself present problems when the lower denture is not stable and retentive, as this situation precludes high masticatory forces. However, the dramatic increase in lower-denture stability provided by implants may render a previously successful complete upper denture less stable; the patient now displaces the upper denture more readily. Implant placement in the upper arch may be impractical or undesirable, and the situation may worsen over time as a result of combination syndrome.

Combination syndrome was first described by Kelly (1972) as a group of specific changes seen in patients with complete maxillary dentures opposed by a mandibular Kennedy Class I removable partial denture. The existence of the "syndrome" has been questioned because of the quality of published evidence (Palmqvist and coworkers 2003); nevertheless, multiple authors have reported one or more of the clinical features, which undoubtedly have a very real impact on patients.

Combination syndrome is characterized by the following features:

- Loss of bone in the anterior maxilla.
- Overgrowth of the maxillary tuberosities.
- Papillary hyperplasia of the palatal mucosa.
- Overeruption of the anterior maxillary teeth.
- Vertical bone loss of the posterior mandibular edentulous ridges.

These changes result in decreased vertical dimension, a reversal of the curve of Spee, an anterior mandibular rotation, and poor denture fit and stability. It has been theorized that the cause may partly be the natural tendency of patients to favor chewing on remaining anterior teeth, as this allows generation of maximal force.

Mandibular overdentures are generally supported by implants in the anterior region with good bone quality and sparse innervation. A similar situation occurs where maximal function is generated anteriorly, and given the lack of periodontal proprioceptive feedback, the forces may be even higher, again resulting in combination syndrome, possibly in as short a period as two years (Thiel and coworkers 1996). Surgical correction is frequently required to address soft-tissue problems, and this may be impractical in an aging patient.

It can be seen that the provision of even "simple" treatment, here in terms of placing two implants and an overdenture, is only part of the equation; the associated overall care considerations can become paramount.

Prevention and management

It is perhaps logical to presume that the rate of both biological and technical complications increases with the age of the prosthesis or the implants. However, the practicality of dealing with these complications may decrease with increasing patient frailty.

When considering the topic of implant therapy in the elderly patient, there are two generic situations:

- The provision of an implant-retained prosthesis in an elderly patient.
- The maintenance of such treatment that was provided when the patient was less impaired.

When considering what treatment to provide in an aged patient, we should be mindful of the fact that previously edentulous patients may have to re-learn old skills or learn new ones to maintain peri-implant health. These two situations are fundamentally different:

- In the former, we have the opportunity to more readily assess existing and possible later functional or cognitive decline; we can design a simple treatment that is easy to care for, has low maintenance requirements and a high degree of reversibility—we can design into our treatment the possibility of adaptation to future needs or the simple resolution of problems arising from technical or biological complications.
- In the latter, there is no possibility of this if the patient already has a complex prosthesis. In a scenario of failing physical or mental health, surgical or prosthetic treatment to address a failing implant or prosthesis could be complex and beyond practicality (Engfors and coworkers 2004).

Removing an integrated implant is not easy, even in a situation of peri-implant bone loss. While instrumentation has been developed to use reverse torque to unscrew an implant, this is not always successful and surgical intervention may be required, with a need for bone removal and consequent morbidity. Such procedures also cause psychological distress, and the loss of a previously comfortable and functional prosthesis as a result of implant loss can affect the quality of life. The ability of elderly patients with declining neuroplasticity to adapt to changes will be compromised; it is quite possible that they simply will not be able to adapt and that this will have consequences for nutrition, self-esteem, and multiple other quality-of-life measurements.

While the provision of implants may be helpful in avoiding a need to adapt to a significantly different situation—for example in providing an implant-retained restoration in the newly edentulous patient, avoiding a denture—we have to think ahead. The management of even simple complications such as retorquing a retaining screw or replacing the resin seal of a screw-retained prosthesis may present difficulty in a geriatric patient. Such procedures may be more difficult in an institutional setting or even impossible, for example in a patient with dementia.

What is considered "simple" treatment may not always be so, particularly if the future maintenance is likely to be more involved. For example, the increasing use of protocols providing a full-arch fixed reconstruction on two short upright implants and two long angled implants has raised interesting questions about how many implants are needed to provide a fixed prosthesis. This technique is often promoted as a "simplified" approach with no need for grafting, and a reduction in cost as fewer implants are used. The implants are loaded immediately, reducing treatment time and giving patients fixed teeth in one appointment, with a result that may be as reliable as any other protocol. Such claims may be very attractive to patients and, consequently, to dentists.

However, careful interpretation of the supporting evidence is required, as there may be a significant potential for technical and biological complications. There are few long-term high-quality data. Some of the supporting evidence is in the form of finite-element analyses, whose applicability to normal clinical conditions is questionable: the uniformity of modelled cortical-bone thickness is inappropriate, as the protocol calls for a significant reduction in crestal alveolar bone, reducing or removing the cortex. In the clinical situation, bone density varies considerably at different locations and no studies model the effect of loosening of one abutment. Effective monitoring of peri-implant parameters is not possible if there is a significant volume of pink prosthetics and a consequent lack of access for probing, and therefore is often not reported.

Given that most of the load on an implant is transferred to the cortical bone in the first 2 mm or so of the implant and that there is abundant evidence that short implants work well (Pierrisnard and coworkers 2003), do we need long implants at all? Removal of such an implant if affected by peri-implant disease may require considerable further surgery.

The reduction in ridge height needed to create space for prosthetic components in this protocol is questionable on several points. Firstly, the major flap elevation involved in degloving a jaw is not a simple surgical procedure. Secondly, the required significant alveolectomy may be a major surgical procedure, particularly in an elderly patient. If such a reduction is required, might there be sufficient bone available for a conventional denture, which is of course very successful in many patients (de Albuquerque Júnior and coworkers 2000; Heydecke and coworkers 2003b)? Also, if implants are lost and the ridge has been surgically removed, there may be no possibility of placing more implants or delivering a conventional denture, as the jaw will have been "iatrogenically resorbed."

Biological complications are more likely to arise in a situation when there is little access for cleaning, as described above (Gallucci and coworkers 2009a). The regular removal of such prostheses for proper access to the implants for cleaning is of questionable value, given that this is often only prescribed on an annual basis. In an elderly patient with limited access to care, poor health, or mental decline, maintenance of proper oral health may be impossible.

The same may apply to the management of technical complications, such as fracture of the prosthesis or loosening of components. In large full-arch reconstructions, even a small fracture of veneering material, causing mucosal ulceration, may require removal of the entire prosthesis for repair or replacement. Many authors have recommended a modular approach, such as replacing every three teeth with a three-unit FPD on two implants (Stanford 2007). This segmented approach allows a simpler, less costly, partial intervention in event of any failure (Gallucci and coworkers 2005).

It has also been suggested that because of the clinical and laboratory complexity and costs associated with these types of prostheses, a maxillary overdenture on four to six implants, typically connected with a rigid bar-and-clip attachment system, may be an alternative solution (Mericske-Stern and coworkers 2002).

By contrast, although implant-retained overdentures may be associated with a more frequent need to adjust or replace the retentive elements inside, this maintenance is considerably simpler. The need for maintenance will clearly be related to the age of the prosthesis, although post-placement adjustments appear to be more frequent in the first year (Payne and coworkers 2000), possibly as a result of adaptation on the part of the patient.

However, even the provision of a simpler prosthesis such as an overdenture may give rise to later problems if there is no possibility to remove intraoral components appropriately and easily. One-piece implants with integral prostheses (such as "mini-implants" used for overdenture retention) are useful in providing lower-overdenture stability with minimal surgical intervention and at reduced cost. When functioning well, there can be significant improvements in oral health-related quality of life (OHRQoL) outcomes. However, in a patient with dementia who cannot or will not wear the accompanying denture, the intraoral element can cause significant ulceration and discomfort.

In some situations, patients may well be incapable of telling caregivers that there is a problem; the caregivers themselves frequently fail to recognize that implants are in place, or even that the denture was not a conventional denture. The problem may manifest itself in a reluctance of the patient to take food and drink, due to oral pain and discomfort, which in itself may be misdiagnosed as a difficult behavior resulting from dementia. In a two-piece implant system, removal of the intraoral components is at least possible, even if challenging, and this may resolve the problem as mucosa grows over the implant. Sectioning a one-piece implant for such a patient, even in the clinical setting, may be so impractical as to require sedation.

As patients get older, visual impairment may have an impact on their ability to perform effective oral hygiene; insertion or removal of a denture, identification of cracks or deterioration in the prosthesis and recognition of the need to seek advice may also be affected. Reduced strength and manual dexterity may also have an effect on how well they can unclip a removable prosthesis. Systems that allow for changes in the method or degree of retention allows us to adapt the prosthesis to their needs.

All maintenance and repair requires access to the dentist and implies additional cost, so it is important to design into both the surgical and prosthetic aspects features that allow for adequate plaque control and reversibility. In addition, and when appropriate, a timely conversion of a complex prosthesis to a prosthesis with these features while patients are still able to seek treatment may prevent later difficulties.

There are many key elements to planning implant therapy, and it is impossible to list them all. However, examples of simple considerations that may help reduce biological and technical complications include:

Planning for hygienic maintenance

- Ensuring adequate interimplant distances to allow access for cleaning with interdental brushes.
- Designing the prosthesis with readily identifiable access points for interdental brushes of a prescribed size; such brushes can be adapted to compensate for reduced grip strength, manual dexterity, or to facilitate use by a caregiver if the patient is unable to use them. Floss is not likely to be used effectively or at all in such circumstances.
- Creating convex mucosal surfaces on fixed prostheses, with clearance to prevent soft tissue trauma when cleaning.
- Structured professional aftercare programs are necessary, and oral health education of caregivers will be required as well.

Planning for overdenture patients

- Ensuring maximal anteroposterior spread of implants; this gives better stability, reduces the possibility of combination syndrome, and increases the opportunity for replacement of a failed implant while maintaining adequate implant spacing.
- Using milled bars with distal extensions also reduces the chance of combination syndrome; milled bars are more rigid and are less likely to fracture.
- Considering maxillary implant placement to reduce chance of combination syndrome.
- Designing dentures with appropriate occlusion at the correct vertical dimension and with adequate extensions. Implants do not make a bad denture into a good denture.
- Regular recalls for occlusal adjustment and relining.
- Labeling of denture with patient identifiers.
- Use of two-piece implant systems with a range of retentive components that allow for adjustment of the retentive force; also that allows for removal of abutment and "submergence" of the implant if necessary.

Planning for fixed prostheses

- Plan the treatment according to the patient's capacity to accommodate the necessary procedures—if treatment is difficult, will this affect the fit? Misfit and screw-loosening increase the risk of complications due to component wear as well as microbial accumulation.
- Consider the need for later adaptation. Plan implant positions strategically with a view to subsequent conversion to an overdenture.

Conclusions

The provision of implants in older patients, where we can choose a simple approach that can be planned with aging issues in mind, may not necessarily be a problem. The bigger challenge may be how to deal with problems arising with previously successful implants and prostheses in patients who are less fit and able than they were when that treatment was provided. With an increasingly older population and a larger number of very old people, we will more frequently see patients treated with implants that are ailing and prostheses that can no longer be maintained either by the patient (or caregiver) or by the dental professional due to access issues. In addition, there may be medical and psychosocial issues, whose impact is not yet well documented and may be hard to quantify, given the difficulties in performing a multivariate analysis.

Complications will occur; we have a responsibility to try and ensure that they have the least possible impact on the well-being of our patients and that they be, as far as possible, relatively easy to treat.

13 <u>Clinical Case Presentations</u>

13.1 Improving an Existing Implant-supported Denture in an Alzheimer Patient with Bipolar Affective Disorder with Moderate Depression and Dementia

U. Webersberger

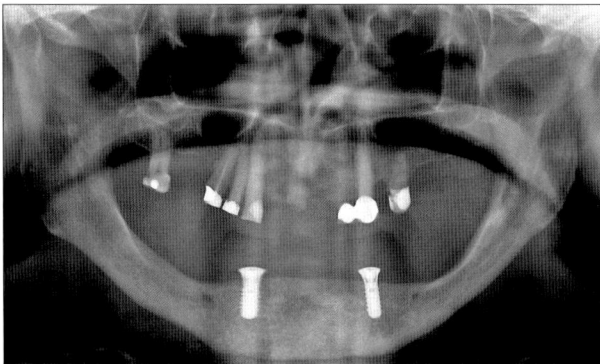

Fig 1 Panoramic radiograph after placement of the two mandibular implants.

An 83-year-old man presented together with his caregiver at the dental department of the Medical University of Innsbruck, Austria with complaints of swelling in the right maxillary canine area and loss of retention of his 5-years-old mandibular denture.

The patient had a significant medical history (20 years) of bipolar affective disorder with moderate depression (F 31.3) and dementia in Alzheimer's disease (F 00.2).

The patient had been in ambulant psychiatric therapy for his depressive illness for the past 20 years. He lived alone and had no children; his sister assisted with daily living. She reported that the patient exhibited compulsive hoarding behavior. In the previous two months, she had noted increasing disorientation and vertigo in the patient. She therefore accompanied him for a medical consultation at the Department of Psychiatry and Psychotherapy of the Medical University of Innsbruck. He was released home after a 6-week inpatient stay. A care allowance was applied and a daily caregiver was organized to help him with his activities of daily living.

The patient's dental history included placement of two Straumann Tissue Level implants (Standard, diameter 4.1, length 10 mm; Institut Straumann AG, Basel, Switzerland) in the interforaminal area 5½ years previously, because the patient experienced eating difficulties due to his ill-fitting lower denture (Fig 1).

After a healing period of 4 months, the mandible received two Straumann Locator attachments and an implant-supported overdenture. Composite fillings were provided in the maxilla. The existing partial denture was left in place because the patient felt comfortable with it.

During this time, the patient showed signs of depression, but was well oriented. With the new mandibular overdenture, he had no more problems eating, swallowing, or speaking. His oral hygiene at the time of insertion was sufficient. After 2 years, Locator replacement males were inserted after a loss of retention in the mandibular denture. After this period, multiple signs of deterioration occurred. Supervision to prevent plaque formation was performed, but daily oral self-care became problematic. The patient became increasingly dependent on assistance. He could not come to a regular dental appointment anymore.

After oral examination and radiographic investigation (Fig 2), the following diagnosis was made:

- Dental abscess resulting from a destroyed maxillary canine.
- Non-salvageable residual dentition.
- Retention loss of the implant-supported mandibular denture because of food impaction in the Locator abutments (Figs 3 to 5).

The patient felt very uncomfortable with the retention loss of his mandibular denture. Given his poor oral hygiene with food impaction around and in the Locator attachments and in the pink retention element of the denture, the patient could no longer insert his denture properly. He was unable to clean the Locator abutments. One reason was that he had lost part of his vision in both eyes and could not see the impacted food. Other reasons included his loss of manual dexterity and his self-consciousness; he felt insecure and was afraid to damage the denture.

After careful evaluation and discussions with the patient and his caregiver, the following treatment plan was proposed:

- Extraction of all remaining teeth.
- Provisional extension of the maxillary partial denture, resulting in a complete denture.
- Modification of the implant-supported mandibular denture with an easy-to handling abutment while maintaining tooth positions.

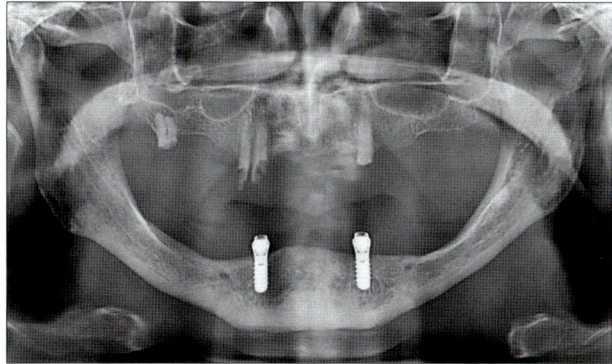

Fig 2   Panoramic radiograph 5 years later.

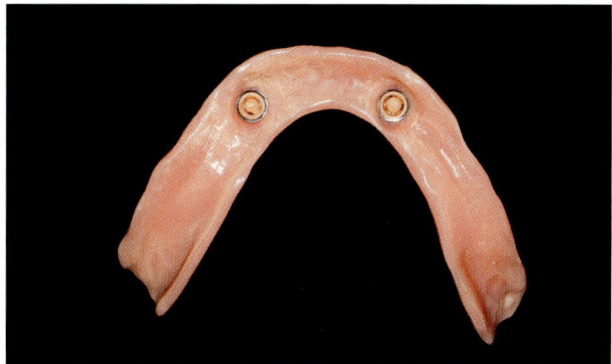

Fig 3   Base of the mandibular denture.

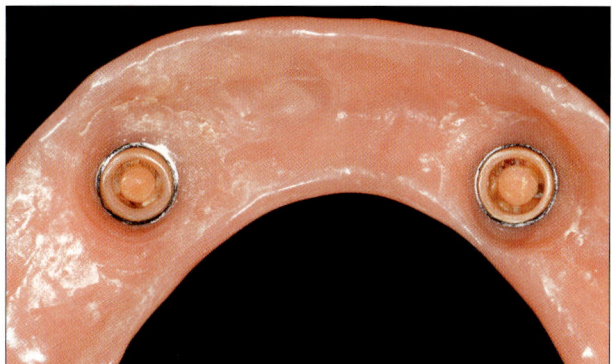

Fig 4   Locator male (in the pink retention element of the denture) with food impaction.

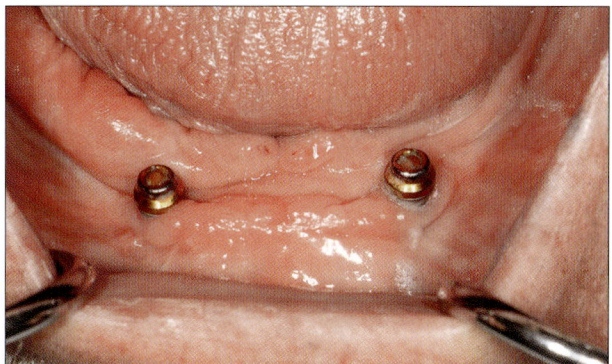

Fig 5   Very poor oral hygiene. Food impaction around and in the Locator attachments.

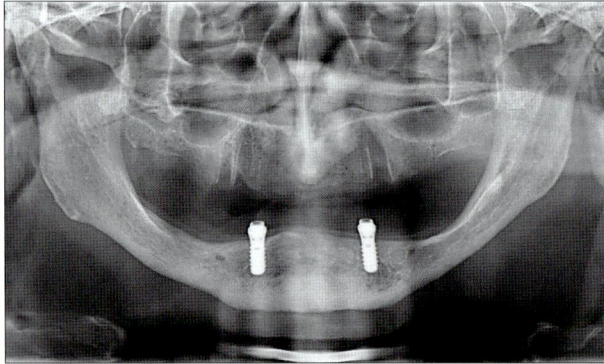

Fig 6 Panoramic radiograph after extraction of the remaining teeth in the maxilla.

The extraction of the remaining teeth in the maxilla (Fig 6) and the insertion of the extended denture proceeded without complications. In the mandible, we decided to keep the denture and merely replace the abutment to keep the changes to a minimum and to spare the patient from having to adapt to a completely new denture. We choose the Straumann Titanmagnetics (Institut Straumann AG, Basel, Switzerland) insert as the new overdenture abutment.

After removing the Locator attachments, the Straumann Titanmagnetics inserts were carefully hand-tightened with the Titanmagnetics insert applicator. The abutments were torqued to 20 Ncm using the Straumann ratchet with torque-control device. Figure 7 shows the Straumann Titanmagnetics inserts placed on the Tissue Level implants.

The maximum torque for tightening the Straumann Titanmagnetics inserts is 15 to 20 Ncm, unlike Locator abutment, for which the torque is 35 Ncm.

After insertion, the positioning cuffs were placed on the Titanmagnetics inserts (Fig 8). They protected the margin of the gingiva and the functional surfaces during polymerization of the Titanmagnetics denture magnet and ensured a resilience of 0.3 mm.

The denture magnets were set into the flat cavity of the positioning cuffs (Fig 9). The mandibular denture was relieved above the magnets. A hollow space was created to let the Titanmagnetics magnets fit correctly under the denture. The fit of the denture was checked in the mouth (Fig 10).

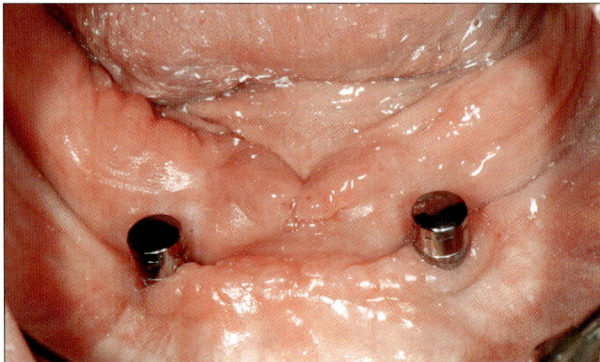

Fig 7 Straumann Titanmagnetics inserts placed on the Tissue Level implants.

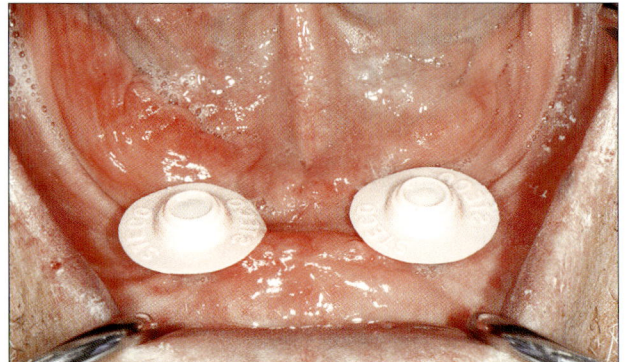

Fig 8 Positioning cuffs on top of the Titanmagnetics inserts.

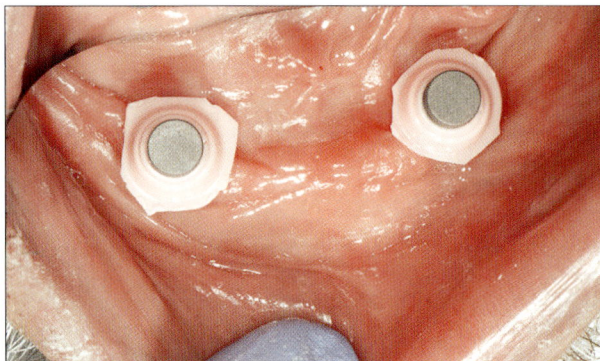

Fig 9 Denture magnets in the flat cavity of the positioning cuffs.

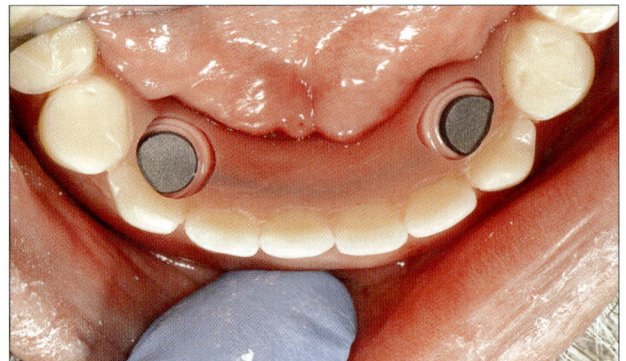

Fig 10 Existing mandibular denture was relieved above the magnets.

The denture magnets were polymerized into the previously created cavities with autopolymerizing methyl methacrylate (Aesthetic Autopolymerisat; Candulor, Wangen, Switzerland). The cold-curing polymer was placed in the cavities on the intaglio side of the denture and placed in the mouth. The patient had to bite hard for about 15 minutes until the polymer had set.

The polymerized magnets in the mandibular denture created a smooth surface, which made it easier to clean for the caregiver and patient using a brush or just running water (Fig 11). The abutments had an even surface, making impaction impossible. Plaque, however, would assemble around the implants and would have to be removed by the caregiver, who had been instructed accordingly.

The patient felt very comfortable wearing the modified denture. Cleaning the Titanmagnetics abutments was no problem for the caregiver. Unfortunately, after a short while the patient became bedridden and could not come to the dental clinic for a check-up. A phone call with the caretaker revealed that the patient still ate with his maxillary denture and helped clean it.

The patient and caretaker were informed that in case of magnetic resonance imaging (MRI) of the head and neck, it was recommended to remove the denture with the magnets. Additionally, the magnetic abutments have to be unscrewed from the implants before an MRI examination of the region (Laurell KA and coworkers 1989; Gegauff and coworkers 1990).

The patient and his caretaker were handed an implant pass to inform the clinic about the type of implant system used and the type of magnets inserted in the event that an MRI was needed.

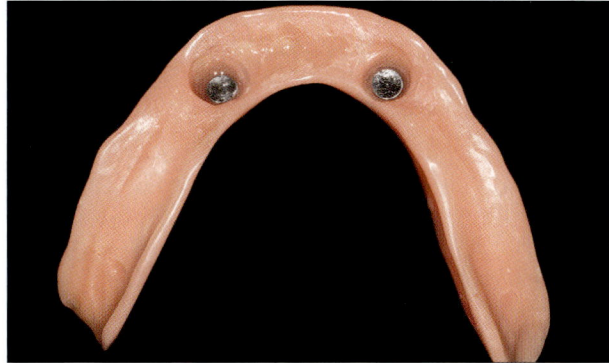

Fig 11   Polymerized magnets in the mandibular denture.

13.2   Maxillary Complete Denture and Mandibular Overdenture on Two Implants with Universal Design

R. Leesungbok

A 78-year-old female patient was referred by the Department of Neurosurgery to the Department of Biomaterials and Prosthodontics of Kyung Hee University Dental Hospital, Gangdong, Seoul, South Korea. The patient was suffering from facial nerve palsy due to an ischemic stroke that had left parts of her eye, chin, lip, tongue, and extremity paralyzed. She had been wearing maxillary and mandibular complete dentures for 10 years, but after the stroke they were not suitable anymore as her mandibular denture became dislodged during function (Figs 1 and 2).

In our aging society, dentures for the disabled and elderly are crucial in terms of patient satisfaction and health-related quality of life. Patients suffer from chronic and severe disorders, and elderly/disabled patients

need special dental care. The provision of dentures using a minimally invasive treatment approach and a universal design are important issues (Leesungbok 2004).

Rules for minimally invasive treatment for the disabled and elderly

- Minimize pain during treatment.
- Minimize the total treatment time.
- Minimize swelling and pain after treatment.
- Minimize the number of implants.
- Load immediately with universal design to achieve immediate oral function.
- Consider fixed prostheses rather than removable prostheses; a fixed prosthesis is the best universal design.

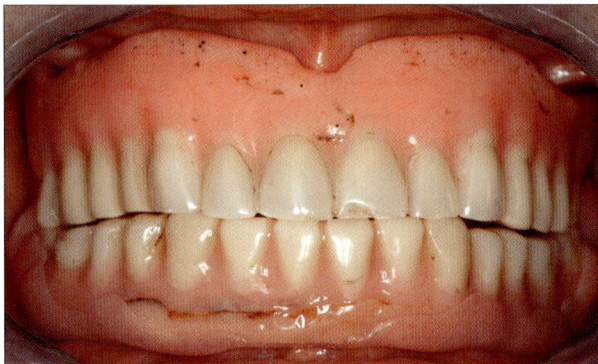

Fig 1   Baseline situation. 78-year-old woman wearing her old maxillary and mandibular complete dentures.

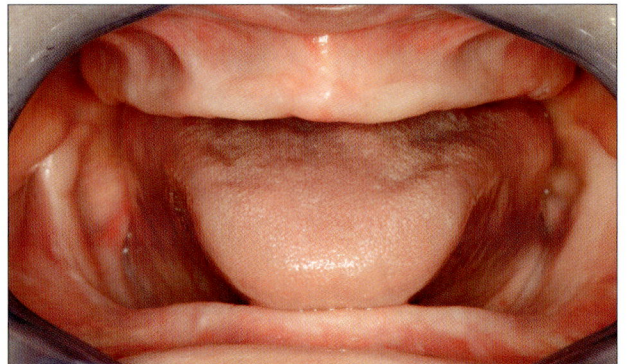

Fig 2   The same patient without the old dentures. Severely atrophied ridges in both jaws.

Universal design strategies for occlusal rehabilitation of the disabled and elderly

- Strategy 1: Fixed restorations on six to eight maxillary and/or four to eight mandibular implants (Fig 3).
- Strategy 2: Overdentures on four maxillary and/or two to four mandibular implants (Fig 4).
- Strategy 3: Maxillary complete denture and mandibular one-piece fixed restoration on four implants (Fig 5).
- Strategies 4a and b: Maxillary complete denture and mandibular overdenture on two implants (Figs 6 and 7).

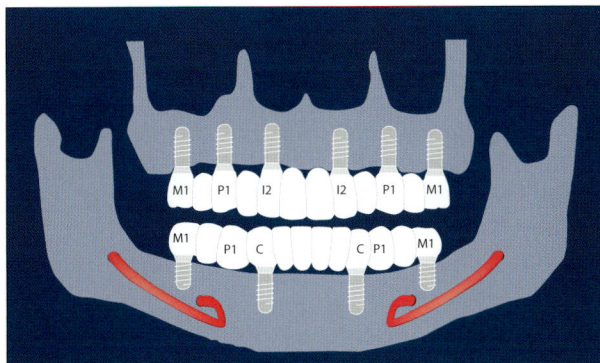

Fig 3   Strategy 1: Fixed restorations on six to eight maxillary and/or four to eight mandibular implants.

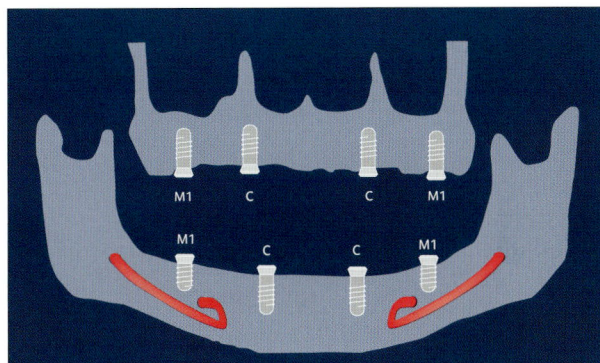

Fig 4   Strategy 2: Overdentures on four maxillary and/or two to four mandibular implants.

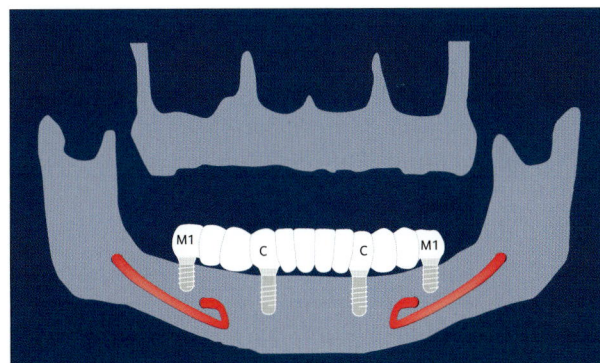

Fig 5   Strategy 3: Maxillary complete denture and mandibular one-piece fixed restoration on four implants.

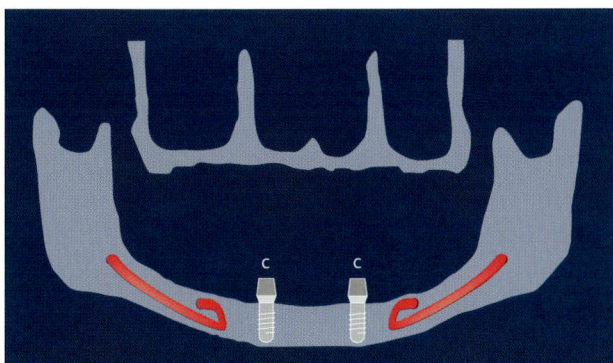

Fig 6   Strategy 4a: Maxillary complete denture and mandibular overdenture on two implants with single abutments.

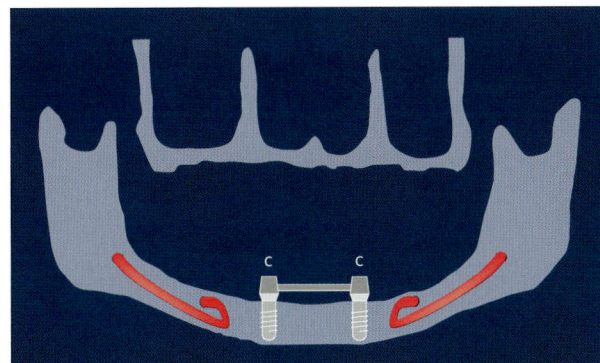

Fig 7   Strategy 4b: Maxillary complete denture and mandibular overdenture on two implants connected with a bar in a severely atrophied mandible.

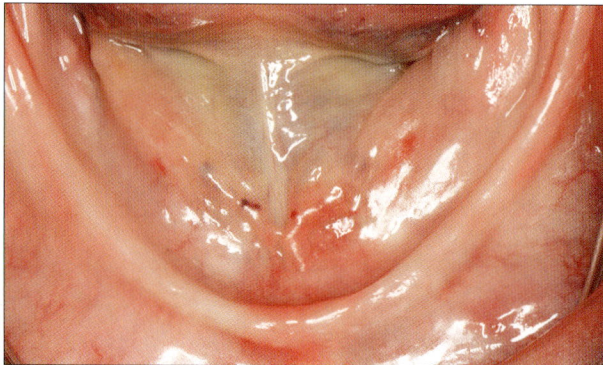

Fig 8 Occlusal view before surgery. Vertically and horizontally atrophied ridge, especially in the mandible.

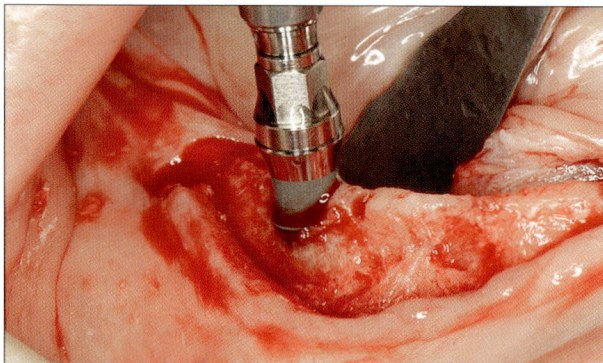

Fig 9 Two implants (Straumann Tissue Level, SLA) were placed on the site of canines after raising a full-thickness flap. One keeper abutment (IP; Aichi Steel, Tokai, Japan) connected to the right implant.

At baseline, the patient presented with severely atrophied ridges, with reduced vertical height and horizontal width in both jaws. According to strategy 4a (Fig 6), in the case of severely atrophied edentulous maxillary and mandibular jaws, a complete maxillary denture and a mandibular overdenture on two implants are recommended as a minimally invasive treatment option, especially for elderly disabled patients (Fig 8).

Surgical and prosthodontic procedure

- Top-down treatment planning—selecting a strategic option for elderly-disabled patient
- Minimally invasive surgery
- Immediate loading with universal design to achieve immediate oral function
- Periodic recalls

In a U-shaped mandibular arch, if two implants are to be placed on the ridge, the sites of canines or first premolars are recommended as implant sites (Fig 9). Two Tissue Level SLA implants (RN, diameter 4.1 mm, length 10 mm; Straumann, Basel, Switzerland) were placed at the canine sites after raising a full-thickness flap. The insertion torque was more than 35 Ncm for both implants. Immediate loading by a removable overdenture is possible with this torque value. One magnetic so-called keeper abutment (IP; Aichi Steel, Tokai, Japan) was connected to the right implant at a torque of with 25 Ncm (Fig 10). The other keeper abutment (also IP) was connected on the left implant at a torque of 25 Ncm. The flap was sutured completely (Fig 11).

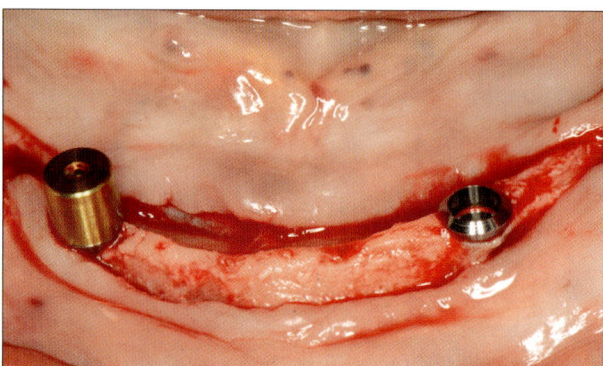

Fig 10 Two implants (Straumann Tissue Level, SLA, RN, diameter 4.1 mm, length 10 mm) were placed on the site of canines after raising a full-thickness flap. One keeper abutment (IP; Aichi Steel, Tokai, Japan) connected to the right implant.

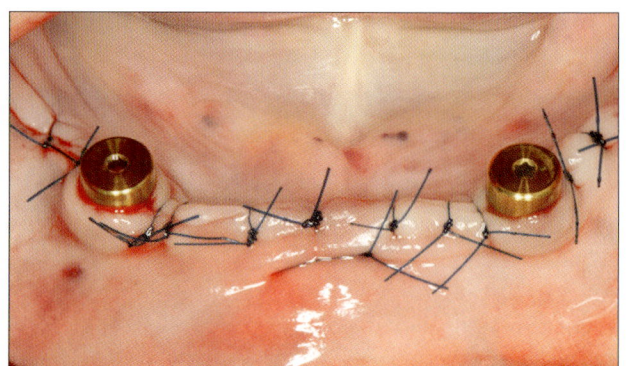

Fig 11 The other keeper abutment (also IP) connected on the left implant. Sutured flap.

Figure 12 shows a flexible and self-adjusting magnetic attachment (Magfit-SX 800; Aichi Steel). Rubber dam was placed over the keeper abutment to block out the undercut area and as a separator. Magfit-SX 800 attachments with spacers were placed on the keeper abutments (Fig 13).

Pink acrylic resin was poured into the voids of the prepared overdenture (Fig 14). The overdenture was positioned exactly and held in place until the resin has set completely (Fig 15). After the resin had fully set, the overdenture was removed from the mouth. The metal 0.4-mm spacer was removed from the magnetic attachment surface (Fig 16).

The spacers were removed from the attachment, and the mucosal surface was finished as needed (Figs 17 and 18).

Figure 19 shows the situation after insertion of the maxillary complete denture and mandibular magnetic overdenture as a typical example of a universal design for elderly and disabled patients (Fig 19). The patient had suffered from facial paralysis for more than five years (Fig 20). Functional movements, including chewing and wide opening, were tested. The maxillary complete denture and mandibular magnetic overdenture worked very well and were easily handled by the patient, who was highly satisfied with the universal design (Fig 21).

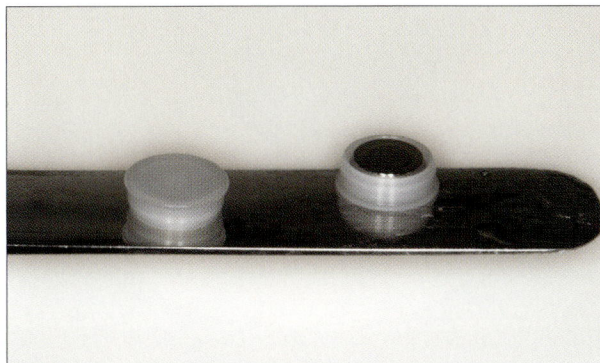

Fig 12   Flexible self-adjusting magnetic attachment (Magfit-SX 800; Aichi Steel).

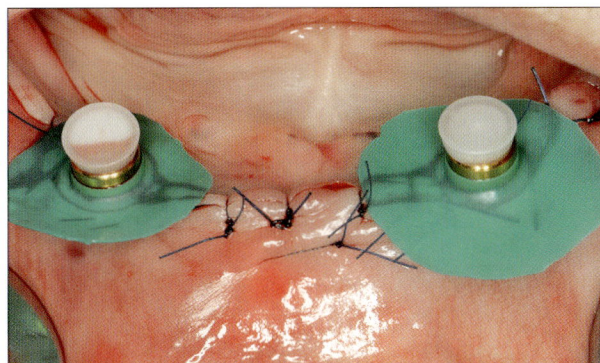

Fig 13   Rubber dam around and Magfit-SX 800 attachments with spacers on the keeper abutments.

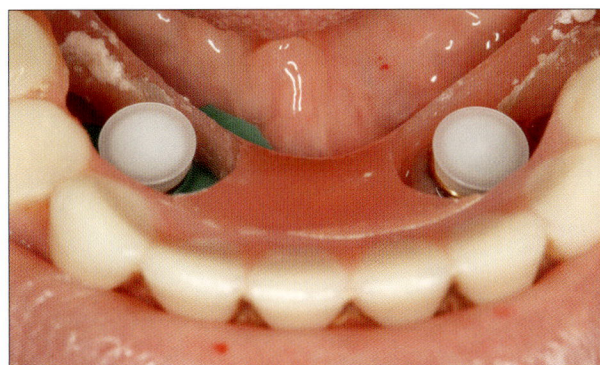

Fig 14   Voids of the prepared overdenture before pouring pink acrylics.

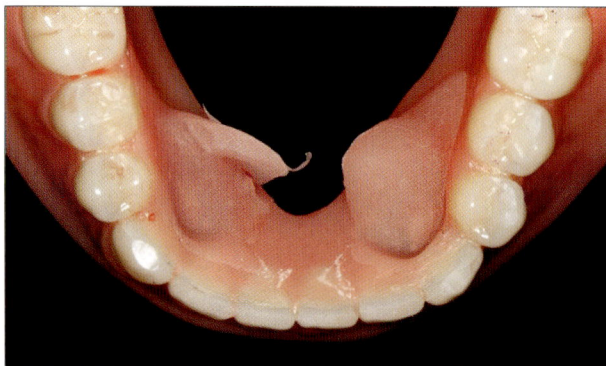

Fig 15   The resin has set completely.

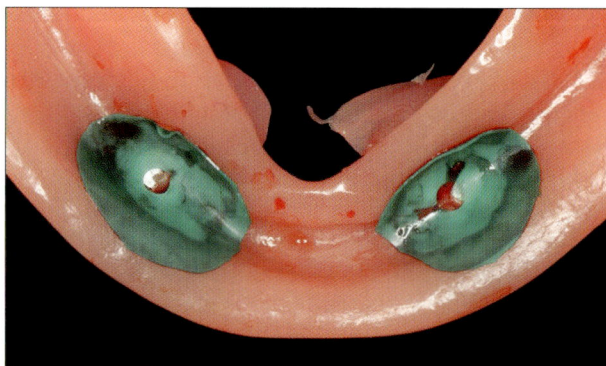

Fig 16   Tissue side of the overdenture before removal of the rubber dam and spacers.

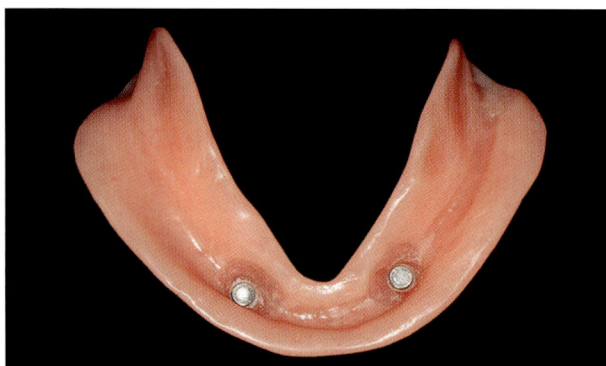

Fig 17   Tissue side of the definite overdenture with rubber dam and spacers removed.

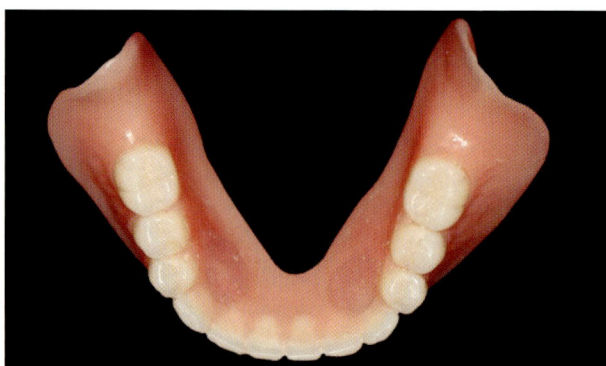

Fig 18   Occlusal view of the definite overdenture after completed finishing and polishing.

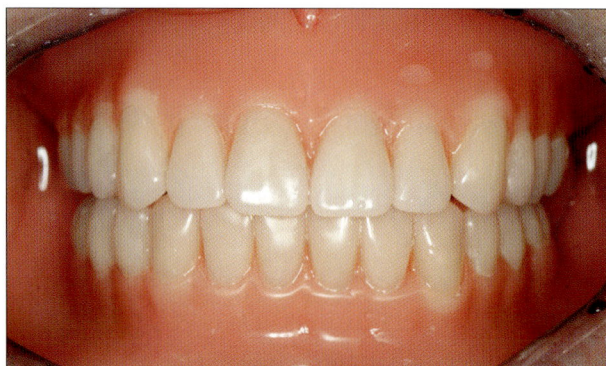

Fig 19   Inserted maxillary complete denture and mandibular magnetic overdenture.

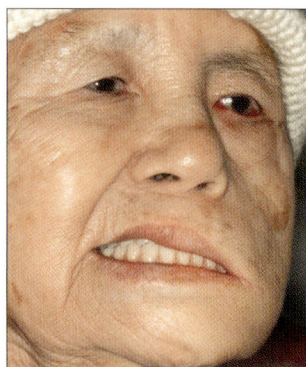

Fig 20   The patient had been suffering from a facial paralysis for 10 years.

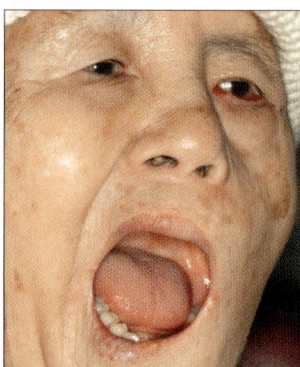

Fig 21   Maxillary complete denture and mandibular magnetic overdenture in situ.

Figure 22 is a panoramic radiograph taken directly after the placement of the two implants in the mandible. There were no complications at the six-year follow-up (Figs 23 and 24).

Discussion

Prevalence of complete or partial edentulousness. Fully edentulous patients are becoming less frequent thanks to advancements in dental health and dental care. According to the National Oral Health Survey released in South Korea in 2000, 26.8% of patients aged 65 to 74 years presented with a fully edentulous maxilla, 19.63% with a fully edentulous mandible). In 2006, the corresponding figures had decreased to 21.6% in the maxilla and 14.3% in the mandible—a drop of more than five percentage points in just 6 years.

As dental implants become increasingly popular, implant overdentures in fully edentulous cases have been shown to give greater patient satisfaction and better function than conventional complete dentures. The number of fully edentulous patients has been steadily declining, while the number of partially edentulous patients has been rising and the period of partial edentulism has been prolonged—and the treatment paradigm for partial edentulism is changing.

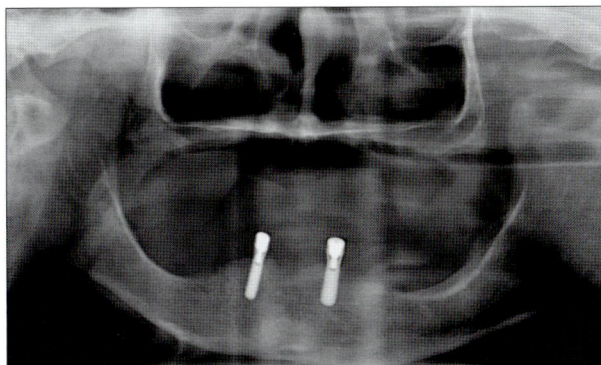

Fig 22   Panoramic radiograph taken directly after the placement of the two implants in the mandible.

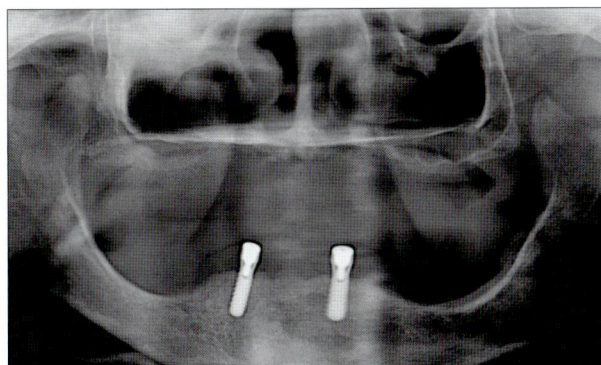

Fig 23   Follow-up panoramic radiograph after 6 years of wearing the mandibular magnetic overdenture supported by the two implants.

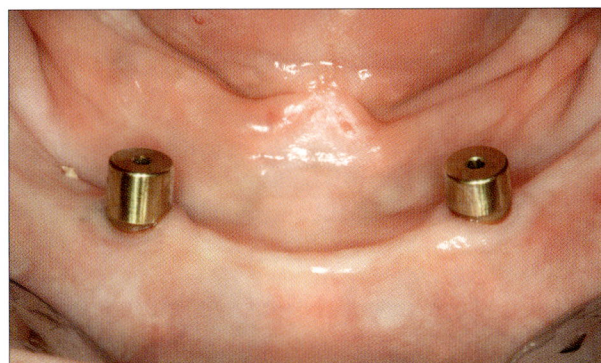

Fig 24   Six-year follow-up. Keeper abutments for the mandibular magnetic overdenture as a universal design.

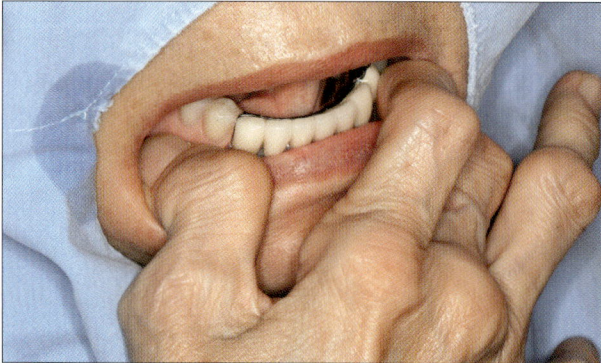

Fig 25   Dentures for the disabled and elderly play a crucial part in patient satisfaction and oral health-related quality of life.

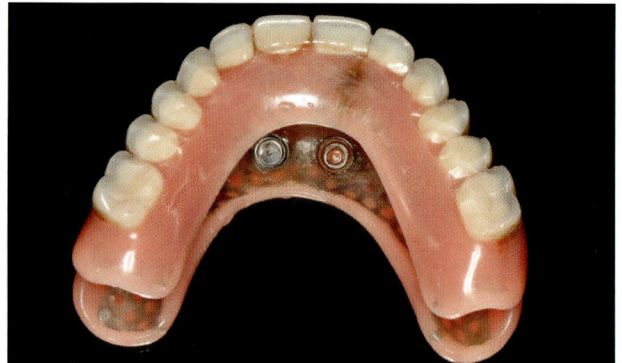

Fig 26   An 82-year-old elderly disabled patient had worn this implant-supported maxillary overdenture made at a local dental clinic 2 years previously.

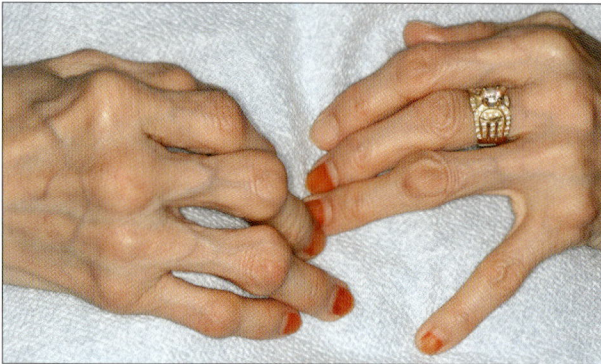

Fig 27   Dental care and denture treatment with a universal design should be considered especially for elderly or disabled people.

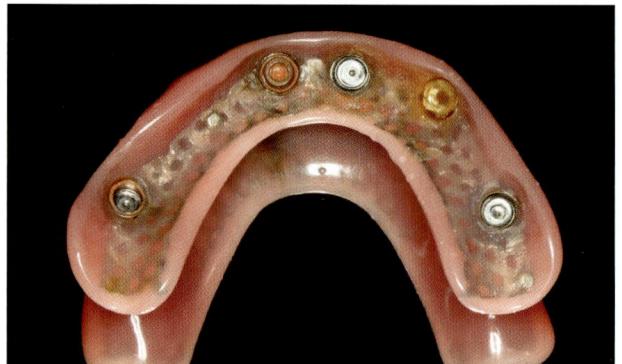

Fig 28   This overdenture had originally contained 5 Locator retentions. Only one retentive device remained because the patient mishandled the denture during insertion/removal due to her manual handicap.

Universal design. The philosophy of universal design refers to the design that can be used for everyone. Devices, facilities, and equipment designed barrier-free can be readily used by non-disabled people (nurses, assistants, family members, friends, etc.) as well as by disabled people. Universal design makes dental appliances accessible to everyone without difficulty, regardless of possible disabilities (North Carolina State University 1997; Harpur 2013; Figs 25 to 28).

The seven principles of universal design are:

1   Equitable use
2   Flexibility in use
3   Simple and intuitive
4   Perceptible information
5   Tolerance for error
6   Low physical effort
7   Size and space for approach and use

Magnet-retained overdentures for the disabled and elderly. The production quality and the physical properties of the materials generally depend greatly the skill and precision levels of the manufacturer. Great skill and expertise are required to manufacture friction-type mechanical retainers. And while the friction between the metal and the elasticity of the metal/plastic retainer components may initially show high performance level, these retainers wear out after many insertion/removal procedures or exhibit damage or deformation due to physical fatigue. Some components are highly durable, but this cannot conceal the fact that there will be a functional decline. Moreover, they can be especially difficult to use by elderly or disabled patients (Riley and coworkers 2001). The author has used many types of the magnetic attachments clinically during the past 20 years and defines magnetic attachments as "retentive devices on prostheses using magnetic attractive force formed between the magnet (magnetic assembly) and the stainless-steel keeper."

There are three different types of devices that use magnetism clinically for retention in dentistry (Fig 29):

1   Devices that use repulsion between same-name magnetic poles with an open magnetic circuit.
2   Devices that use attraction between different-name magnetic poles with an open magnetic circuit (Fig 29a).
3   Devices that use a stainless-steel keeper that attaches to the magnet with a closed magnetic circuit (Figs 29b-c).

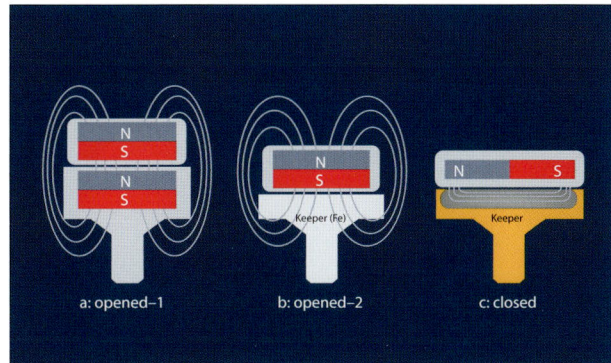

Fig 29   One type 2 device and two type 3 devices. (a) Magnet and magnet, using attraction between different-name magnetic poles, open magnetic circuit. (b) Magnet and keeper, open magnetic circuit. (c) Magnet and keeper, closed magnetic circuit.

The repulsion method (type 1) is infrequently used in orthodontics at this point. Type 2 has been tested widely by researchers—but a pair of magnets requires much space that is unnecessary clinically, raises the issue of protecting the main magnet, and does not necessarily double the attractive force when the two magnets are attached physically (Fig 30). Therefore, as in type 3, one side of the magnet should be used with a keeper. The keeper itself is not a magnet, but when placed in a magnetic field it is magnetized, with the two components attracting each other; this design minimizes the vertical height. When the keeper is removed from the magnetic field, it becomes an ordinary bit of stainless steel again, rather than acting as a magnet (Maeda and coworkers 2005a; Hasegawa and coworkers 2011; Figs 31 to 33).

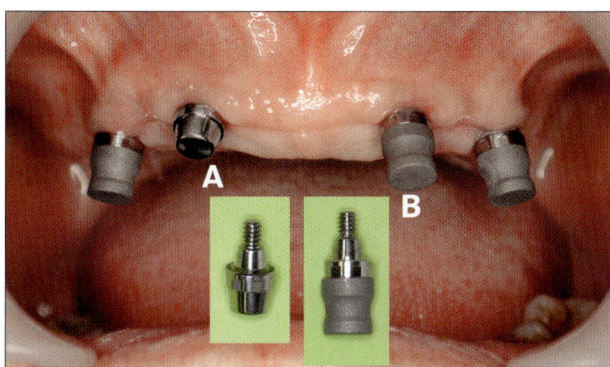

Fig 30   A pair of magnets (Steco, Hamburg, Germany) used as in type 2 requires unnecessarily much space. A = magnetic abutment; B = magnetic cap.

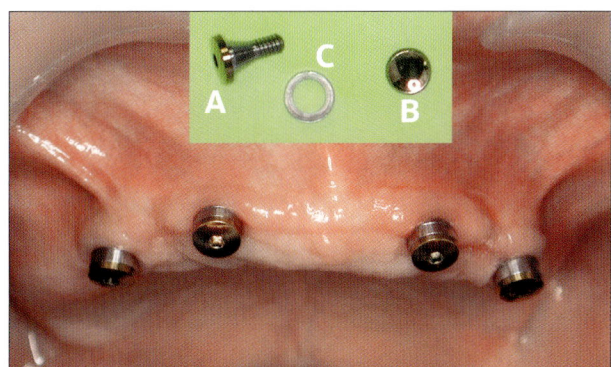

Fig 31   In type 3, one side of the magnet (Magfit, Aichi Steel) is used with stainless-steel keeper. A = stainless-steel keeper abutment; B = magnetic assembly (magnet encapsulated by stainless steel); C = stainless-steel keeper ring.

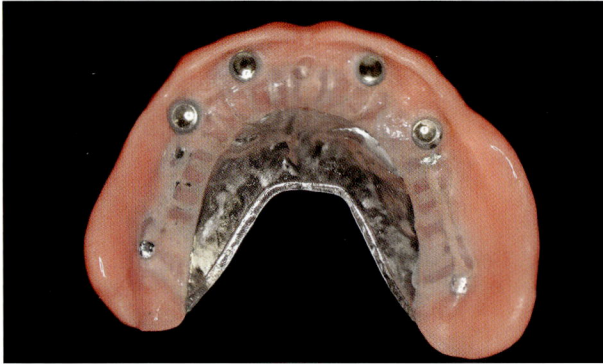

Fig 32   Mucosal surface of a typical universal-design overdenture with magnetic attachments for the patient in Figure 31.

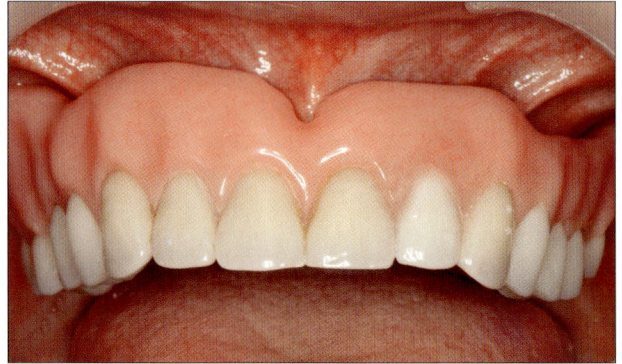

Fig 33   No complications at the 8-year follow-up. Facial view of the same universal-design overdenture as in Figure 32.

For many years, aluminum-nickel-cobalt magnets with open magnetic fields have been used in dentistry as retentive devices, but success had been limited because these magnets were susceptible to corrosion by saliva and because their retentive force is weaker than the initial retention offered by mechanical attachments.

In recent years, magnets made from alloys of the rare-earth elements samarium and neodymium have gained in popularity, since they provide a stronger magnetic force per unit size and can be hermetically encapsulated by stainless-steel housings to resist corrosion and tarnishing in the intraoral environment. Due to the greater attractive force (8 – 10 N), despite their smaller volume and because they are free of corrosion, magnetic attachments have the potential for increased durability and have been shown to be superior to other popular mechanical retentive devices (ball and socket, bar and clip attachments) for removable prostheses on implants (Akin and coworkers 2011).

Double crowns, highly functional as retainers, also require a high level of technical skills to make. Technicians encounter challenges such as having to ensure a careful balance or perform delicate soldering on most precision attachment systems. The magnetic attachment used as a denture retainer is not only a good substitute for the mechanical-frictional retainers, but also offers other practical advantages based on the specification of the magnet presented here:

- It does not show damage or abrasion as mechanical retainers do and can thus be used for prolonged periods without a decrease in retention.
- It is flexible in denture design and manufacturing, since the direction of force is not strictly fixed.

- It has an esthetic appearance, since it is embedded into the denture.
- It is easy to handle and to keep clean, especially for elderly or handicapped patients, as the denture design is not complex.
- Because the attractive force weakens rapidly when the magnetic assembly and keeper create a gap on the attached surface as the range of normal oral function is exceeded, the risk of harmful stress to the tooth or implant can be reduced effectively compared to other mechanical retainers.
- It is easy to repair damaged components of the magnetic attachment by simply exchanging them.

Conclusion

Since dental implants were first used as artificial roots to support restorations in edentulous sites, treatment planning for prostheses has changed significantly. Where there used to be no alternative but to employ removable dentures on the distal-extension side of a partially edentulism jaw, dental implants have created a revolutionary tooth-replacement option for those patients. Dental implants in a partially or completely edentulous alveolar ridge have revolutionized our treatment options for removable dentures and evolved into a new treatment paradigm where natural teeth and implants coexist in the same mouth.

In a case study at the Department of Biomaterials and Prosthodontics of Kyung Hee University Dental Hospital, Heki and Gangdong, Seoul, South Korea, the universal design resulted in greater patient satisfaction than conventional dentures or overdentures with frictional-type retainers.

13.3 Improving a Centenarian's Quality of Life

M. Schimmel

In 2007, a 97-year-old patient presented for treatment at the Geneva Dental School. His dentist had retired. Like many elderly patients, he was left without regular dental care. He lived on a geriatric ward, as he was partly dependent on help with most of the activities of daily living (ADL), such as getting dressed, washing, taking a shower, or climbing stairs. However, he was able to go to the bathroom and get up from bed on his own (ADL score 80, min. 18, max. 126; a low score signifies a high degree of dependency) (Lawton and Brody 1969). He was not bound to a wheelchair, but used a walker. Moreover, he was socially highly active—his family visited on a regular basis and he often went to the restaurant with his friend, who was some 20 years younger. His cognitive function did not seem to be impaired in a normal conversation, although his MMSE score was only 21/30 at that time (Folstein and coworkers 1975). The patient was a retired pharmacist, and his latest passion was astronomy.

His medical history revealed a myocardial infarction 15 years before the first visit; he received dilatation of the coronal vessels in 1992 and 1996. In 2002, he suffered from transitional stroke symptoms, which at the time were attributed to a sclerosis of the right carotid artery. Consequently, the affected artery was dilated and a stent placed. He also suffered from bilateral glaucoma and cataract. These medical conditions resulted in a long list of daily medications: paracetamol (1,500 mg/day), spironolactone (a diuretic), clopidogrel (a platelet-aggregation inhibitor), molsidomin (a coronary vasodilator), acetazolamide (a treatment for glaucoma), macrogol (a laxative), omeprazole (a treatment for gastroesophageal reflux disease), pravastatin (a statin), torasemide (a loop diuretic), carteolol (a glaucoma treatment and non-selective beta blocker), nitroglycerin (a coronary vasodilator), and a carbamide ointment.

The patient was very happy about the prospect of improving his unsatisfying dental situation. He took pleasure in his frequent visits to the Dental School, as this interrupted his daily routine on the ward.

His dental history revealed the extraction of his last mandibular tooth and insertion of a complete conventional denture two years before. The removable partial prosthesis (RPP) in the maxilla had been made 5 years before the first consultation.

The patient's oral health-related quality of life (OHRQoL) was moderately reduced, with an OHIP-EDENT score of 25/60 (where a high score means a low OHRQoL) (Allen and Locker 2002). Regarding his satisfaction with his dental prostheses, he claimed that they were easy to clean and that he liked their esthetics. He stated in the Denture Satisfaction Questionnaires (Rashid and coworkers 2011) that he was moderately satisfied with them overall but had difficulties speaking, eating white bread, hard cheese, raw carrots, dried sausages, apples, and steak—primarily because of the unstable lower denture. He would mostly swallow those food items unchewed.

The intraoral examination revealed a cantilever bridge in the maxilla, a ball attachment on the root of tooth 23, and a residual root of tooth 25 (Fig 1). The mandible was edentulous, but with a healthy mucosa. Denture hygiene was improvable, with a score of 9 out of 15 for the max-

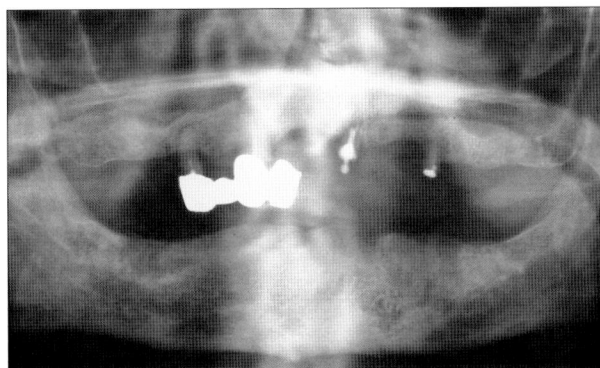

Fig 1   Baseline panoramic radiograph. Two hopeless teeth (15 and 22) and two other teeth that could support an overdenture. The interforaminal bone height was sufficient to accommodate two implants.

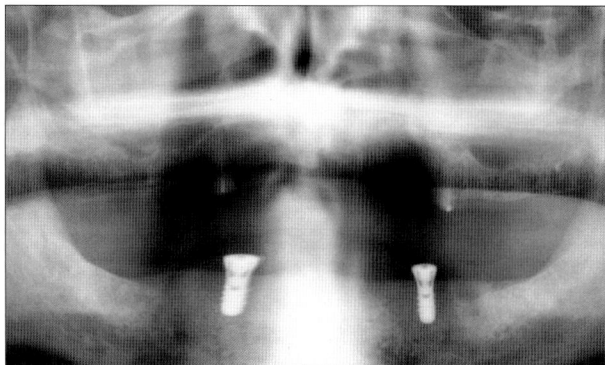

Fig 2   Two short implants were placed and left to heal transmucosally.

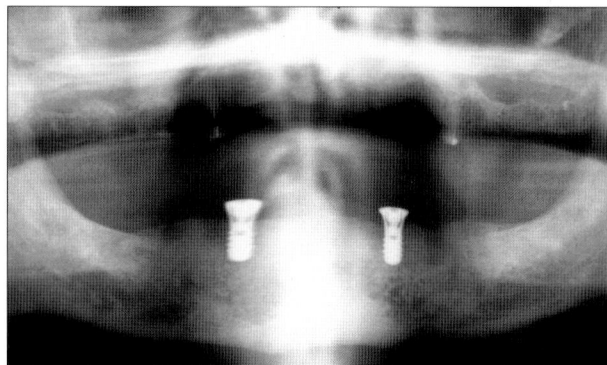

Fig 3   Implant 33 had not osseointegrated, probably due to premature loading. A replacement implant was placed slightly mesially of the original surgical site.

illary prosthesis; as he never wore his mandibular denture, no denture plaque index was recorded here. The saliva flow rate (SFR) after a 2-minute collection period was low at 2 ml stimulated and 1 ml unstimulated.

Taking the radiological findings into account, it was decided to transform the remaining maxillary RPD into a root-supported overdenture on roots 23 and 25. The maxillary denture was to be relined conventionally.

In October 2007, teeth 15 and 22 were extracted. The remaining two roots in the maxilla were decapitated and covered with a hybrid composite resin. The RPP was transformed into a root-supported overdenture by adding the missing teeth and relining the denture with polymethyl methacrylate using an indirect technique. The same procedure was applied to reline the mandibular complete denture (CD) in a second stage.

One year after this treatment, the patient did not feel he had seen the improvement he had hoped for. He desired to receive implants to stabilize his mandibular prosthesis.

The surgical procedure (standard protocol for transgingival healing) was performed in mid-December 2009. Two interforaminal implants were placed at sites 33 and 43 (Straumann SLA, RN, diameter 4.1 mm, length 8 mm; Institut Straumann AG; Fig 2) according to the standard protocol (Payne and coworkers 2010).

Seven days after the surgery, the sutures were removed and the mandibular prosthesis modified to avoid mechanical interference with the healing abutments. The patient was advised not to wear his mandibular denture during this initial healing period. It was agreed to load the implants and connect the abutments after a 6- to 8-week period (Gallucci and coworkers 2014).

In February 2009, the patient presented for the agreed procedure. He reported that he had not worn his dentures during the entire healing period (7 weeks). He had enjoyed a four-week holiday in a Hotel in the Swiss Mountains and, therefore, wanted to rule out any complications with the implants. But when loading implant 33, it became obvious that osseointegration had not taken place and, therefore, the implant was removed. During the same visit, another 8-mm Straumann implant (SLA, 4.1 mm RN) was inserted slightly mesially of the original site (Fig 3). The patient was instructed not to wear his mandibular complete denture for two weeks. The sutures were removed after 7 days.

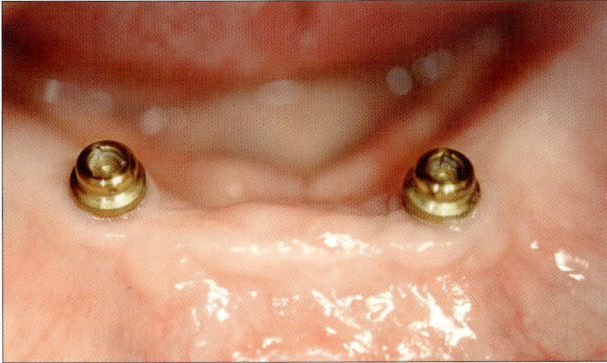

Fig 4 The implants were loaded using Locator attachments.

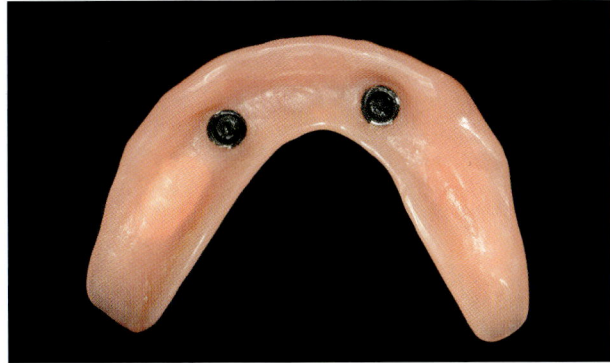

Fig 5 Even the insert with the lowest retentive force of the Locator system was too strong for the patient to handle. Therefore, the patient was discharged with the laboratory inserts, which have an acceptably low retention but cannot withstand the intraoral environment for long.

At the end of March 2009, the patient was seen for implant loading. This time, both implants were osseointegrated and the mandibular complete denture was transformed into an implant-supported overdenture (IOD) using Locator attachments (Zest Anchors, Escondido, CA, USA; Figs 4 to 6). Again, the patient had not worn his dentures for 6 weeks to avoid complications.

After stabilization of the mandibular prosthesis by two Straumann implants and Locator abutments, the patient was extremely pleased with his oral appearance and function. The OHIP-EDENT score dropped to 1/60, indicating a highly improved OHRQoL. In the Denture Satisfaction Questionnaire, he indicated maximum satisfaction with the IOD. He had no more problems speaking and stated that he would even eat hard cheese or dried sausages without any difficulty; his capacity to eat white bread, steak, apples, and salad had improved. The patient felt that he now chewed his food properly before swallowing. However, the three-month control revealed insufficient implant hygiene, and instructions were given to ameliorate the oral-hygiene situation. His SFR had improved and was stable at 3 ml stimulated and 1.5 ml unstimulated. At the one-year control, the denture hygiene was quite good, with scores of 4/15 and 2/15 for the maxillary and mandibular prosthesis, respectively.

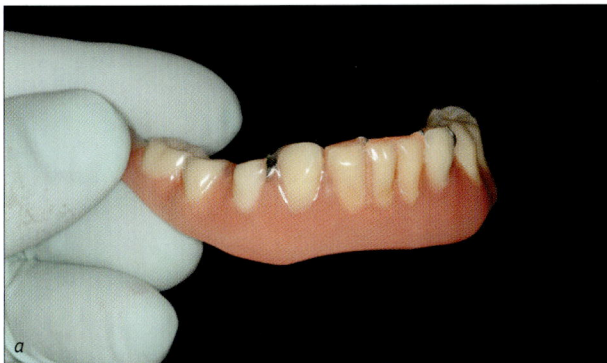

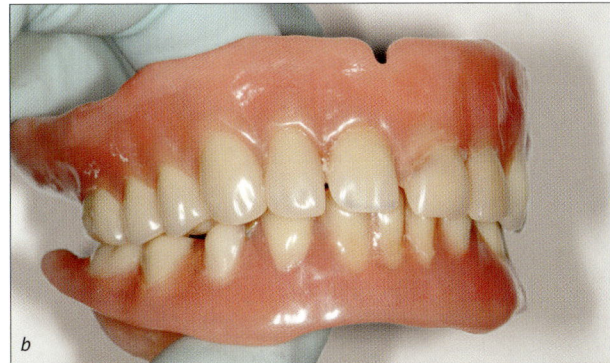

Figs 6a-b The converted prosthesis was old and worn, but the patient was well adapted to functioning with it. In very old patients, compromises often have to be accepted in terms of denture design, as adaptive capacity decreases with age.

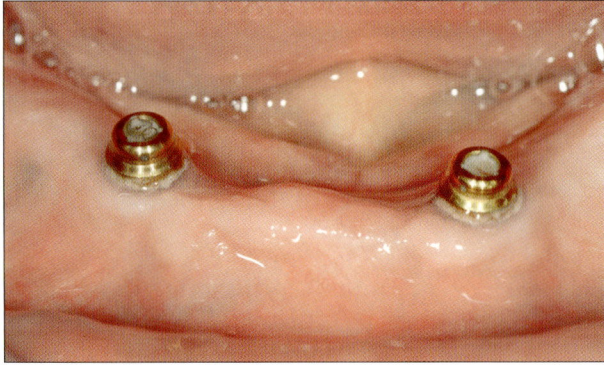

Fig 7   There was always plaque around the attachments and in the central retentive hole. The inflammatory signs were surprisingly weak.

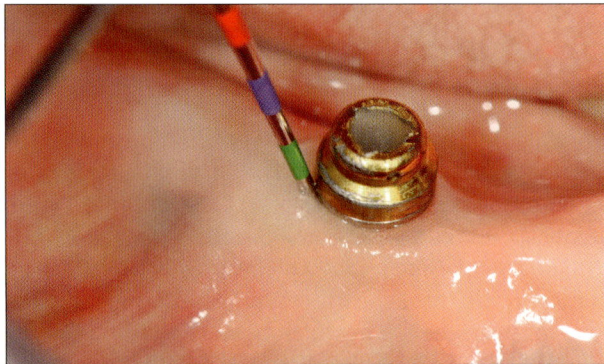

Fig 8   Central hole obturated to prevent food impaction. Despite high plaque scores, there were no clinical signs of peri-implantitis.

Plaque was always present, but the plaque score was remarkably low when taking into account his dependency for ADLs (Fig 7). Still, the implant probing depths never exceeded 2 mm at any site, even after 4 years of the IOD in situ.

The low inflammatory response corresponded to the stable peri-implant bone, as noted in the radiographs.

At the one-year appointment, it was evident that residual food remained in the central holes of the Locator-abutments. Thus, the hole was obturated with temporary inlay material (Telio; Ivoclar Vivadent, Schaan, Liechtenstein; Fig 8). The red Locator inserts without a central pin were provided to retain the prosthesis.

Figures 9a-d show the follow-up radiographs taken 2009 through 2012.

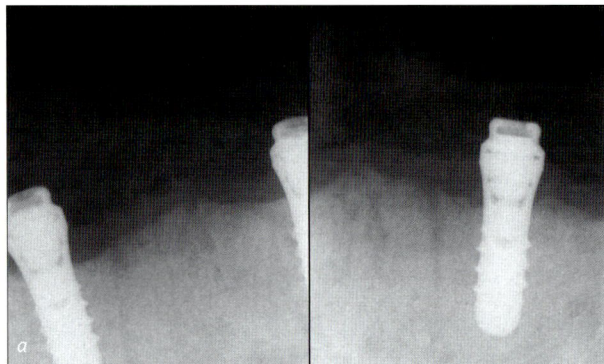

Figs 9a-d   Stable peri-implant bone conditions and no signs of peri-implantitis around sites 43 and 33 on these follow-up radiographs taken 2009 (a), 2010 (b), 2011 (c), and 2012 (d).

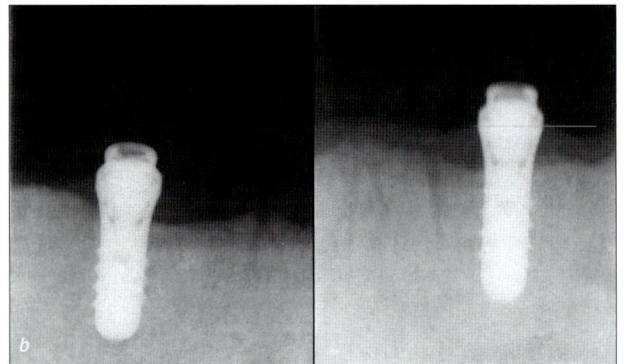

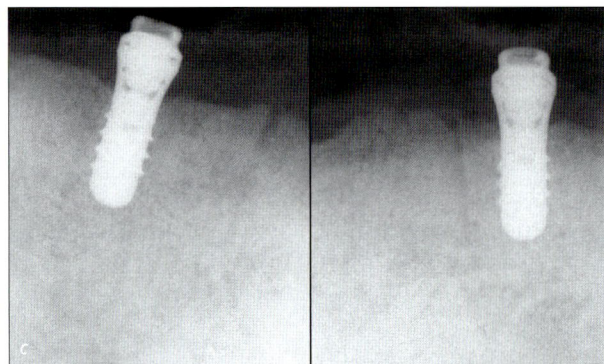

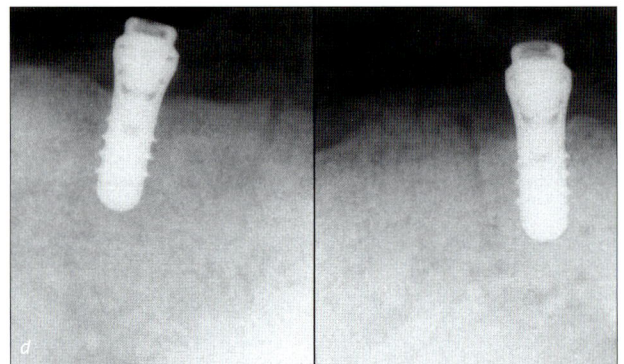

The patient was last seen at the dental clinic at age 101 (Fig 10). His cognitive functions had further declined, and he had a MMSE score of 18/27. He was almost blind by that time and highly dependent in his ADLs. However, he was still eating by himself and had remained socially active. His OHIP score was still low at 13/60, and he reported being very satisfied with his denture. He enjoyed hard cheese but would still not eat carrots, apples, steak, or salad.

The patient passed away at the age of 103. He had benefited from implant therapy for over five years and never regretted the decision.

Disclosure

The patient had participated in an ITI-funded RCT on the stabilization of complete dentures in dependently living older adults (Müller and coworkers 2013). The effect of denture abstention on masseter muscle thickness has been published as a case report (Schimmel and coworkers 2010).

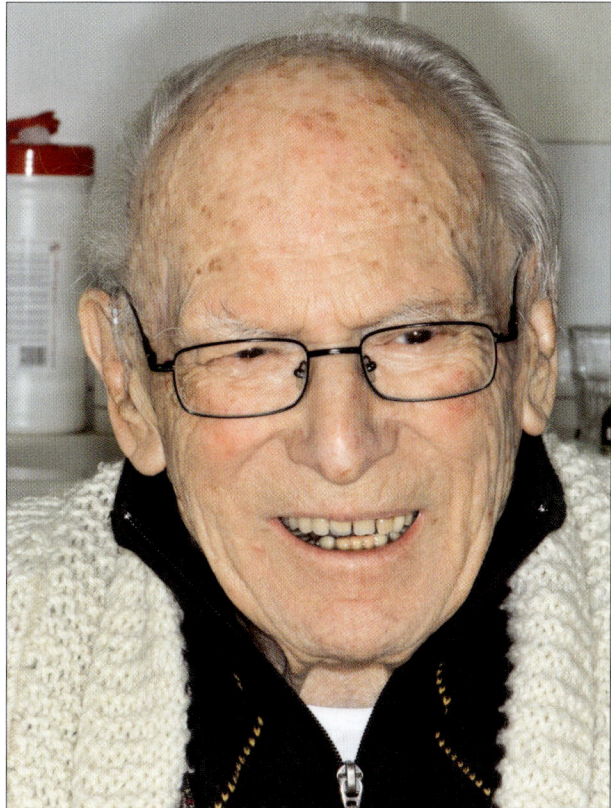

Fig 10   The patient at age 101.

13.4 Oral Rehabilitation of an Elderly Edentulous Patient with Osteoarthritis Using an Implant-supported Mandibular Prosthesis with Locator Abutments

G. McKenna

A 78-year-old man was referred to the dental hospital by his general dental practitioner. He was a non-smoker but was taking a number of medications as prescribed by his general medical practitioner, including atorvastatin-calcium for high cholesterol, lisinopril and hydrochlorothiazide for hypertension, warfarin as an anticoagulant, and metformin for the management of type 2 diabetes. The patient also suffered from osteoarthritis in both hands (Fig 1). The patient was edentulous in the maxilla and partially dentate in the mandible. A mandibular acrylic partial lower denture had been recently delivered but was poorly tolerated.

On presentation, an extraoral examination revealed nothing adverse. Intraorally, the soft tissues were healthy, with little evidence of oral dryness. The remaining mandibular dentition consisted of teeth 34–44 and the retained roots of teeth 45 and 48. The teeth were heavily restored, and teeth 34–31 all showed grade 2 mobility. A panoramic radiograph was taken (Fig 2). An initial treatment plan called for extracting the teeth with a hopeless prognosis and constructing a well-fitting mandibular partial denture after a suitable period of healing.

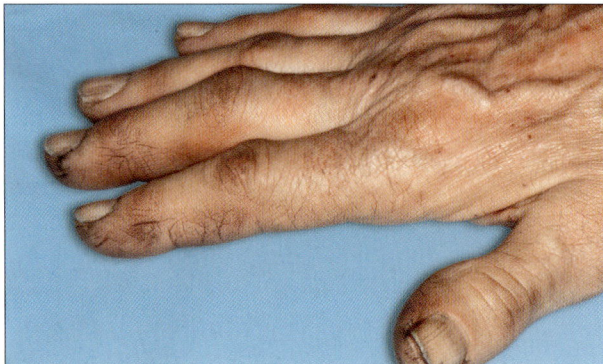

Fig 1 Patient's hand.

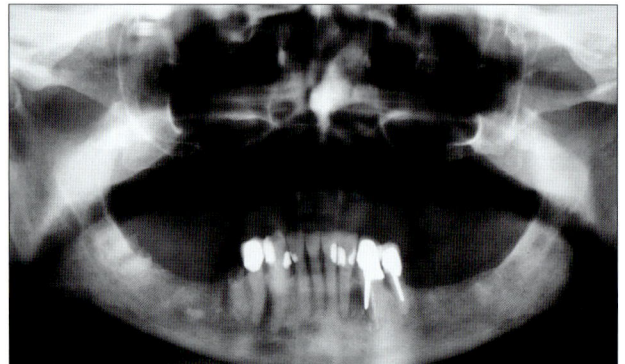

Fig 2 Panoramic radiograph at the initial presentation.

Twelve months after this treatment, the patient returned, reporting difficulties in wearing his mandibular partial denture. A clinical examination and a panoramic radiograph revealed that tooth 44 had decoronated and that recurrent caries was present in teeth 41 and 42. The remaining mandibular incisors now showed grade 2 mobility (Fig 3), and their prognosis was very poor.

The hopeless prognosis for the remaining teeth was discussed with the patient and a revised treatment plan developed. This included:

- Extraction of the remaining teeth and provision of a mandibular complete immediate denture.
- After 6 months of healing, placement of two implants at sites 33 and 43 under intravenous sedation with midazolam.
- Provision of an implant-retained maxillary overdenture on Locator abutments (Straumann, Basel, Switzerland).
- Provision of a new maxillary complete conventional denture.

Eight weeks later, the maxillary denture was completed and delivered. The remaining natural teeth in the mandible were extracted atraumatically under local anesthesia. Healing of the extraction sockets was unremarkable (Fig 4).

Under intravenous sedation, a full-thickness mucoperiosteal flap was raised with relieving incisions. Two tissue-level implants (Straumann Regular Neck, SLActive, diameter 4.1 mm, length 12 mm; Institut Straumann AG, Basel, Switzerland) were placed at sites 33 and 43 in accordance with the treatment plan. Localized guided bone regeneration (GBR) was used to cover the exposed implant threads on the buccal side with autologous bone chips harvested using a bone scraper (HuFriedy, Chicago, Illinois, USA) supplemented with DBBM bone substitute (Bio-Oss; Geistlich Pharma, Wolhusen, Switzerland). The augmentation site was covered with a non-crosslinked, porcine-derived, resorbable collagen membrane (Bio-Gide; Geistlich Pharma). As significant primary stability was achieved at the time of implant placement, transmucosal healing abutments were placed. A panoramic radiograph was taken to confirm the positioning of the two implants (Fig 5).

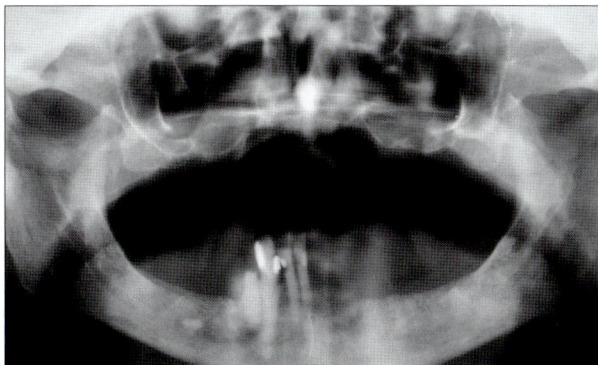
Fig 3 Panoramic radiograph 12 months after the initial referral.

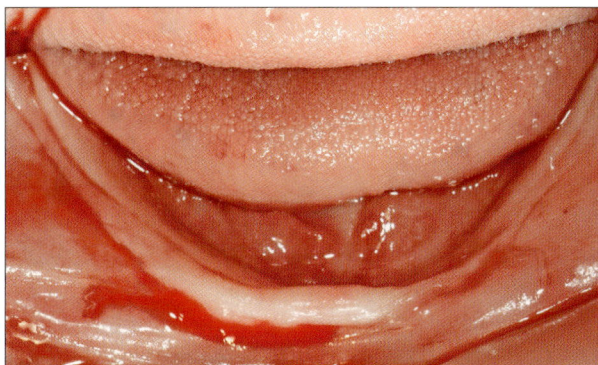
Fig 4 Lower edentulous ridge 6 months after the extractions.

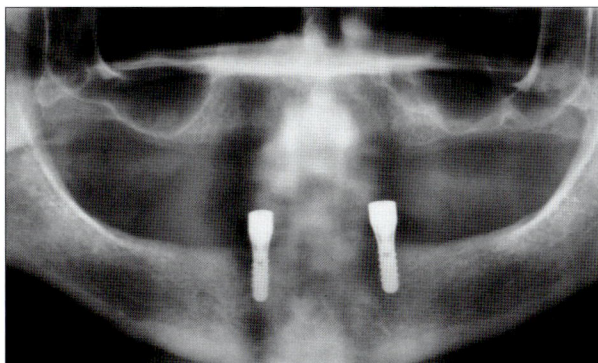
Fig 5 Panoramic radiograph to confirm optimal placement of implants 33 and 43.

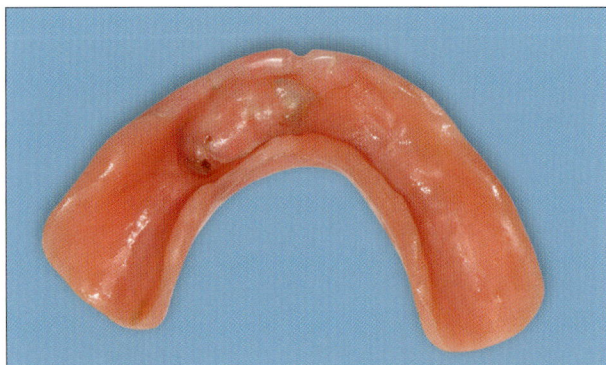

Fig 6   Mandibular complete denture modified to accommodate implants.

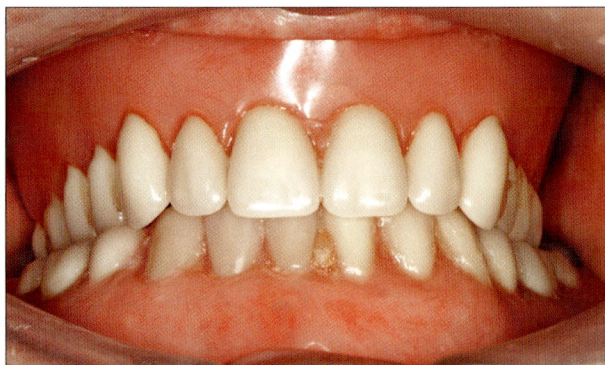

Fig 7   Modified dentures in situ.

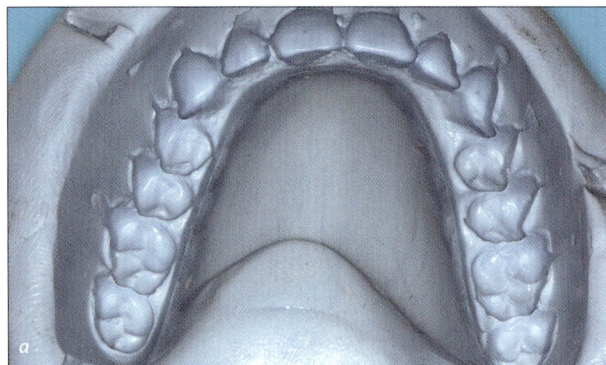

Figs 8a-b   Copy impression for the maxillary complete denture.

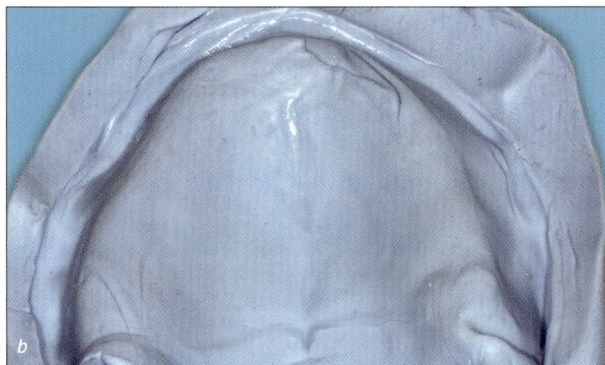

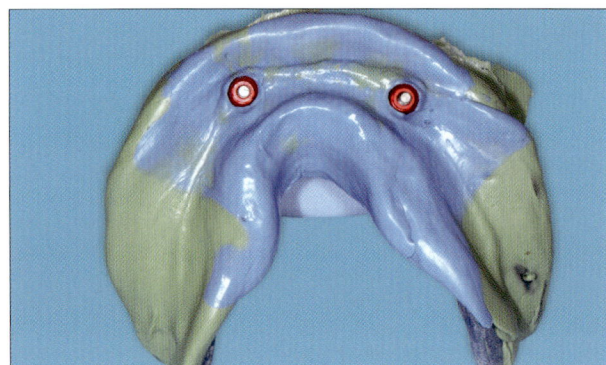

Fig 9   Fixture-level impression of the mandibular implants in a custom tray.

In order to accommodate the transmucosal healing abutments, the fitting surface of the patient's existing mandibular complete denture was modified to prevent loading of the implants (Figs 6 and 7).

Construction of the definitive prostheses began 3 months after implant placement. As the patient was very pleased with the appearance and esthetics of the existing maxillary denture, a copy denture was constructed by taking an impression of the existing prosthesis in silicone putty (Aquasil Putty; Dentsply, Surrey, UK) (Fig 8). A mandibular conventional denture was prescribed and a fixture-level impression was taken in polyvinylsiloxane (Aquasil Putty and Ultra; Dentsply) in a custom tray with impression copings (Straumann RN impression copings) (Fig 9).

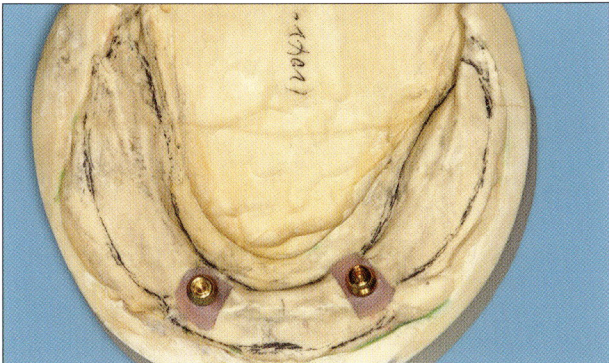

Fig 10 Mandibular working model with Locator abutments (height 4.0 mm) in situ.

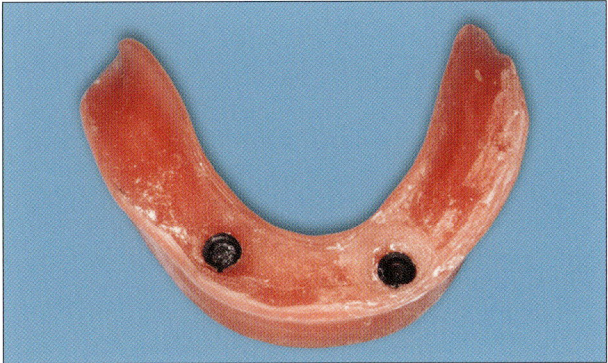

Fig 11 Maxillary bite record.

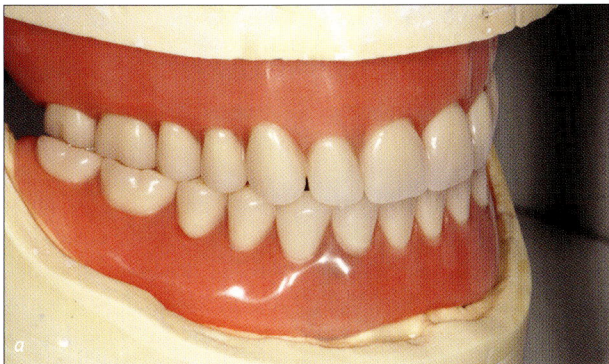

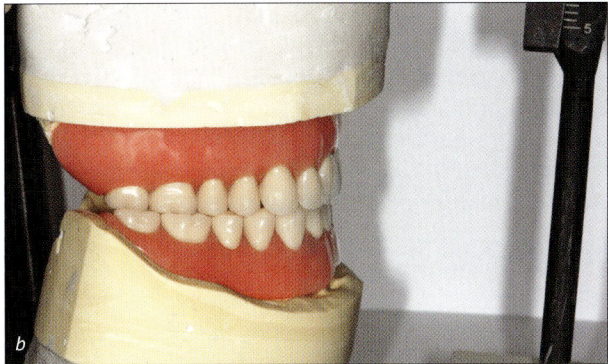

Figs 12a-b Denture try-in on semi-adjustable articulator.

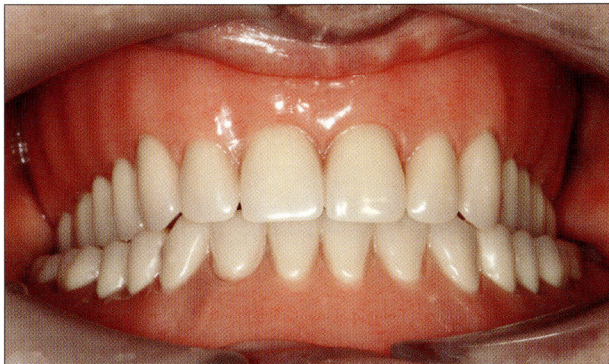

Fig 13 Maxillary and mandibular prostheses at try-in.

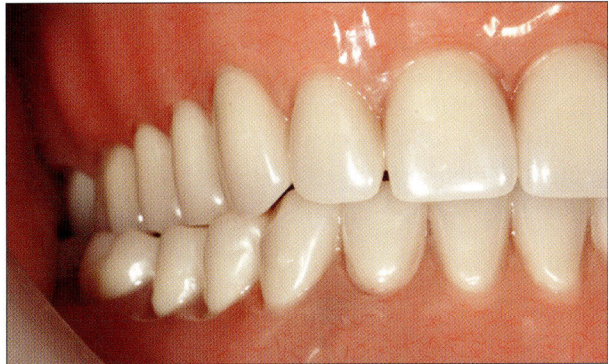

Fig 14 Right-side occlusion of the definitive prostheses.

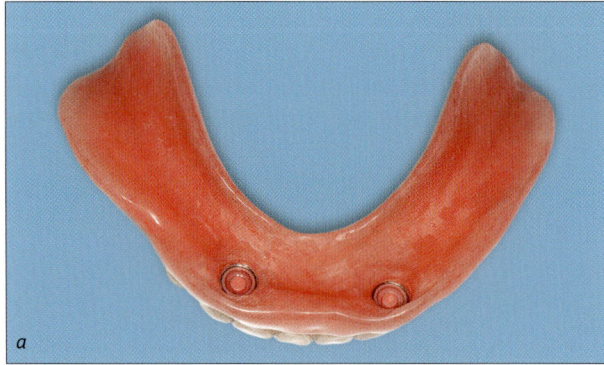

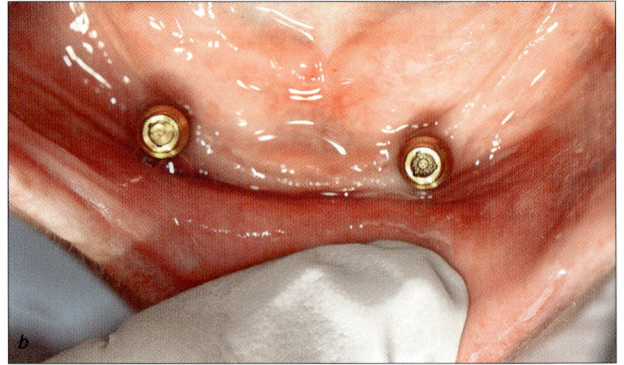

Figs 15a-b   Mandibular implant-supported overdenture with pink male Locator inserts.

A working model was constructed from the impression and Locator abutments placed to retain the mandibular denture (Fig 10) due to the patient's medical condition (osteoarthritis in both hands). A mandibular bite record was constructed and the jaw registered (Fig 11).

The jaw registration facilitated construction of the definitive prostheses on a semi-adjustable articulator (Denar Anamark Plus; Whip Mix Europe, Dortmund, Germany) (Fig 12). The mandibular prosthesis was provided with a bilateral buccal crossbite to add to the available tongue space and improve patient comfort.

The definitive prostheses were inserted and instructions provided on the insertion and removal of the implant-supported mandibular overdenture (Figs 13 and 14). To facilitate accommodation of the new mandibular prosthesis, pink inserts were provided (Locator male, light retention, 1.36 kg) (Figs 15a-b).

The patient was recalled at 6-monthly intervals during the 18 months since the treatment. Minimal maintenance was required; the Locator inserts were changed on one occasion. The patient was very pleased with the result, as was his wife (Fig 16). He noted a significant improvement in chewing, speech and self-confidence and reported that he had "returned to playing bridge with his wife and her friends." He was placed on a yearly recall, with maintenance also provided by a dental hygienist working with his general dental practitioner. A repeat panoramic radiograph was taken 24 months after implant placement, which shows approximately 2 mm of horizontal bone loss associated with the left implant (Fig 17). However, no clinical signs of inflammation were observed.

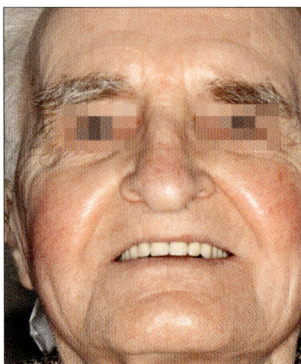

Fig 16   The patient wearing his maxillary complete denture and mandibular implant-supported overdenture at the 12-month review.

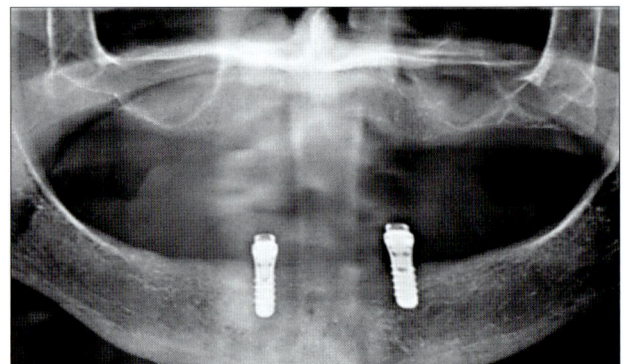

Fig 17   Panoramic radiograph 24 months after implant placement (Locator inserts in place).

13.5 Maxillary Implant-supported Full-arch Removable Dental Prostheses for a Geriatric Patient: Sequencing the Treatment for an Optimal Outcome

A. Dickinson

A 90-year-old, essentially healthy woman requested assistance following what she determined was the loss of a dental restoration from a maxillary anterior tooth. She also complained of pain associated with tooth 11.

The patient was assessed as relatively fit and healthy. She took medications for mild hypertension and to prevent angina attacks (atenolol and diltiazem). She had a form of arthritic joint degeneration affecting several joints; especially in her hands and fingers. When required she used an NSAID (meloxicam) for pain management.

She reported living alone in a care facility that allows for independent living, with domestic support when and if necessary and primary medical triage when required.

The initial clinical examination (Figs 1 to 6) and evaluation revealed the following:

- Grade 3 mobility and pain in tooth 11 with labial swelling and involvement of the sinus tract associated with the apical area of this tooth.
- Fractured crown of tooth 13.
- Unsatisfactory upper RPD with cast-metal base (not shown).
- Reduced occlusal vertical dimension.
- Heavily restored remaining maxillary anterior teeth.
- Periodontally hopeless remaining two maxillary molars (teeth 18 and 28).
- Reduced mandibular dentition (teeth 35 to 45 only).
- Mandibular teeth periodontally and functionally stable.

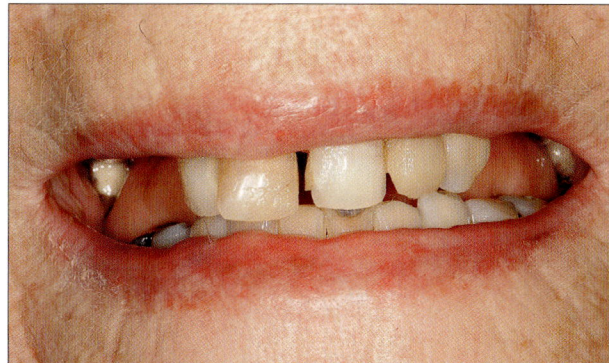
Fig 1 Preoperative smile demonstrating tooth display.

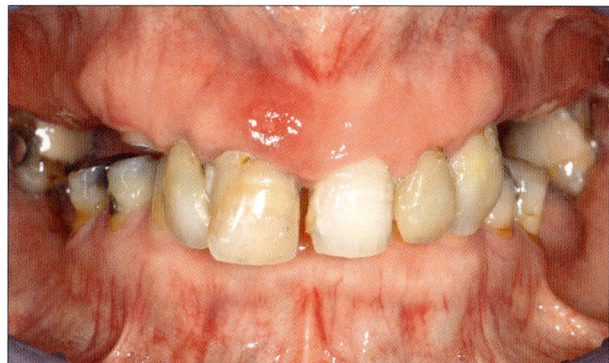
Fig 2 Preoperative facial view in intercuspal position. Reduced vertical dimension of occlusion and labial pathology associated with tooth 11.

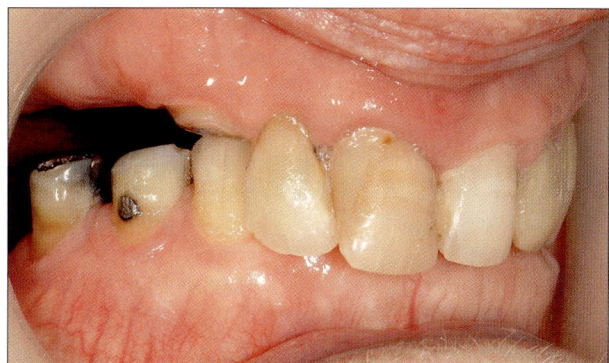
Fig 3 Right-side view with the jaw in maximum intercuspation.

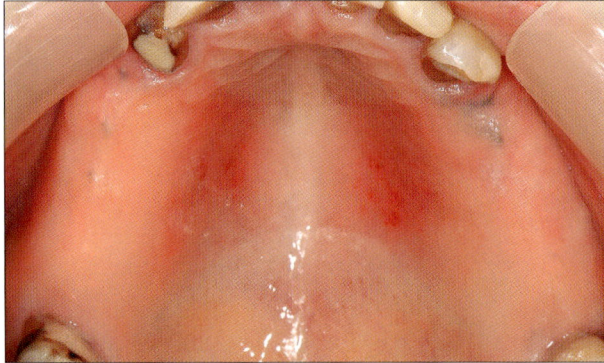

Fig 4   Occlusal view of the maxillary arch.

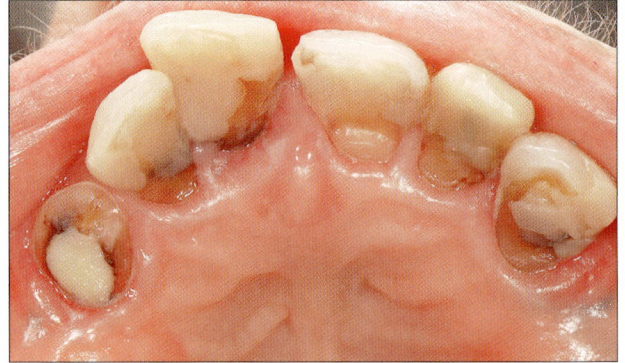

Fig 5   Preoperative occlusal view of the remaining maxillary anterior teeth.

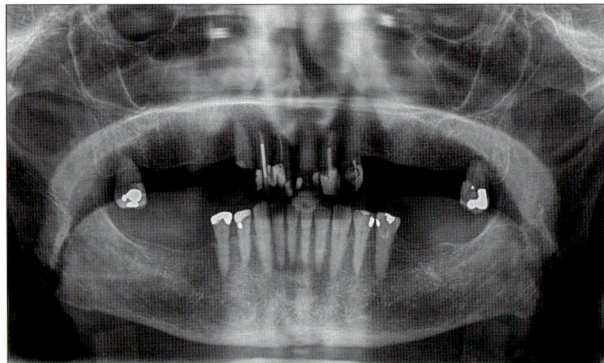

Fig 6   Panoramic radiograph taken after the initial presentation.

Case analysis and preoperative planning

Mounted casts were prepared. The desired increase in vertical dimension and the planned tooth positions were diagnostically evaluated. A CBCT (Figs 7a-d) was taken without a radiographic template, as the desired implant positions were unlikely to be in question.

A broad discussion was undertaken with the patient and her immediate family. Various therapeutic options were considered and the advantages and disadvantages of each discussed. Emphasis was placed on eliminating of the existing disease and on a solution to the several structural and functional problems identified by the patient, as well as those brought to the patient's attention.

The goal was to provide an outcome that would be broadly based on the therapeutic objectives described by Chen and Buser (2008).

Primary objectives

- Successful esthetic and functional outcome.
- Esthetic outcome with long-term stability.
- Low risk of complications during healing and function.

Secondary objectives

- The least number of surgical interventions.
- The least possible pain and morbidity.
- Short healing and overall treatment time.
- A cost-effective treatment.

With specific reference to this patient, and because of her age, greater emphasis was placed on the reduction of pain and morbidity in combination with a cost-effective therapeutic outcome, in preference to focusing on reducing the number of surgical interventions and the overall length of the treatment.

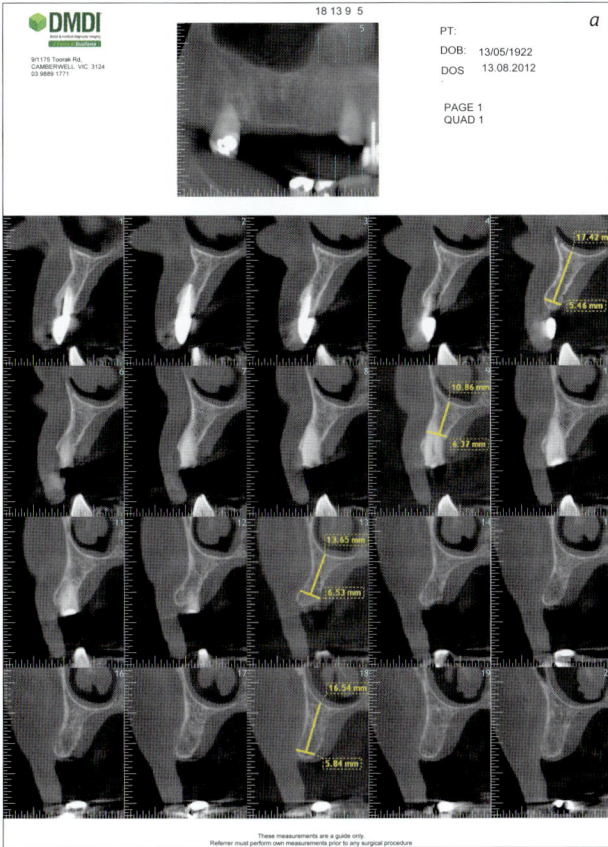

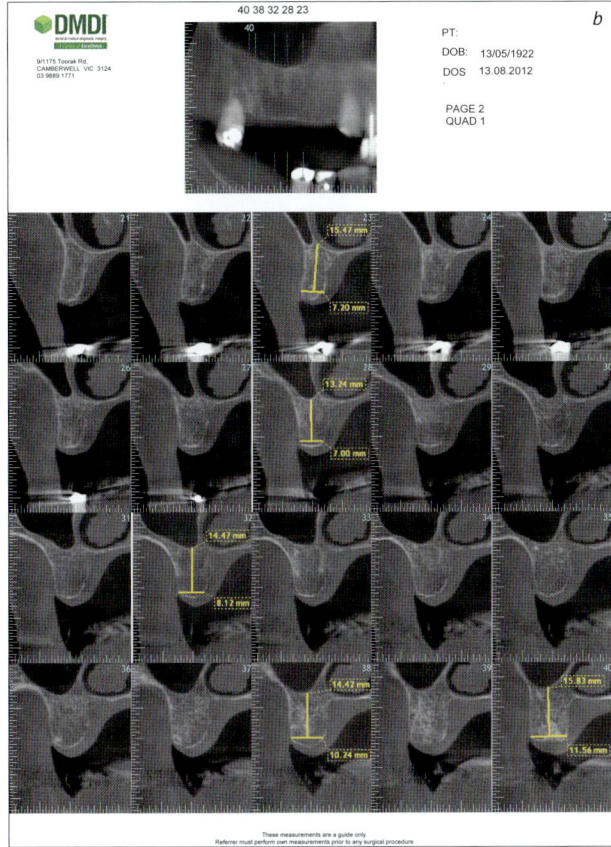

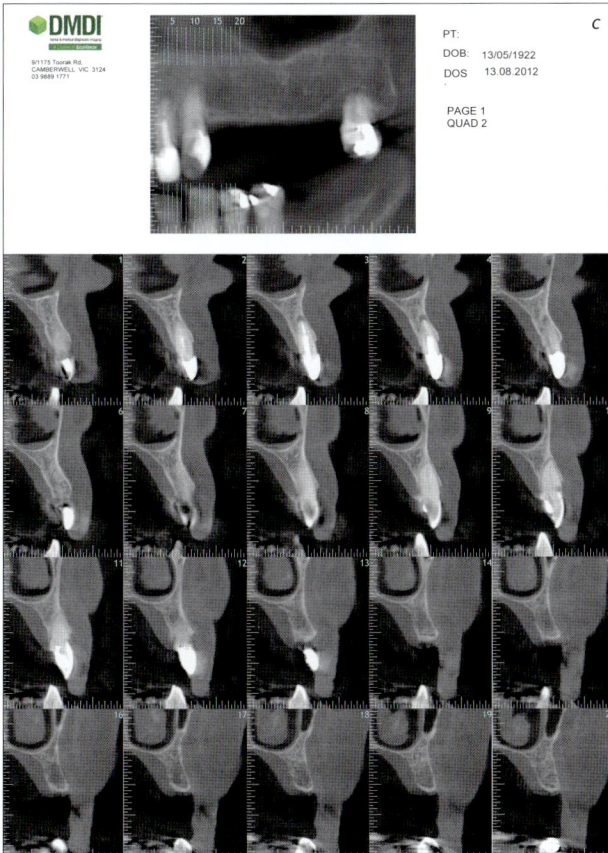

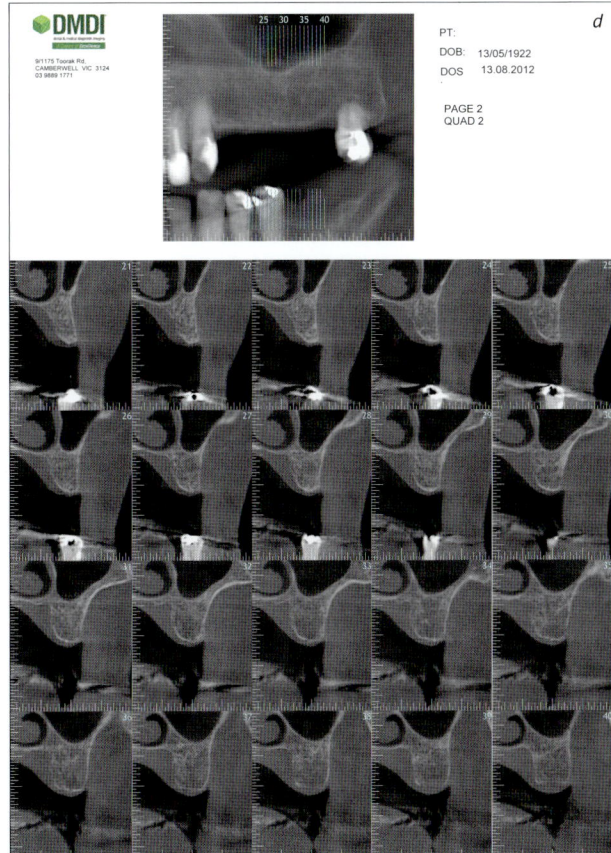

Figs 7a-d   CBCT sections. (a-b) First quadrant, pages 1 and 2. (c-d) Second quadrant, pages 1 and 2.

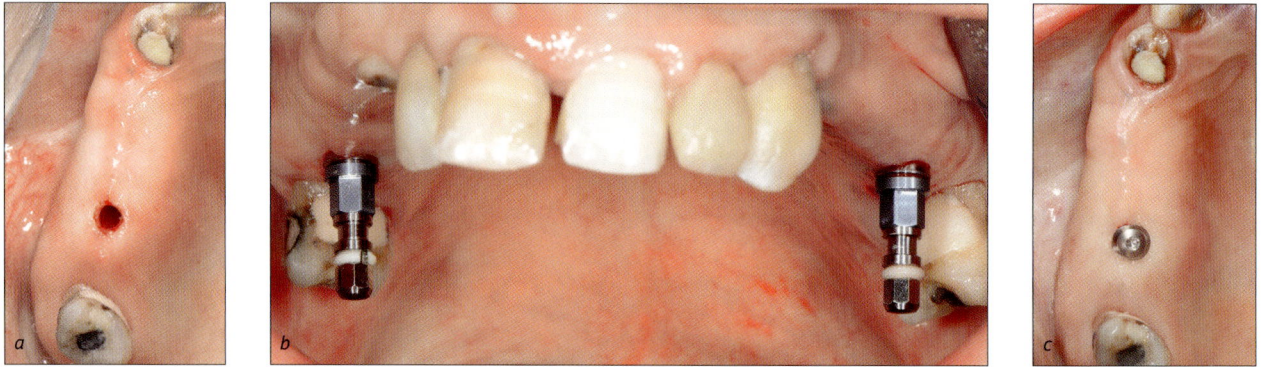

Figs 8a-c   Placement of implant 16. Flapless procedure utilizing a punch incision and placement of a tissue-level SLActive implant providing for a placement that closely paralleled the previously placed implant 26 (courtesy of Dr. Stephen Chen).

The treatment sequence is of great importance in geriatric patients. Emphasis had to be placed on the elimination of disease and the restitution of a healthy and functional oral status, while introducing changes in a manageable time frame and aiming to reduce the need for a transitional prosthesis that may require significant adaptation by the patient.

The therapeutic goal was to transition the patient, in manageable stages, from her debilitated residual maxillary dentition to a complete maxillary prosthesis retained via single retentive elements attached to four dental implants. A surgical and prosthetic treatment sequence was selected that would achieve the desired outcome, but reduce the patient's adaptive requirements.

Treatment plan

The surgical and prosthetic treatment was undertaken using a staged protocol (sequence). This would provide for the early elimination of disease while maintaining function and acceptable esthetics and with the expectation of achieving a reduction in the physiological and psychological adjustments required of the patient.

Initial treatment steps

- Extraction of teeth 13 (root), 23 and 11 (pain).
- Transitional acrylic RDP with anterior palatal coverage to allow for an immediate increase in the vertical dimension of occlusion.
- Placement of two implants:
  Implant 16: Straumann RN S SLActive, length 12 mm (Figs 8a-c)
  Implant 26: Straumann RN S SLActive, length 10 mm (Figs 9a-e)
  (both Institute Straumann AG, Basel, Switzerland)
- Retention of the periodontally hopeless teeth 18 and 28 to allow for continued retention of the transitional RDP.

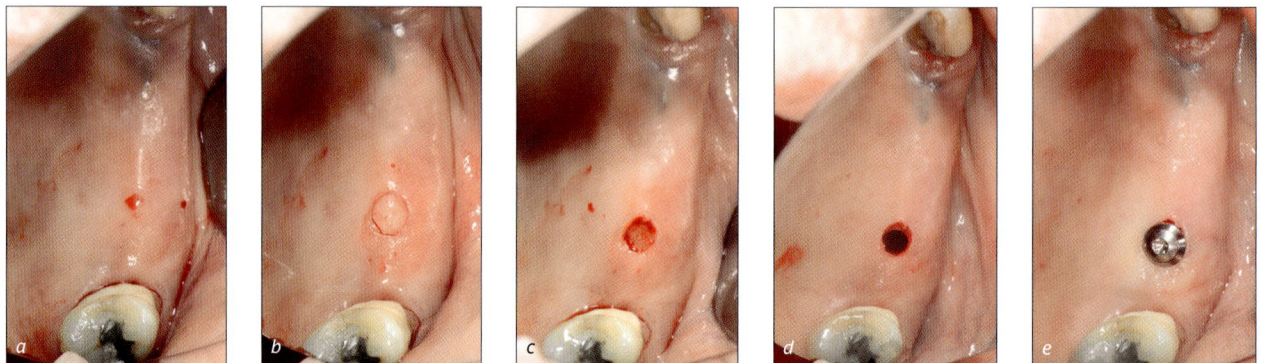

Figs 9a-e   Placement of implant 26. Flapless procedure using a punch incision and placement of a tissue-level RN SLActive implant (courtesy of Dr. Stephen Chen).

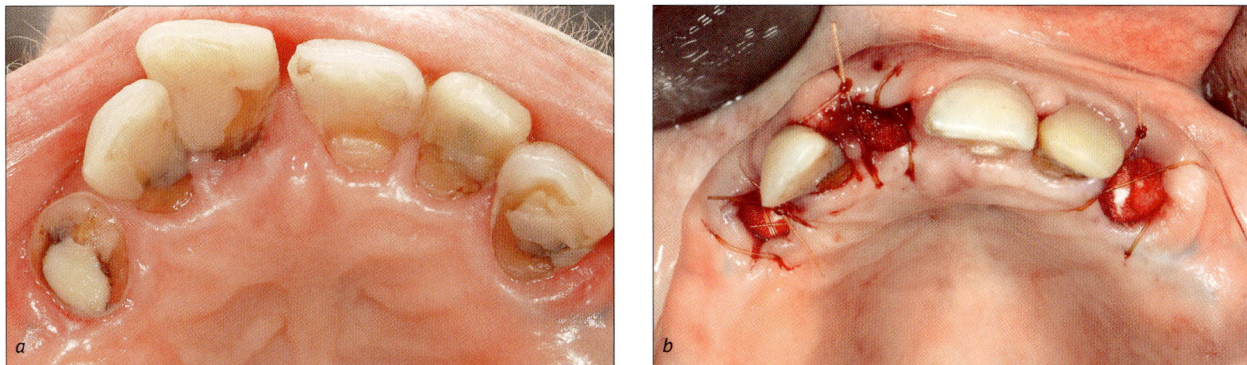

Figs 10a-b   Extraction of teeth 13, 11, and 23 at the time of implant placement in the posterior maxilla (courtesy of Dr. Stephen Chen).

The implant sites were managed with a flapless approach utilizing a punch entry through the alveolar mucosa to prepare the osteotomy site based on the CBCT findings. Both implant sites were prepared to allow for a near-parallel placement of the tissue-level implants (RN).

The extraction of teeth 13, 11, and 23 (Figs 10a-b) was completed at the time of implant placement in the posterior maxilla (Figs 11a-c). This allowed for the definitive management of the infected tooth root of tooth 11,

which had a hopeless prognosis, as well as the fractured root of tooth 13 and the intact tooth 23. The latter two extraction sites were identified for subsequent placement of implants in a type 2 surgical protocol.

The transitional acrylic RDP was modified to facilitate its immediate postsurgical delivery.

The patient stabilized and the initial healing of the implants in the 16 and 26 sites was completed.

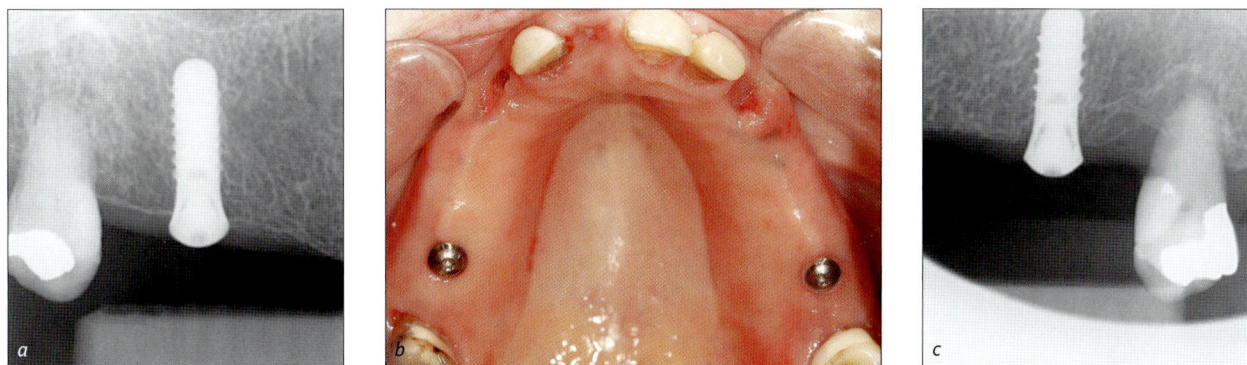

Figs 11a-c   Implants 16 and 26 and extraction of teeth 13, 11, and 23, teeth 18 and 28 still being retained at this point.

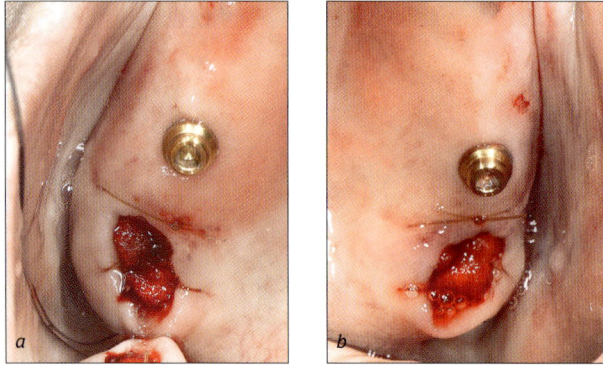

Figs 12a-b   Having placed the Locator abutments on the previously inserted tissue-level RN implants 16 and 26 and modified the transitional acrylic denture, the two remaining molars 18 and 28 were extracted (courtesy of Dr. Stephen Chen).

Intermediate treatment steps

- Locator attachments placed on posterior implants (Figs 12a-b).
- Extraction of teeth 18 and 28 (Figs 12a-b).
- Modification of the transitional acrylic RDP incorporating direct pick-up of the female housing and retentive element within the denture.
- Placement of two further implants (type 2 protocol):
  Implant 13: Straumann RN S SLActive, length
  10 mm (Figs 13a-c)
  Implant 23: Straumann RN S SLActive, length
  10 mm (Figs 13a-c)
  (both Institute Straumann AG, Basel, Switzerland)

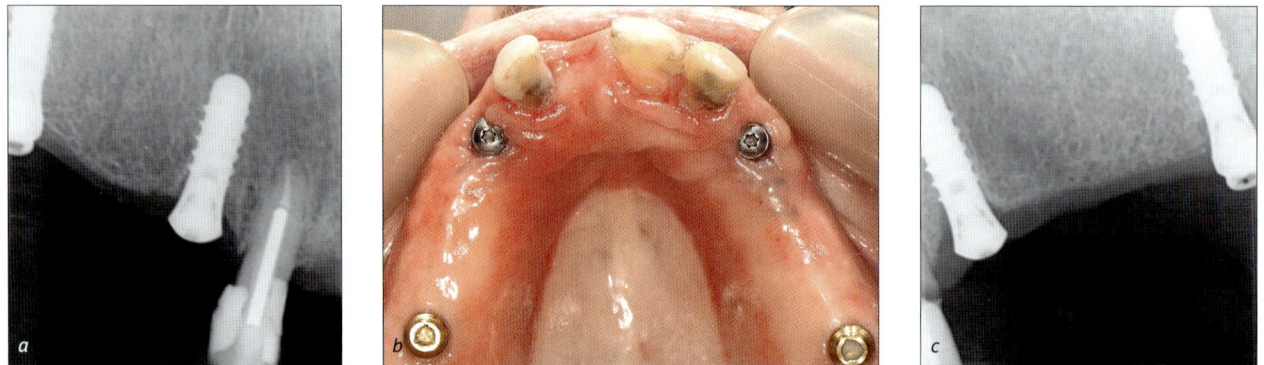

Figs 13a-c   Eight weeks later: implants 13 and 23 and Locator attachments.

Following an adequate period of healing and successful integration of implants 13 and 23, the final prosthetic steps were undertaken.

Final treatment steps

- Placement of the additional two Locator attachments.
- Fabrication of the metal-reinforced maxillary complete implant-supported RDP (Figs 14a-b and 15a-b).
- Extraction of the remaining three teeth (12, 21, and 22; Figs 16a-b).

- Immediate placement of the definitive prosthesis.
- Relining of the appliance following three months of post-extraction healing and function.

The definitive maxillary implant-supported complete RDP included a cast Co-Cr framework for improved rigidity. Because of the shape of the residual maxillary arch that provided adequate lateral resistance, full palatal coverage was not required.

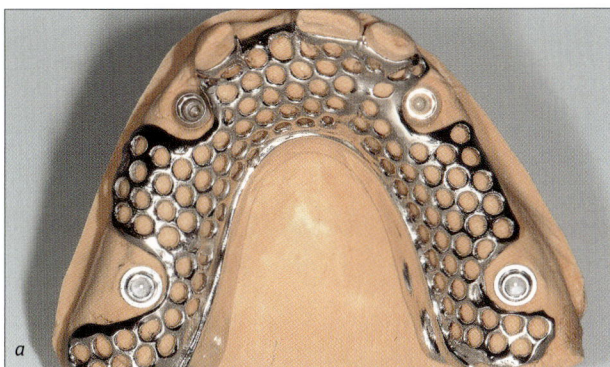

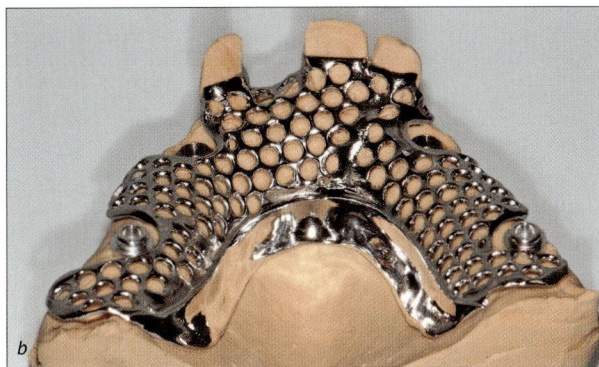

Figs 14a-b   Cast Co-Cr framework for inclusion in the maxillary implant-supported complete RDP. No full palatal coverage.

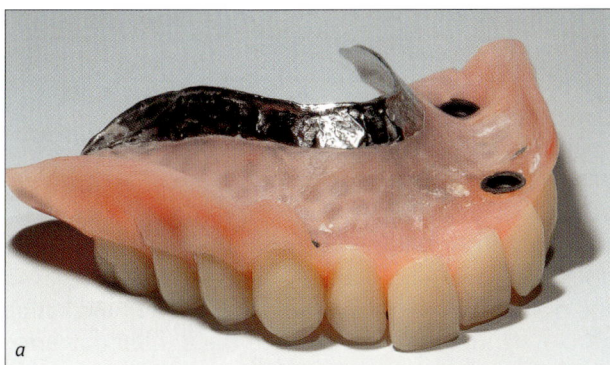

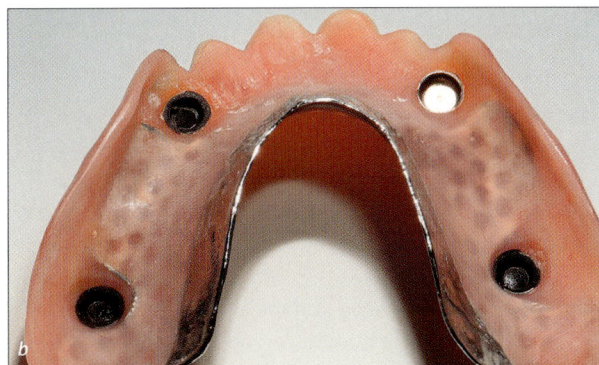

Figs 15a-b   The processed maxillary removable prosthesis.

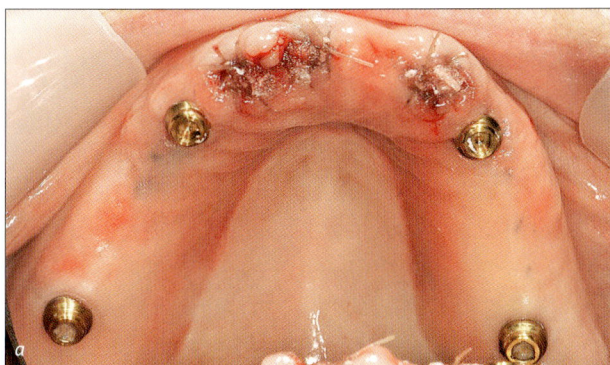

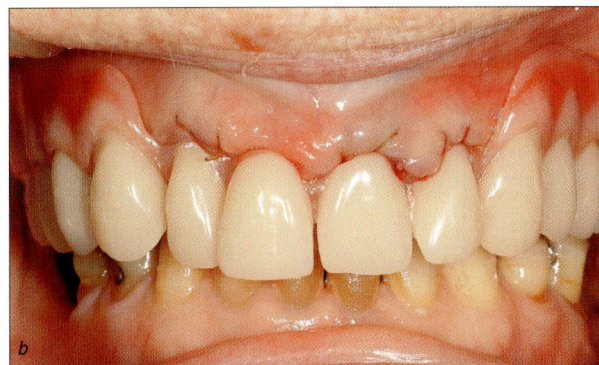

Figs 16a-b   Six weeks after implant placement in the anterior maxilla. Locator attachments on tissue-level implants 13 and 23 and extraction of teeth 12, 21, and 22 with immediate prosthetic delivery.

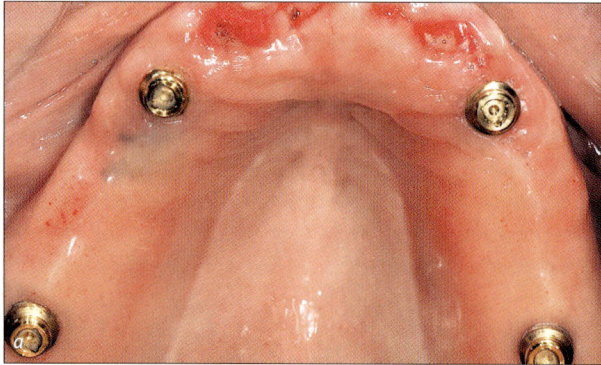

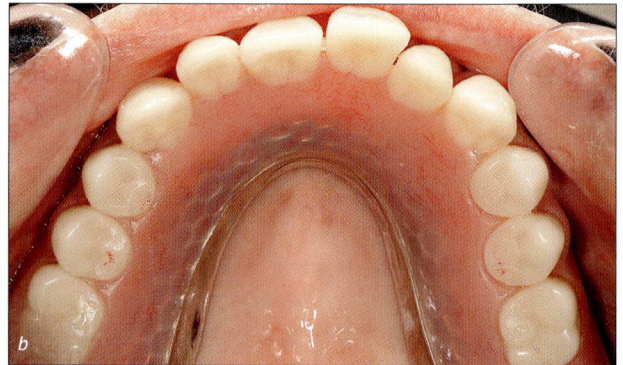

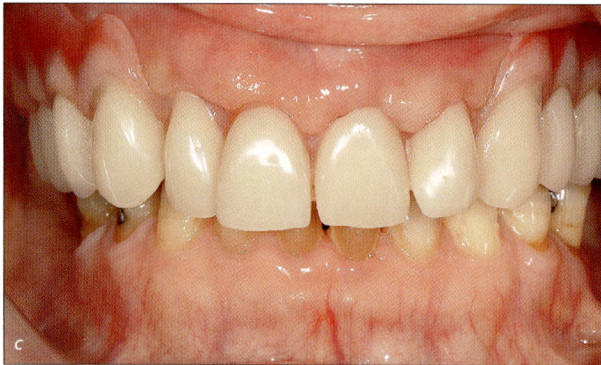

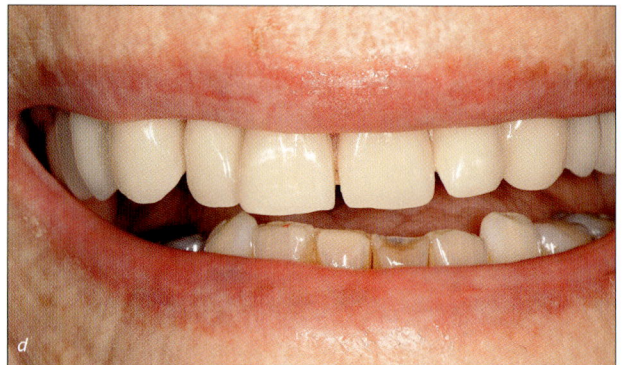

Figs 17a-d   Review two weeks after extraction.

The processed maxillary RDP (Figs 17a-d) incorporated no flange on the facial aspect in the anterior sextant. Only three black processing males were retained in the appliance at the time of insertion to allow for ease of placement and removal.

This protocol allows time for the patient to become accustomed to the correct insertion and removal technique for the prosthesis after delivery. The commencement of the buccal flanges in the cuspid areas also provides a point of reference for the patient to apply her fingers or a smooth implement to dislodge the prosthesis.

Conclusion

The use of four dental implants to support an implant-supported removable dental prosthesis is a clinically well-documented procedure (Gallucci and co-workers 2009b). In geriatric patients, emphasis is best directed to the sequencing of the therapeutic stages in the transition from an unstable and poorly functioning natural dentition or prosthesis to the desired outcome. Time should be allowed for the required adaptation to the changing oral environment and function. Consideration must be given to the requirements for ongoing maintenance by patients themselves and to the possibility of such maintenance becoming the responsibility of third-party care providers.

13.6 Mandibular Overdenture Supported by a CAD/CAM-milled Bar with Long Distal Extensions on Two Conventionally Loaded Implants

M. Srinivasan

An 87-year-old man was referred to our Division of Gerodontology and Removable Prosthodontics at the University Clinics of Dental Medicine, Geneva, Switzerland for dental implant therapy. He was retired and led a very active social life, keeping himself busy in the company of his many grandchildren and with frequent travels to Italy.

The patient's past medical and drug histories revealed that he suffered from angina, asthma, and arthritis of the knee. He was allergic to penicillin. His regular prescription medications included anti-anginal and anti-asthmatic drugs, along with occasional non-steroidal anti-inflammatory drugs for joint pain. Otherwise, he was a healthy patient who occasionally consumed alcohol on social occasions and did not smoke.

A detailed dental history revealed that he had lost his teeth to chronic adult periodontal disease (Fig 1) and had had an edentulous maxilla for over 20 years.

The two remaining mandibular teeth (32 and 33) supported an overdenture (Fig 2), but were failing. The patient was unhappy with his mandibular denture and its poor retention and instability.

A mandibular implant overdenture supported by two interforaminal implants was planned at the Division of Stomatology of the University of Geneva. Two Straumann tissue-level implants (Straumann Standard Plus RN SLActive, Ti, diameter 4.1 mm, length 8 mm; Institut Straumann AG, Basel, Switzerland) were placed; the remaining two teeth were simultaneously extracted (Fig 3).

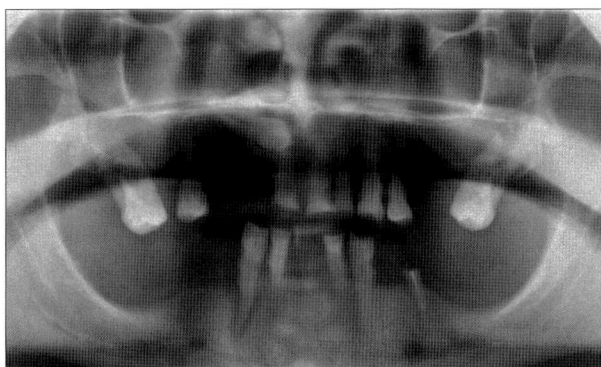

Fig 1   Baseline panoramic radiograph showing a failing dentition.

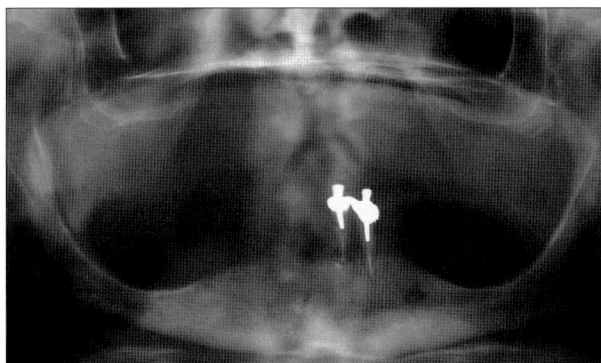

Fig 2   Panoramic radiograph. Two remaining teeth supporting a mandibular overdenture before implant therapy.

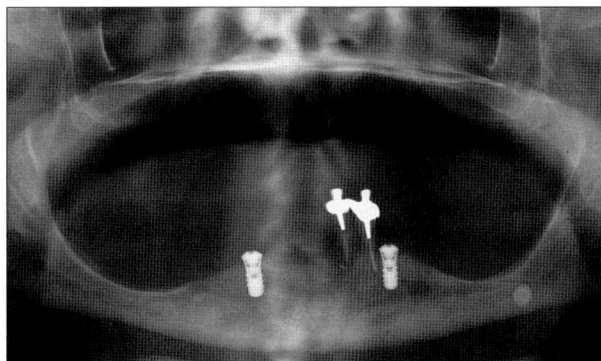

Fig 3   Immediate postoperative panoramic radiograph showing implants 43 and 34.

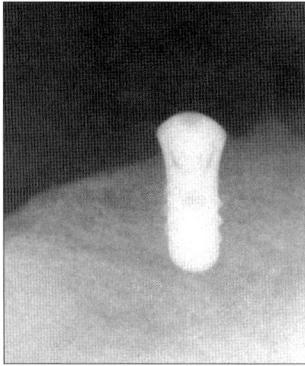

Fig 4a Periapical radiograph at 8 weeks showing the successful implant 43.

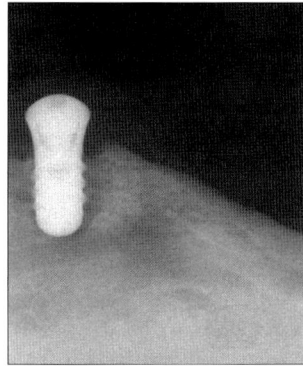

Fig 4b Failing implant 34.

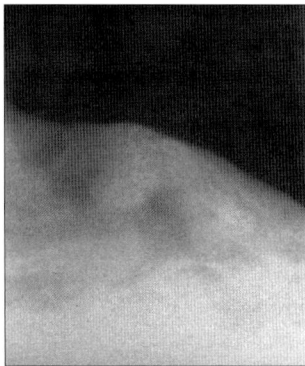

Fig 5a Implant 34 lost 15 weeks after placement.

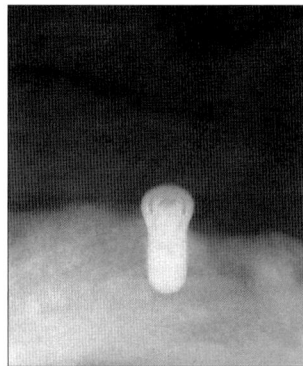

Fig 5b New implant placed at the adjacent site 33.

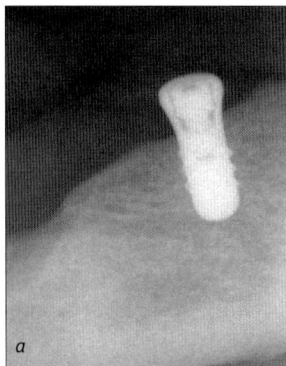

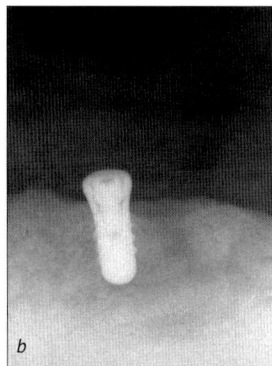

Figs 6a-b Periapical radiographs 12 weeks after placement of the new implant 33. Both implants integrated well and were ready to be loaded.

A conventional loading protocol was planned. During the healing phase, clinical examinations and radiographs revealed an uneventful integration of implant 43 (Fig 4a), whereas implant 34 was failing (Fig 4b). The reasons for this failure remained speculative, but there was no evidence in the literature that the patient's age could have played a role. We therefore suspected that the presence of the endodontically and periodontally compromised residual teeth in the direct vicinity of the implantation site might have been implicated (Listgarten and coworkers 1991; Mombelli and coworkers 1987; Mombelli and coworkers 1988; Mombelli and Lang 1992; Rosenberg and coworkers 1991).

The adaptation of the overdenture during the healing phase was performed alio loco; the possibility could not be excluded that an insufficient relief of the overdenture at the implant site might have resulted in premature loading of the implant. Implant 34 was ultimately lost before loading (Fig 5a) and a new implant was placed at the adjacent site 33 (Fig 5b). After allowing 12 weeks of healing for the second implant, the implants were ready to be loaded (Figs 6a-b). A mandibular implant-supported overdenture on two retentive anchors with Dalbo-PLUS

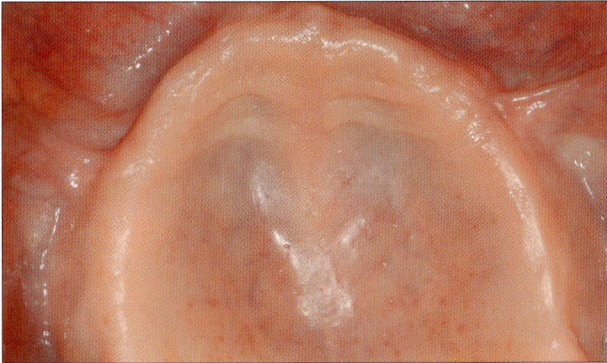

Fig 7   Intraoral view of the edentulous maxilla.

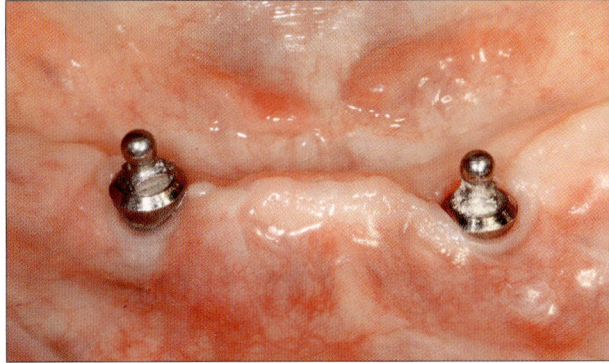

Fig 8   Intraoral buccal view. Implants with existing retentive anchors. Implant shoulders at different levels.

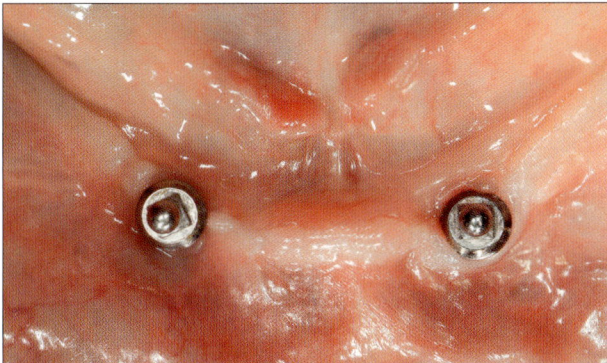

Fig 9   Occlusal view. Mild axial discrepancy of the implants.

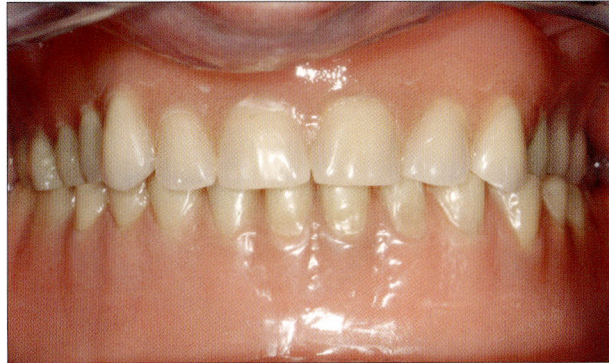

Fig 10   Old dentures with the lips completely retracted.

attachments (Cendres+Métaux SA, Biel, Switzerland) was finally delivered; the existing maxillary conventional complete denture was relined. The patient had undergone this treatment before being referred to us.

At the initial consultation at our clinic, the patient was still unhappy with his mandibular denture (Figs 7 to 10). He complained that the mandibular implant-supported overdenture was not retentive and unstable. He was also unhappy with the esthetics of the maxillary denture, as his upper teeth were not visible when he smiled and that the "pink portions" of the maxillary dentures were too obvious. He consulted for an improvement but rejected any further surgery for more implants or other invasive treatment options.

Detailed intraoral and radiographic examinations revealed a severely resorbed maxilla and mandible. The available bone was Cawood class VI in the anterior and posterior maxilla, while in the anterior and posterior mandible it was Cawood class V and VI, respectively (Cawood and Howell 1988; Fig 11). The available bone height in the mandibular interforaminal region was estimated at 17 mm.

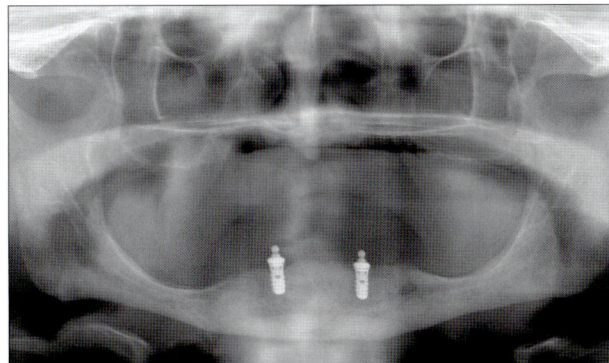

Fig 11   Panoramic radiograph 15 months after loading. Severely resorbed maxilla and posterior mandible. The implants seem to have preserved the bone in the mandible.

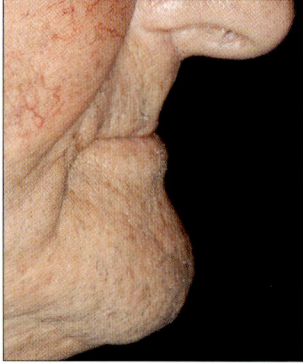

Fig 12 Extraoral profile view, without the prostheses in situ. Concave profile suggesting a need for lip support.

Extraoral examinations without the prostheses in situ revealed a concave profile and a need for soft-tissue support (Figs 12 to 14). With the prostheses in situ, inadequate lip support, a discrepancy between the lip, and smile lines along with an inharmonious tooth display were observed (Figs 15 to 18). The teeth in the existing prostheses were worn and their resin bases exhibited discoloration (Figs 19a-d).

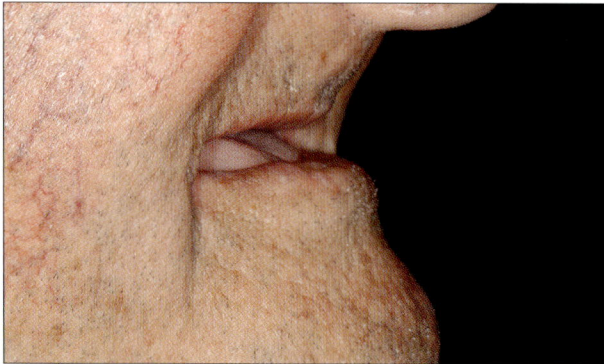

Fig 13   Profile view of smile without the prostheses in situ.

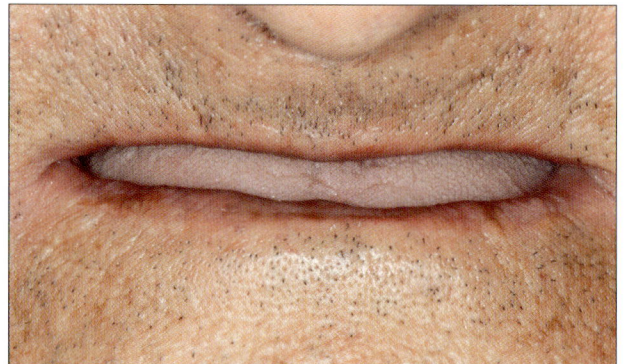

Fig 14   Frontal view of smile without the prostheses.

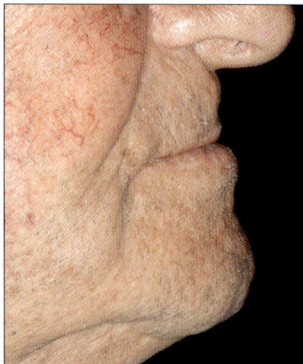

Fig 15   Extraoral profile view with the old prostheses in situ. Lack of adequate upper-lip support.

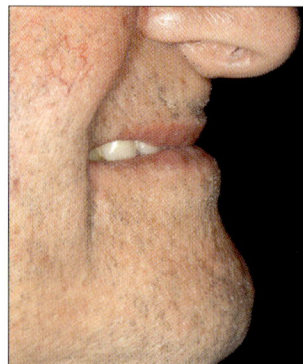

Fig 16   Profile view of the smile with the old prostheses in situ.

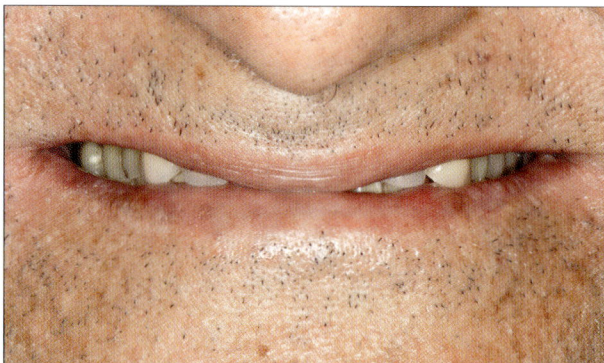

Fig 17   Lip line with the existing dentures.

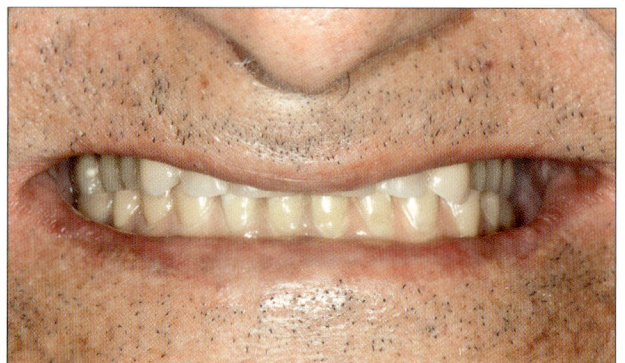

Fig 18   Frontal view of a full forced smile with the old dentures.

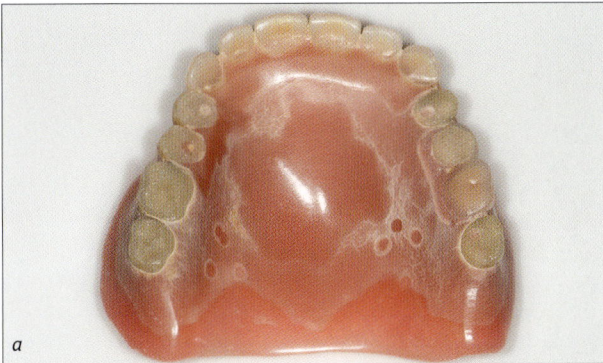

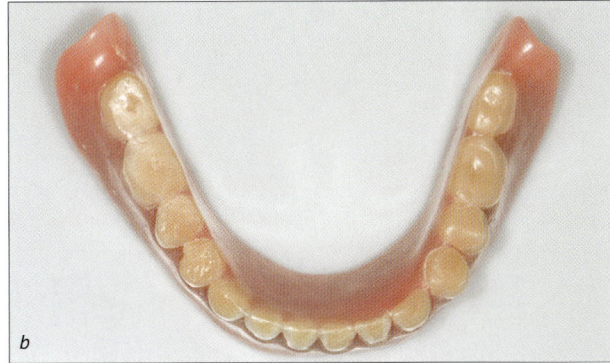

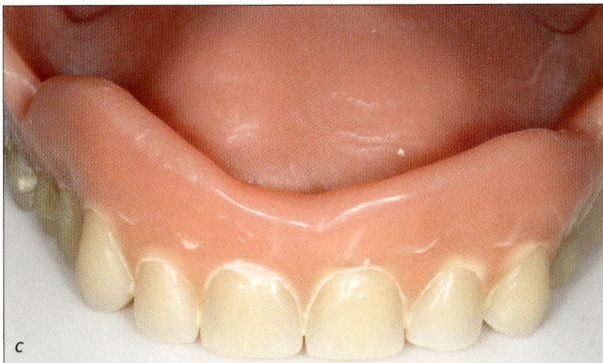

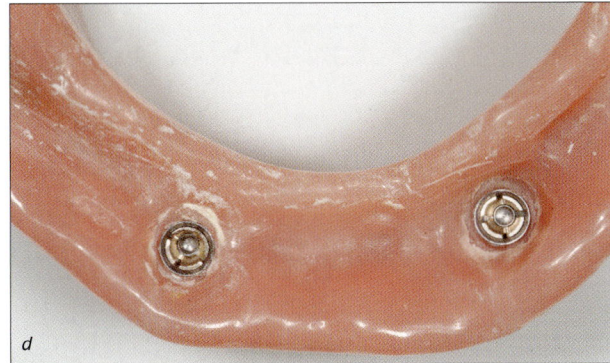

Figs 19a-d   Old prostheses with severely worn teeth and resin discoloration, warranting a remake.

An assessment of the complexity of the case using the SAC tool classified the case as advanced and complex in the surgical (Chen and coworkers 2009) and restorative (Dawson and coworkers 2009) categories, respectively (Figs 20a-b).

Figs 20a-b   SAC assessment tool. The case was assessed as an advanced surgical case and a complex restorative case.

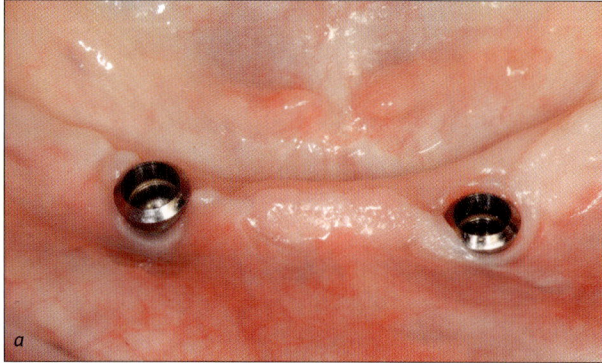

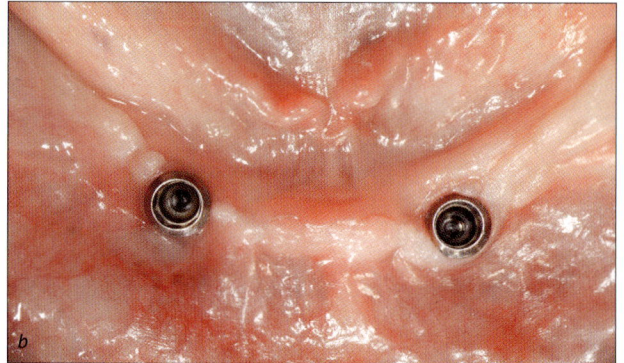

Figs 21a-b   Buccal and occlusal views of the implants after removing the retentive anchors and before the definitive impressions.

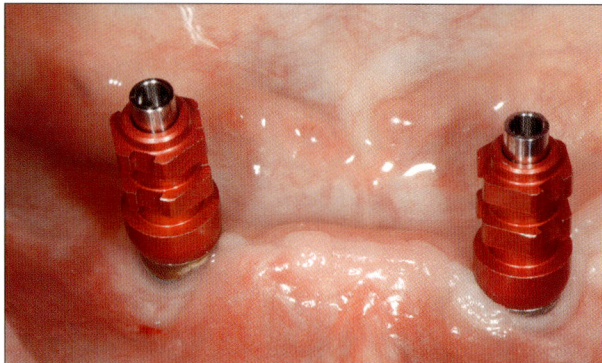

Fig 22   synOcta impression posts mounted on the implants.

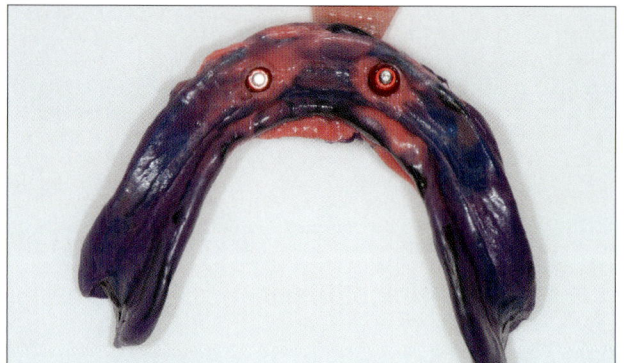

Fig 23   Impression taken with a rigid elastomeric impression material (polyether).

A minimally invasive treatment option was offered to the patient. The proposed treatment plan took into account the various clinical and economic factors along with the patient's desires and expectations. The plan involved utilizing the existing implants and excluded placement of additional implants or further surgery. The spherical anchors were to be replaced by a CAD/CAM-milled titanium bar with long distal extensions for the mandibular implant-supported overdenture. The design of the bar, in particular the length of the extensions, went beyond our usual protocol in geriatric dentistry and was part of a randomized clinical trial performed at the Division of Gerodontology and Removable Prosthodontics.

The research protocol was approved by the local ethics committee, and the patient signed informed consent forms on possible risks, as this treatment concept is novel and not yet documented by long-term evidence. The concept aims to prove the functional improvement of long extensions on CAD/CAM bars for overdentures in terms of masticatory performance as well as oral health-related quality of life (OHRQoL) and patient satisfaction. Further interest focuses on posterior bone resorption in comparison to two-implant overdentures retained by ball attachments, as the larger support area of this novel concept may have a protective effect on the bony structures of the posterior alveolar ridge. For this patient, both maxillary and mandibular prostheses were to be remade.

The treatment phase began with preliminary alginate impressions to obtain custom resin trays. The retentive anchors were removed and master impressions were taken (Figs 21a-b to 23) with polyether impression material (Impregum; 3M ESPE, Seefeld, Germany) using screw-retained synOcta impression posts (Institut Straumann AG, Basel, Switzerland). Master casts were poured and occlusal rims fabricated on acrylic bases.

All conventional clinical and laboratory procedures for the fabrication of complete dentures were adhered to up to the clinical try-in of the tooth set-up stage.

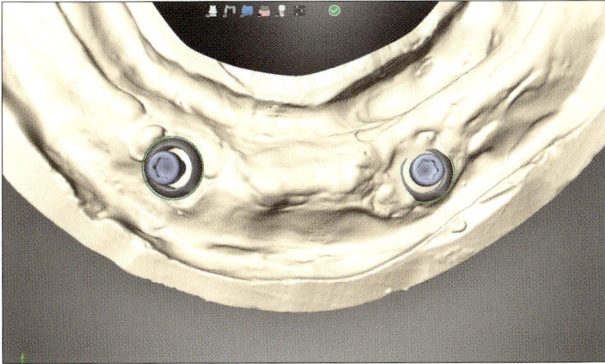

Fig 24   Scan of the mandibular master cast.

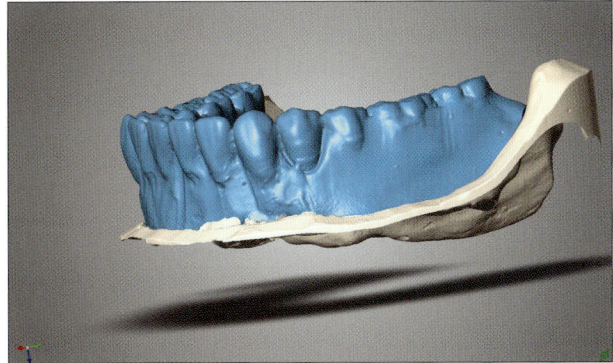

Fig 25   Scan of the tooth set-up.

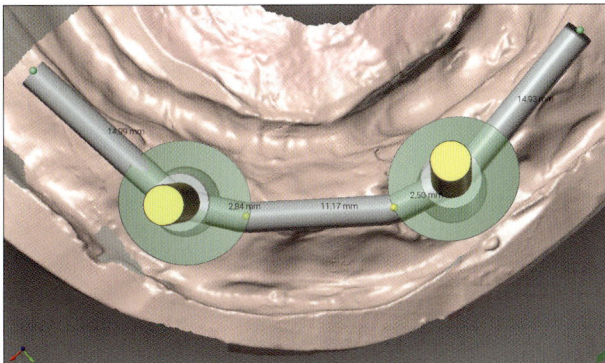

Fig 26   Designing the CAD/CAM-milled bar with long distal extensions in the CARES software.

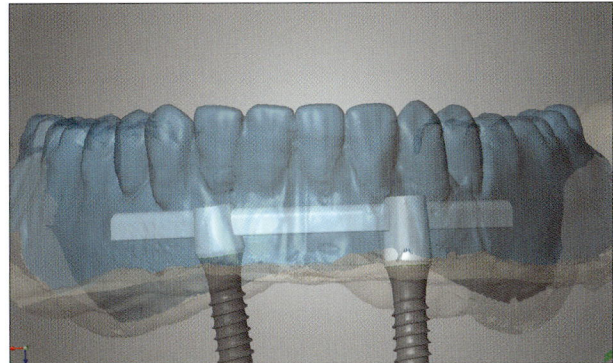

Fig 27   Verifying the bar design against the scan of the tooth set-up.

After the clinical try-in, the mandibular model and the mandibular denture set-up were scanned with an in-lab scanner (Straumann CARES Scan CS2; Institut Straumann AG) using the dedicated software (Straumann CARES Visual Design software; Institut Straumann AG). The CAD/CAM-milled bar with long distal extensions was then designed and fabricated using the validated digital workflow (Straumann CARES Visual 8.5 Validated Workflow; Institut Straumann AG; Figs 24 to 30a-b). The bar was then clinically verified for fit (Figs 31a-b). After the try-in, the dentures were definitively processed and delivered (Figs 32a-d).

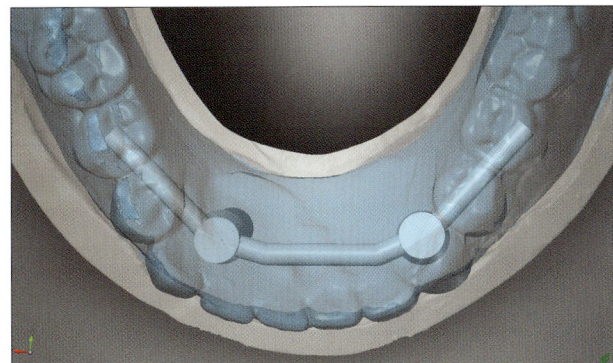

Fig 28   Occlusal view showing the extensions of the designed bar.

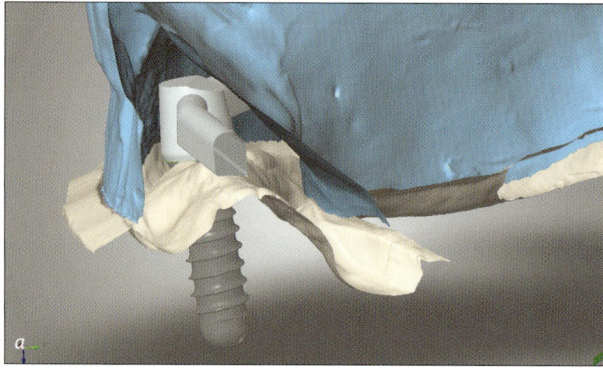

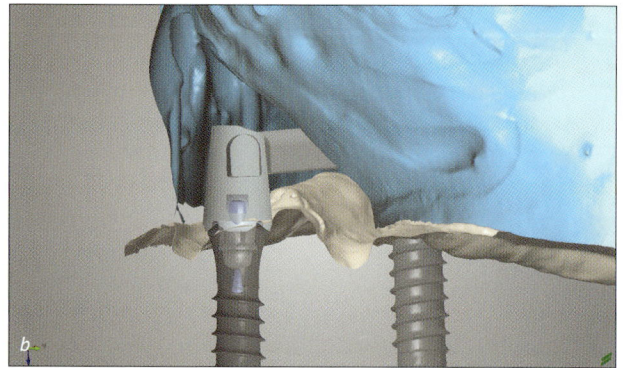

Figs 29a-b   Cross-sectional views. Adequate space between the bar framework and the denture base.

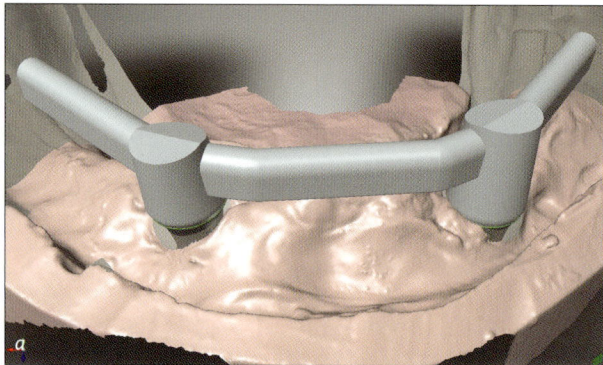

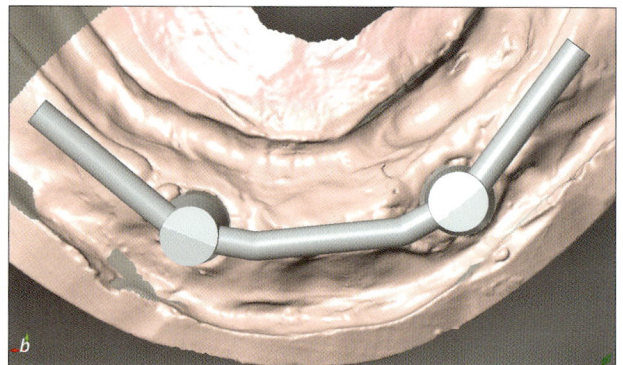

Figs 30a-b   Buccal and occlusal views of the final design of the bar before the milling process.

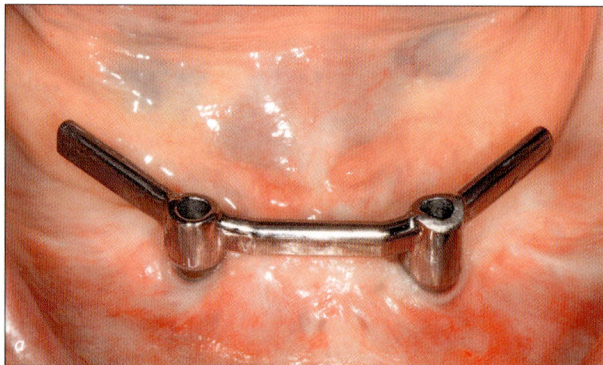

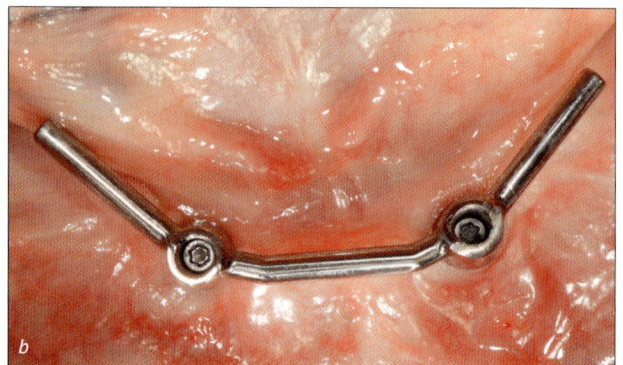

Figs 31a-b   Try-in of the CAD/CAM-milled bar (buccal and occlusal views).

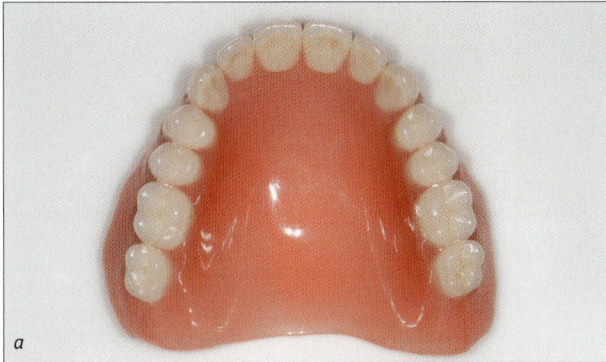

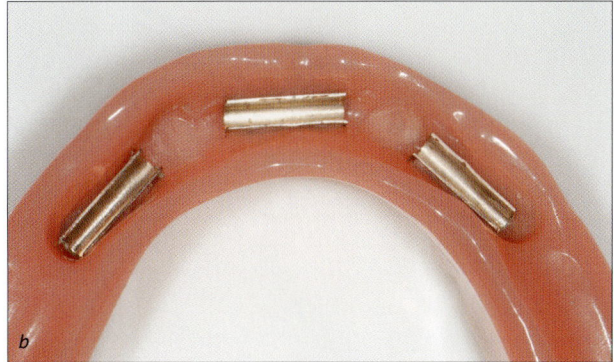

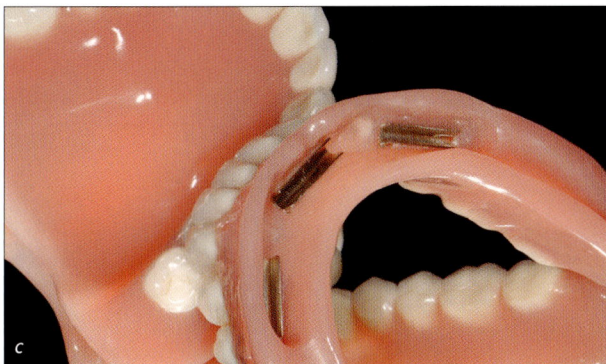

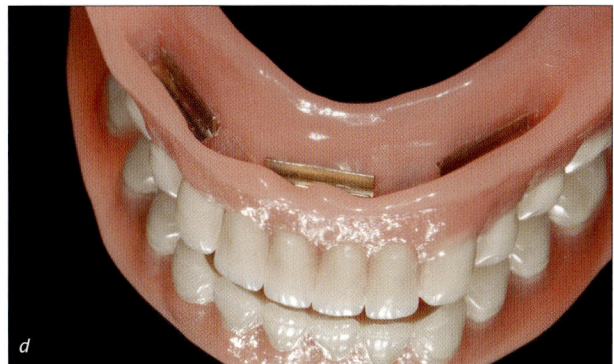

Figs 32a-d   Finished prostheses.

At delivery, the CAD/CAM-milled bar was first tightened on the implants to 35 Ncm using the Straumann ratchet and torque control device (Institut Straumann AG, Basel, Switzerland). The screw access channels on the milled bar were plugged with a polytetrafluoroethylene tape (Teflon; DuPont, Wilmington, DE, USA) and then sealed using a light-curing provisional resin cement (Telio CS In-lay; Ivoclar Vivadent, Schaan, Liechtenstein) (Moraguez and Belser, 2010) (Figs 33 to 35). The finished maxillary and mandibular prostheses were verified for fit, reten-tion, stability and esthetics at the time of insertion, and patient satisfaction was duly noted (Figs 36 to 38a-d).

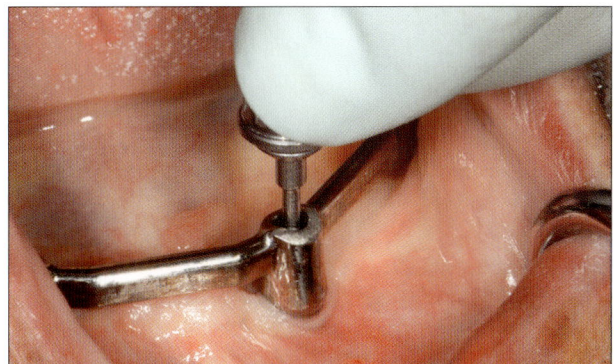

Fig 33   CAD/CAM-milled bar with screws tightened to 35 Ncm.

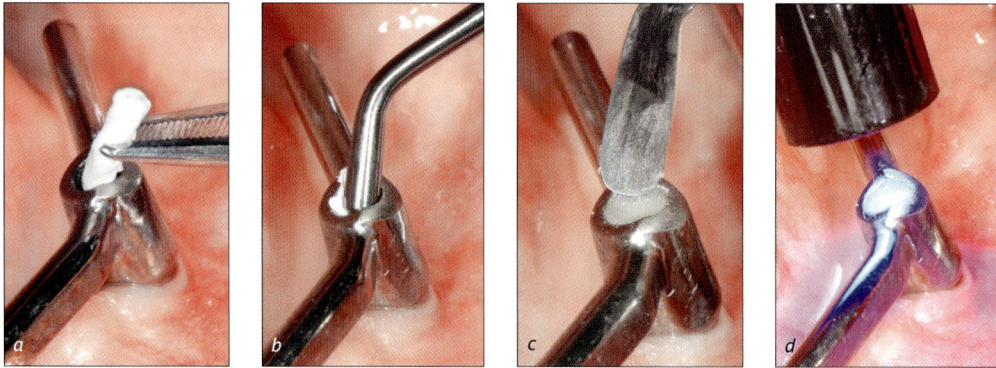

Figs 34a-d   Teflon tape packed into the screw channels. Light-activated provisional resin cement is condensed and polymerized over the Teflon tape.

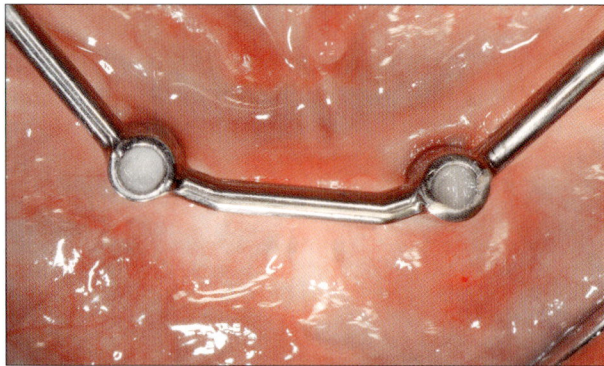

Fig 35   Occlusal view after sealing the screw channels.

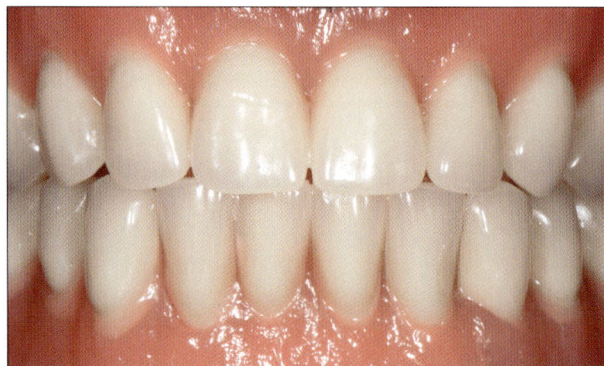

Fig 36   Final prostheses in situ with the lips fully retracted.

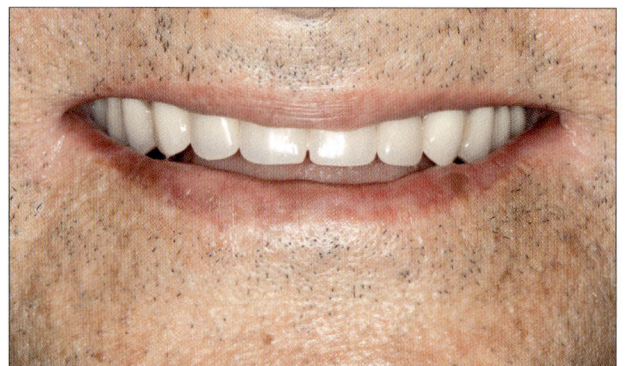

Fig 37   Frontal smile with the new prostheses in situ.

Figs 38a-d   Profile views with the new prostheses in situ showing better soft-tissue support and improved esthetics during smiling. An overall pleasing result and a thoroughly satisfied patient.

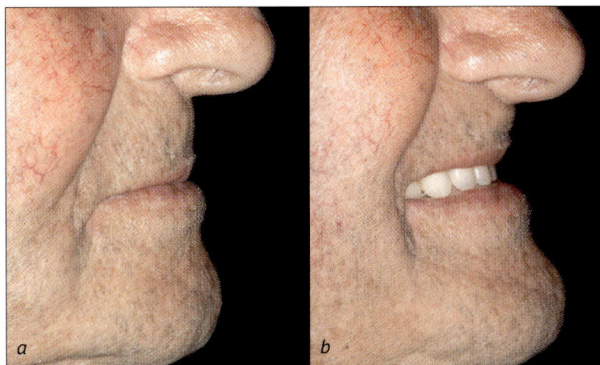

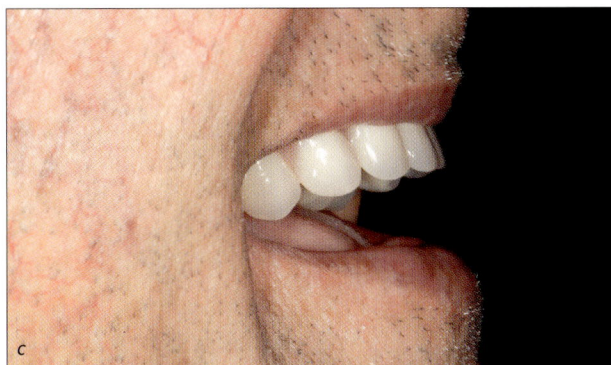

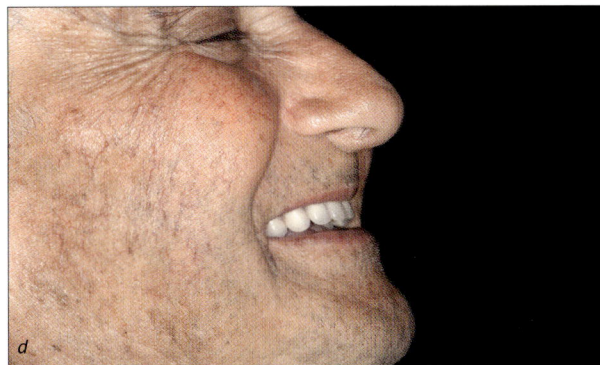

The patient received detailed instructions on the care and hygiene maintenance for the bar and the dentures (Figs 39a-b). The patient was thoroughly satisfied with the result of the treatment.

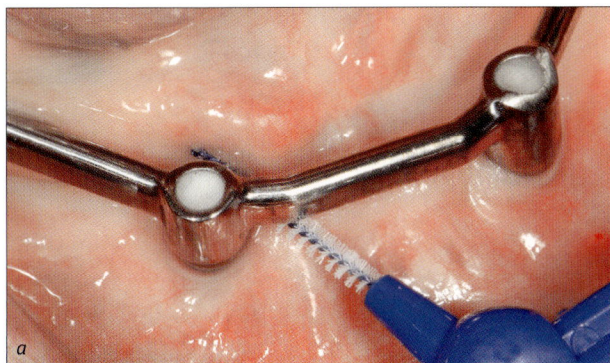

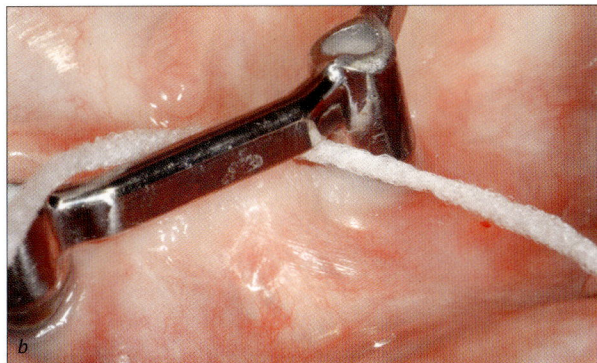

Figs 39a-b   Adequate space for easy maintenance beneath the bar with an interdental brush or dental floss.

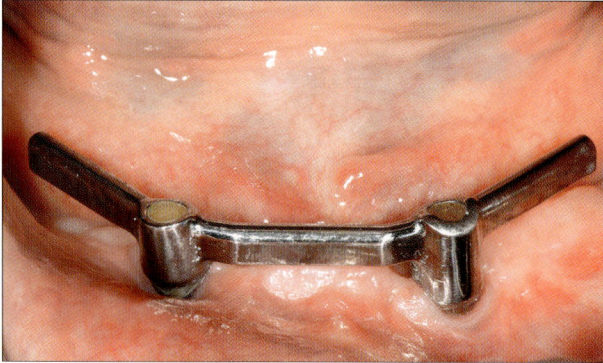

Fig 40   One-year clinical follow-up (buccal view).

At the one-year recall visit, the patient was extremely happy and content with the retention and stability of the mandibular prosthesis (Figs 40 to 43).

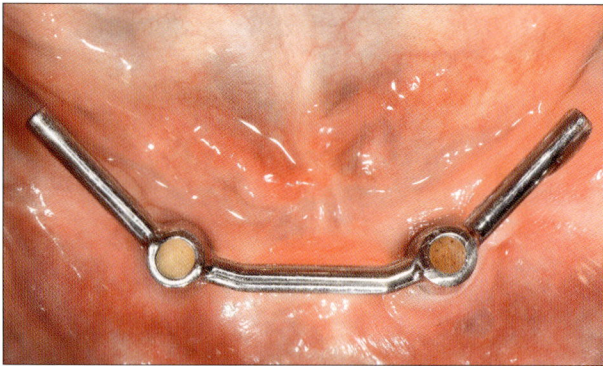

Fig 41   One-year clinical follow-up (occlusal view)

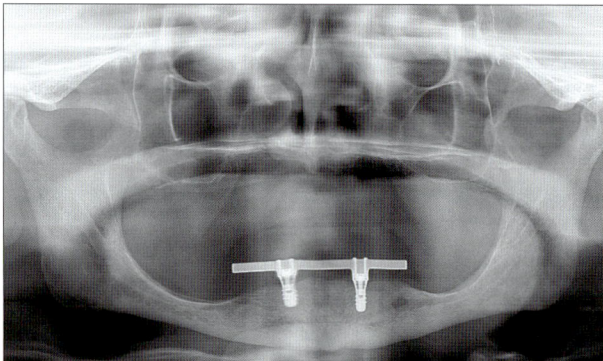

Fig 42   Panoramic radiograph at one year after insertion of the CAD/CAM-milled bar.

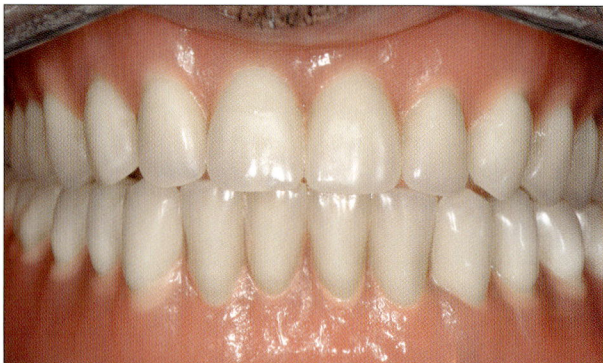

Fig 43   Prostheses in situ with the lips fully retracted at the one-year recall visit.

13.7 Flapless Guided Surgery: Bar-supported Overdenture on Four Implants

R. J. Renting

Guided surgery has become a well-known implantological treatment strategy in recent years. A CBCT scan combined with surgical planning software allows the surgeon to plan the ideal position of the implants before surgery in a digital and three-dimensional environment. With this workflow, the surgeon can recognize and avoid important anatomical structures (Tahmaseb and coworkers 2014).

Guided surgery has a number of advantages if the planning is correct, especially for the medically compromised and geriatric patient, where major surgery should be avoided:

1   Surgery is flapless, so no disturbance of healing needs to be expected.
2   Major augmentation procedures are avoided.
3   The time needed for surgery is reduced to a minimum.

All of these factors are likely to help reduce the pain and discomfort in the postoperative period (Hultin and coworkers 2012) and should be taken into consideration when treating a geriatric patient.

A female patient, born in 1934, medically compromised (Renton and coworkers 2013) (ASA III: history of CVAs, arrhythmia, high blood pressure, type 2 diabetes mellitus, hypothyroid, arthroses, and hyperventilation) presented at our clinic. Her remaining maxillary dentition had had to be extracted some years ago due to multiple periapical infections; since then, the patient had been functioning with a conventional maxillary denture. This denture had been giving her problems in terms of function, eating, and digesting food. She lived at a considerable distance from the clinic. Despite the pain while wearing and using the denture, she kept her spirits and hoped for a different solution. She wished for more comfort and better chewing ability; at the time, she could not visit friends or have dinner in a restaurant with her conventional denture.

Intraorally, the patient presented with a complete mandibular dentition without complaints and sufficient oral hygiene. The maxilla had a flattened aspect and a shallow palate and vestibulum that compromised the retention of the denture (Figs 1a-d). The patient complained about pain when loading the denture. Because of the exerted-force discrepancy between the upper and lower jaws and the difficult status in the maxilla, an implant-supported denture appeared to be the treatment of choice.

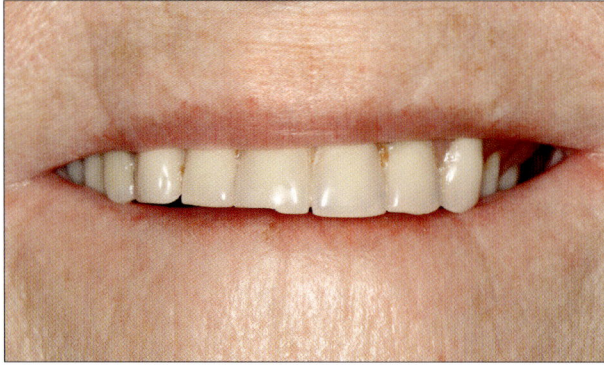

Fig 1a Initial smile line with the maxillary denture.

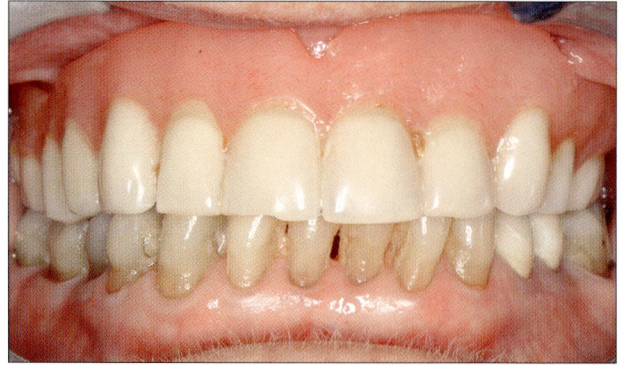

Fig 1b Maxillary denture in maximum occlusion.

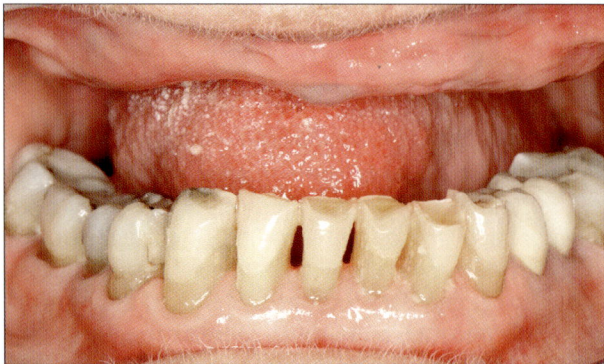

Fig 1c Initial clinical presentation of the edentulous maxilla.

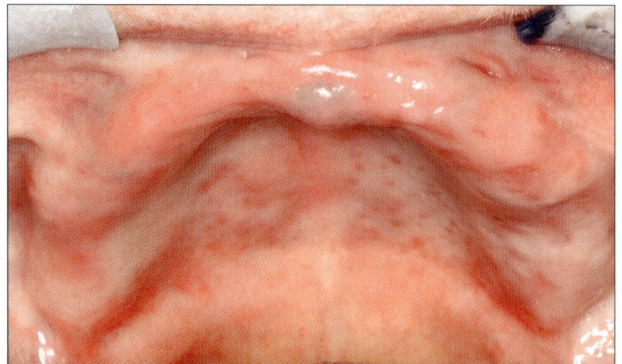

Fig 1d Initial clinical presentation (occlusal view).

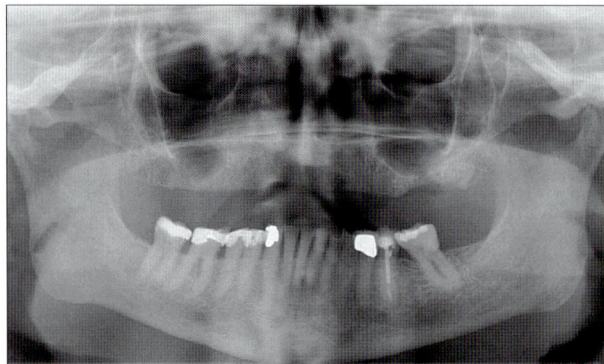

Fig 2 Initial panoramic radiograph.

The panoramic radiograph showed a bilaterally pneumatic maxillary sinus (Fig 2).

Because of the patient's medical condition and history, it was decided to perform the surgery as atraumatically as possible, the goal being to avoid a sinus-floor augmentation. This can be achieved with a flapless guided-surgery workflow.

To be able to perform prosthetically driven digital implant planning, analog information had to be digitized. The first step was a set-up in wax (wax try-in) to analyze and optimize the esthetics and the available intermaxillary space (Figs 3a-b). When the set-up had been approved by the dentist and patient, it was converted to a radiographic template with barium teeth (Israelson and coworkers 2013; Fig 3c).

The analog set-up was now converted into a digital set-up using two CBCT scans and implant-planning software. Two CBCT scans were taken, one of the patient with the scan denture in situ and one of just the scan denture. A lab scanner was used to scan a plaster cast of the maxillary jaw. By superimposing the scans in the coDiagnostiX planning software (Dental Wings, Chemnitz, Germany), a 3D model was created to facilitate prosthetically driven implant planning (Fig 4).

When the planning was completed, a guided surgical guide (drilling stent) was manufactured, in this case by 3D printing (Implantec, Amstetten, Germany). Even though the surgical guide was mucosally supported, this production method still increased accuracy. The main difference was in the positions of the sleeves, which were digitally planned and printed and the surgeon simply clicked metal sleeves in place. This positioning formerly had to be done manually on the plaster cast (Kuehl and coworkers 2015; Schneider and coworkers 2015).

In this case, four implants were planned in the premaxilla region, avoiding the left and right maxillary sinus.

Before the surgery, the fit of the guide was assessed and checked for stability. It is very important to keep the surgical guide immobile while performing the osteotomies. A sufficient width of keratinized mucosa made it possible to perform flapless surgery. Osteotomies where made according to manufacturer's instructions and checked for fenestrations. Four implants were placed (Figs 5a-e): at sites 14, 24 (Straumann SP SLActive Roxolid, diameter 4.1 mm, length 8 mm; Institut Straumann AG, Basel, Switzerland) and 12 and 22 (Straumann SP SLActive Roxolid, diameter 3.3 mm, length 10 mm; Institut Straumann AG). The panoramic radiograph showed the implants in front of the medial sinus walls (Fig 6).

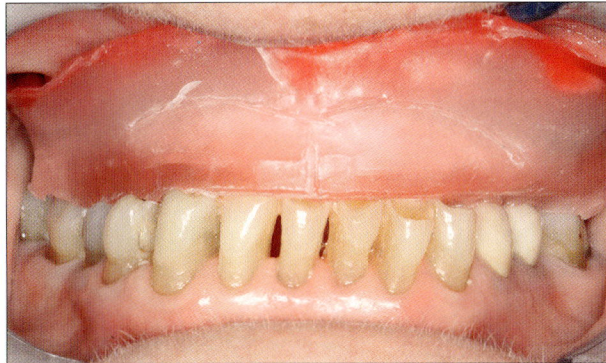

Fig 3a   Diagnostic bite registration.

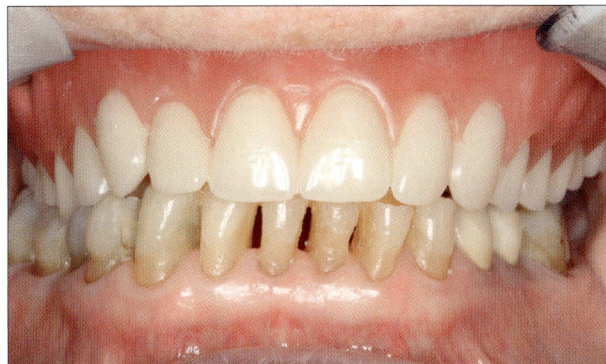

Fig 3b   Diagnostic wax try-in.

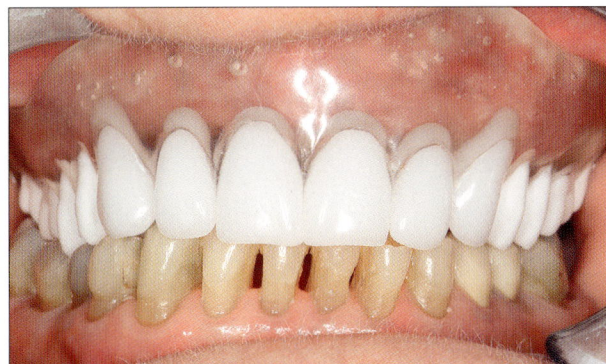

Fig 3c   Radiographic template with barium teeth in situ.

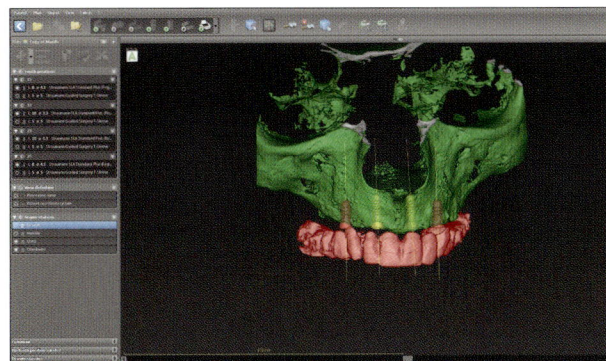

Fig 4   Superimposition of the digitalized information, CBCT scan, and planning (coDiagnostiX; Dental Wings, Chemnitz, Germany).

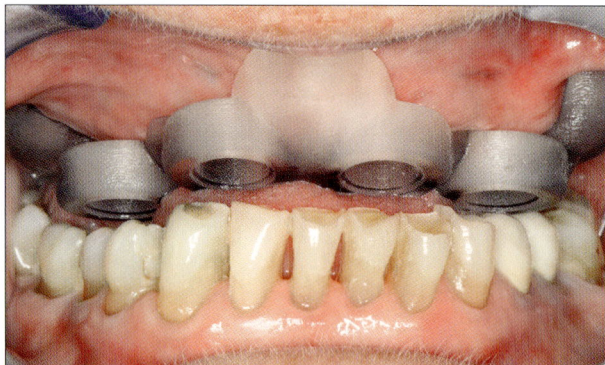

Fig 5a   Frontal view of the 3D-printed surgical guide (Implantec, Amstetten, Germany).

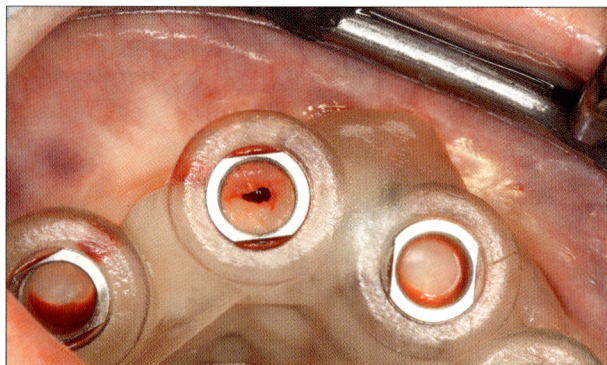

Fig 5b   Occlusal view of the 3D-printed surgical guide complete with guide sleeves.

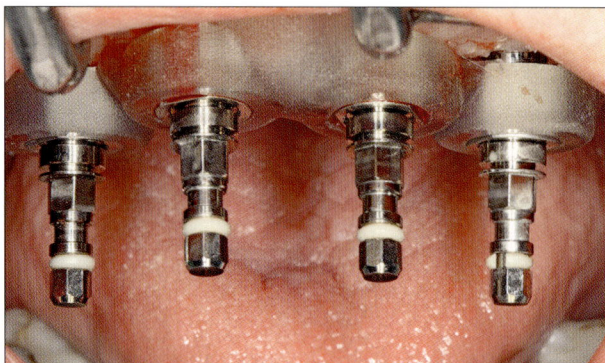

Fig 5c   Frontal view of implant with pick-ups inserted through the guide (guided surgical system: Institut Straumann AG, Basel, Switzerland).

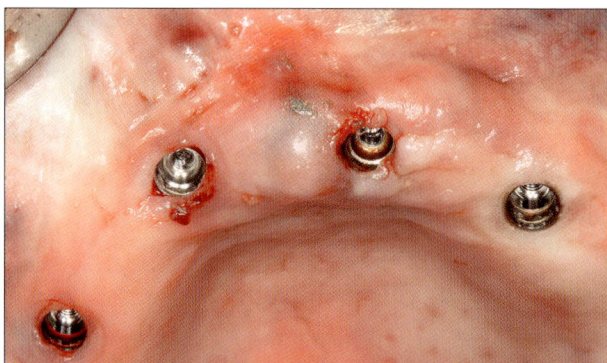

Fig 5d   Occlusal view directly after implant placement.

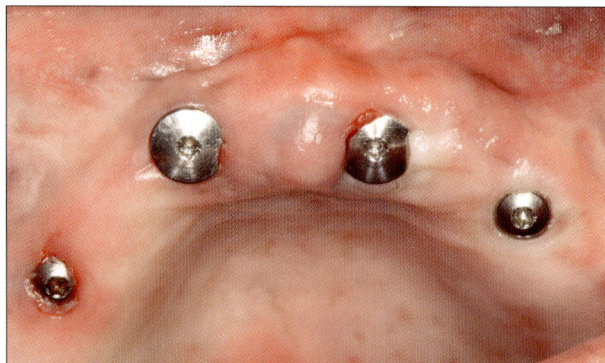

Fig 5e   Occlusal view after placement of healing abutments.

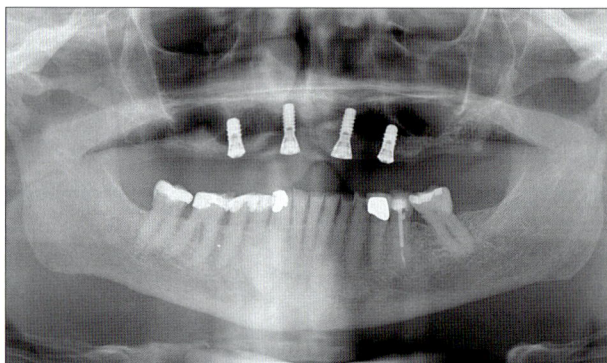

Fig 6   Panoramic radiograph after implant placement.

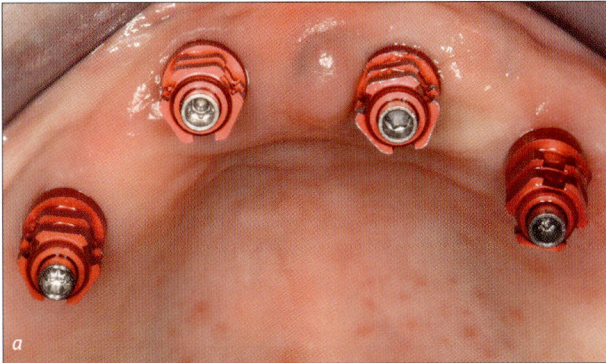

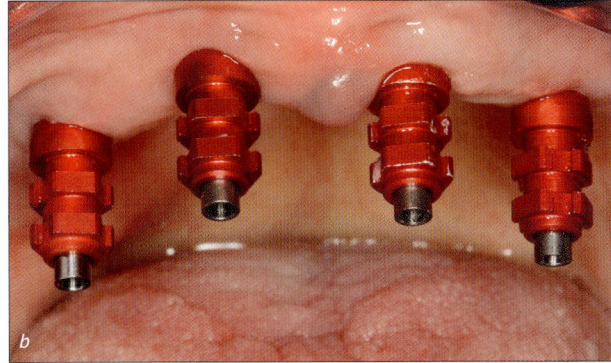

Fig 7a-b   Occlusal and frontal view of impression copings.

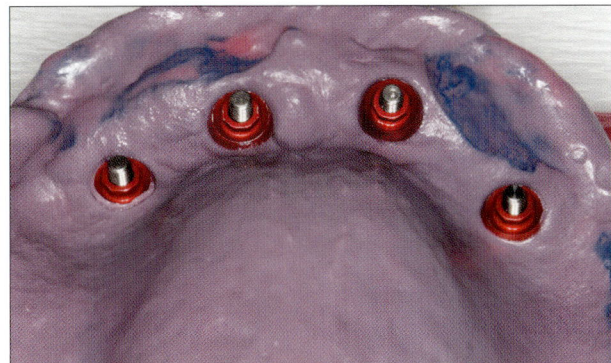

Fig 7c   Impression (Impregum; 3M ESPE, Seefeld, Germany) with impression copings.

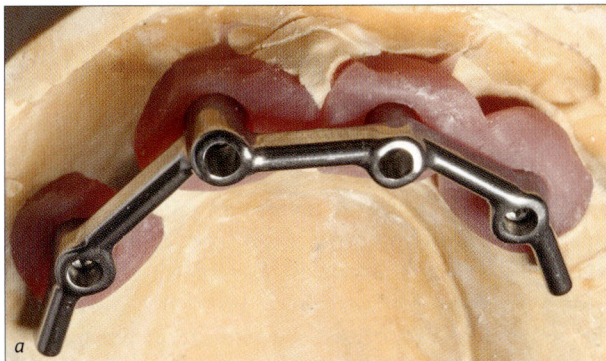

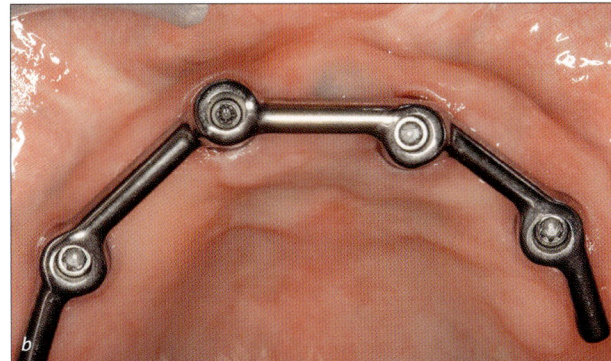

Fig 8a-b   Milled splinted bar on cast model and occlusal view.

After the recommended healing period, the four implants were loaded. The previous set-up was checked again and a conventional impression was taken (Figs 7a-c). A splinted bar on the four implants was chosen to support an overdenture (Figs 8a-c).

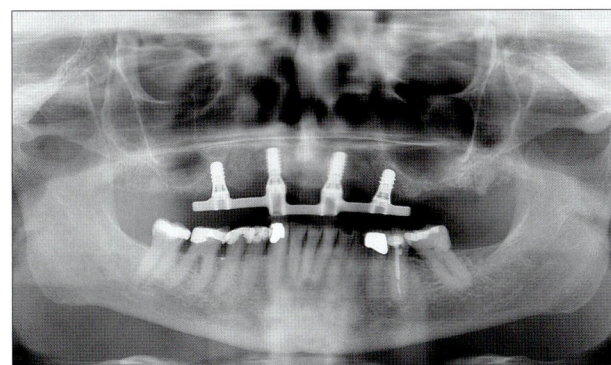

Fig 8c   Panoramic radiograph after placement of the bar on the implants.

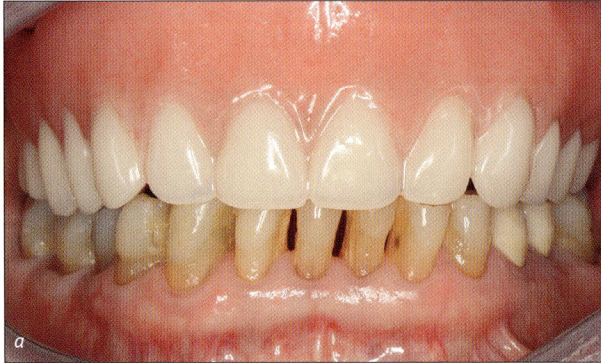

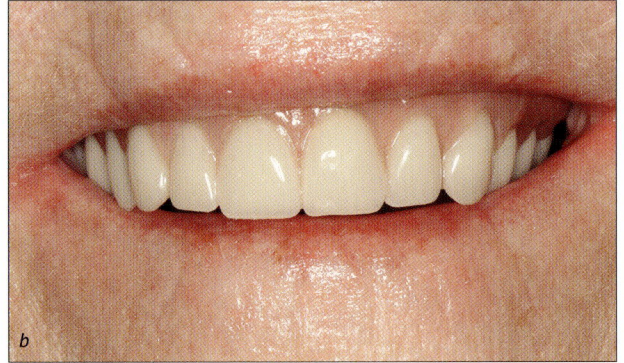

Fig 9a-b   Frontal view and smile at prosthetic delivery.

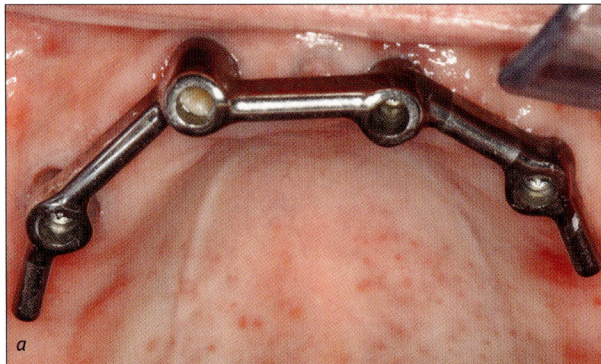

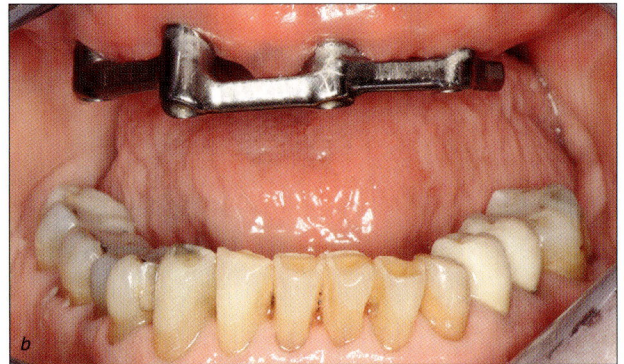

Fig 10a-b   Occlusal and frontal views at the 12-month follow-up.

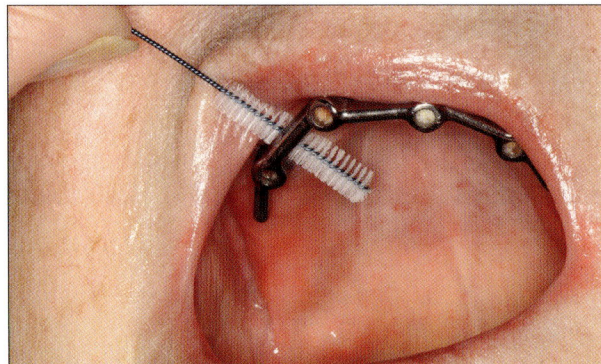

Fig 11   The patient demonstrating her daily maintenance.

Thanks to the guided planning, the surgeon was able to avoid elaborate sinus augmentation surgery and keep surgical entries, treatment time, and morbidity to a minimum. This also meant reduced postsurgical maintenance, resulting in fewer clinical visits. No adjustments had to be made in the patient's medication. No implants were placed in augmented bone, resulting in an osseointegration time of 3 instead of 6 months. All these factors are of great benefit to a geriatric patient with this kind of medical status.

After getting used to the new denture (Figs 9a-b), the patient felt much more confident in social events; her chewing comfort improved, and she was able to eat solid food again. Figures 10 to 14 shows the situation at the 12-month follow-up.

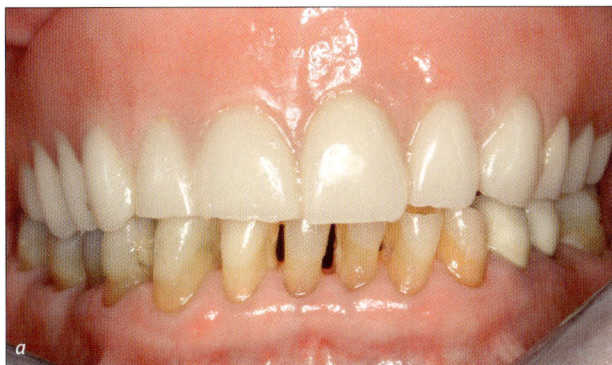

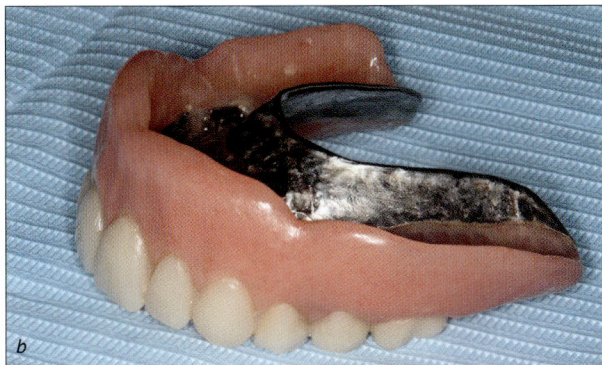

Fig 12a-b   The occlusion and a view of denture at the 12-month follow-up.

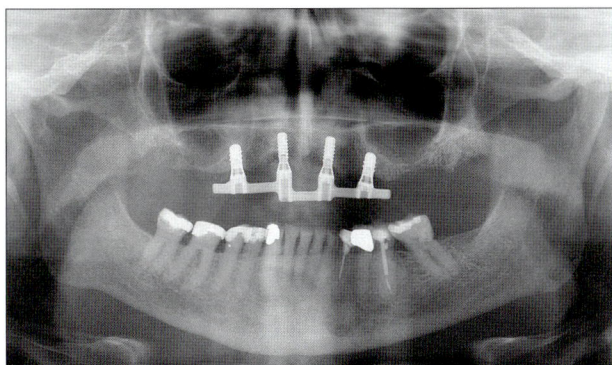

Fig 13   Panoramic radiograph at the 12-month follow-up.

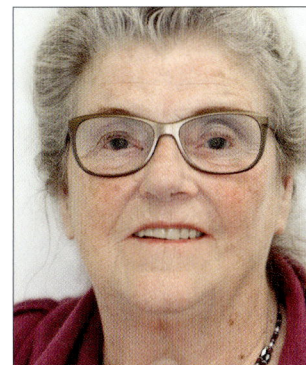

Fig 14   Frontal view one year after prosthetic delivery.

Acknowledgment

The author wishes to thank Dr. W. D. C. Derksen for his help with the planning software.

13.8   Prosthodontic Solution for Two Angulated 6-mm Implants Supporting a Removable Partial Denture in a 74-year-old Patient

U. Webersberger

A 74-year-old woman was referred to the Department of Maxillofacial Surgery at the Medical University of Innsbruck, Austria with retention loss of her upper and lower dentures and resulting pain from the flabby ridge in the maxilla.

Her general medical history included common bradycardic arrhythmias (AV block, 1st degree), bronchial asthma, and type 2 diabetes. She was under the regular control of her general practitioner, who prescribed her a number of medications including: Amilostad (Stada, Bad Vilbel, Germany) for hypertension, Singulair (MSD, Kenilworth, NJ, USA) and Symbicort turbohalers (AstraZeneca, London, UK) for bronchial asthma, metformin for the management of type 2 diabetes, and simvastatin for high cholesterol.

Her dental history included a chin osteotomy 25 years previously. The wires of the chin osteotomy were still in place (Fig 1). To prevent bone resorption, the alveolar defect in the molar area had been filled with bone-graft material during the chin osteotomy after extraction of the molars (Figs 1, 19, and 20). At that time, the patient also became edentate in the maxilla. She was used to dentures, but had been suffering from her hurting flabby ridge in the maxilla for 20 years.

The patient was well oriented. She was living with her husband, had two children and grandchildren, and enjoyed a fulfilling life.

An immediate radiographic evaluation of the remaining alveolar bone height in the mandible was performed without a study model and radiographic ball-bearing template. Instead, the diagnostic X-ray measurement balls were directly incorporated in the existing removable partial denture (RPD) (Fig 2). The method is simple and enables the busy practitioner to obtain an immediate radiographic diagnosis and to inform the patient about the available alveolar bone height at the planned implant site at the first visit.

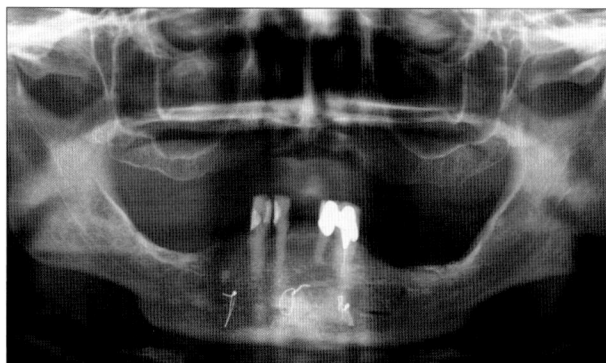

Fig 1   Baseline panoramic radiograph. Wires from a previous chin osteotomy still in place.

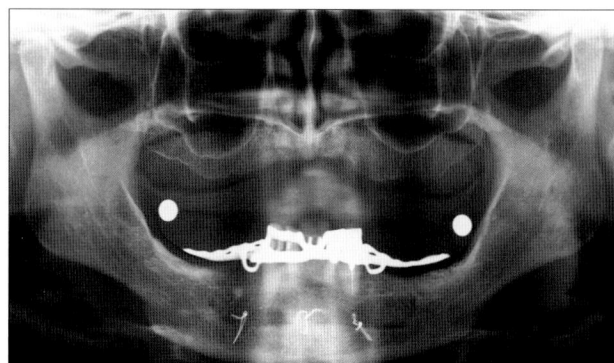

Fig 2   Panoramic radiograph with measurement balls in the distal part of the existing removable partial denture.

The following dental diagnoses resulted after oral examination and radiographic investigation (Figs 1 and 2):

- Completely edentulous maxilla opposing a Kennedy class I partially edentulous mandible (bilaterally).
- Advanced atrophy in the anterior maxilla and posterior mandible.
- Lack of retention and stability of the complete maxillary denture resulting from the flabby ridge.
- The remaining mandibular dentition was considered salvageable.
- Retention loss of the mandibular partial denture.

A staged treatment approach to maximize the esthetic and functional treatment outcome with surgical hard-tissue augmentation in both jaws was discussed with the patient but was declined. She liked the esthetics of her maxillary denture, she just felt very uncomfortable with the retention loss resulting from the painful flabby ridge. Discussions revealed that she had concerns about extensive surgical procedures. She was aware that without additional distal implant support, the retention and stability of the mandibular RPD could not be improved.

After careful evaluation and discussions with the patient, the following treatment plan was decided on:

- Maxillary vestibuloplasty.
- Provisional relining of the maxillary denture.
- Insertion of two angulated implants at sites 37 and 47.
- Restoration of the remaining teeth with composite fillings.
- After healing, definitive relining of the maxillary denture.
- Implant-supported RPD with resilient implant attachments.

Oral hygiene and conservative treatment of the remaining mandibular teeth with composite fillings proceeded without complications. After maxillary vestibuloplasty surgery with a free mucosal flap harvested from the cheek, two 6-mm Tissue Level SLA implants (Institut Straumann AG, Basel, Switzerland) were placed at sites 37 and 47 (Fig 3).

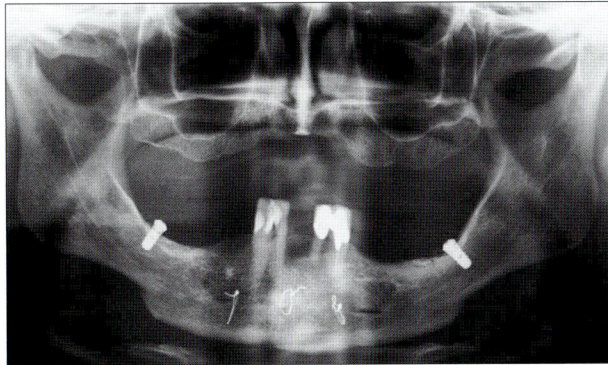

Fig 3   Panoramic radiograph view after placement of two implants in the mandible.

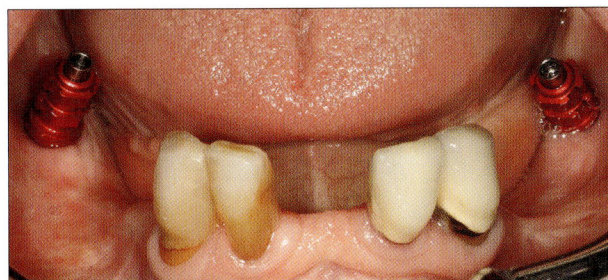

Fig 4   Straumann open-tray impression posts on the Tissue Level implants.

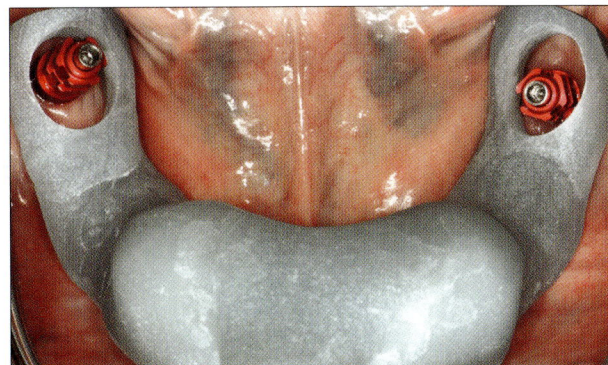

Fig 5   Occlusal view of the open impression tray.

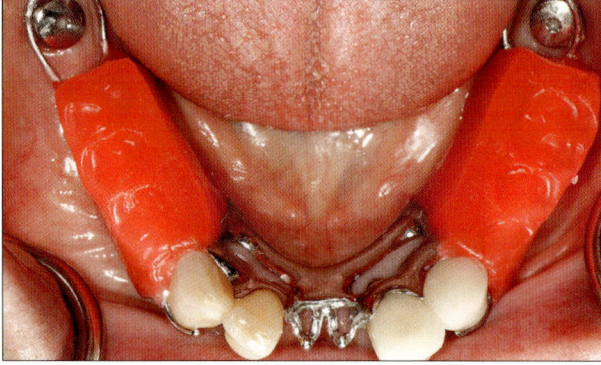

Fig 6   *Occlusal rim of the framework after determination of the jaw relationship.*

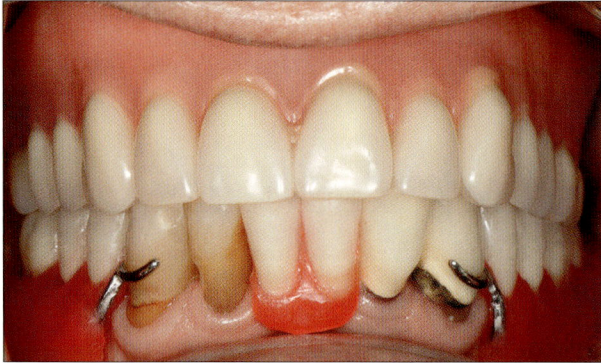

Fig 7   *Trial mandibular denture.*

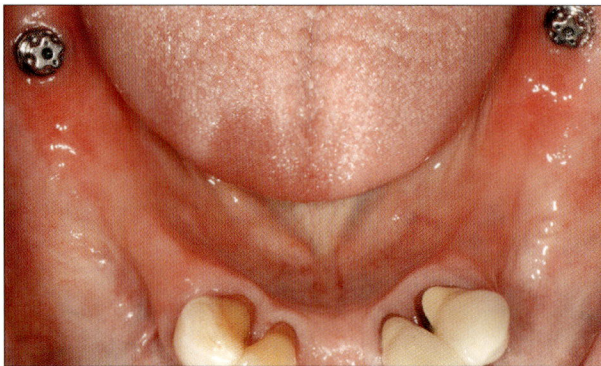

Fig 8   *Occlusal view. Mandible with torqued SFI abutments.*

After the vestibuloplasty, the intaglio surface of the maxillary denture was relieved and relined with a soft relining material (Coe-Comfort; GC Europe, Leuven, Belgium). Two months later, the border of the existing complete denture was molded using impression compound (KerrHawe, Bioggio, Switzerland) to duplicate the contour and size of the vestibule. A functional impression was then taken using Permlastic polysulfide (KerrHawe). The new denture base was reprocessed at the dental laboratory with heat-polymerizing acrylic resin. Another two months later, two impression posts were inserted in the mandible (Fig 4), and an open-tray impression was taken in silicone (Affinis; Coltene, Altstätten, Switzerland) with a custom open acrylic-resin tray (Fig 5).

Figures 4 and 5 demonstrate the mesial angulation of the implants in the molar area. The available implant attachments allow restoring non-parallel implants diverging by up to 40°. However, even more compensation was needed here. This problem could not be resolved with the originally planned Locator attachment. Because of the great divergence, we decided to use the new SFI-Anchor D60 abutment (Institut Straumann AG, Basel, Switzerland), which provides 50% more angulation compensation: implant divergences of up to 60° can be compensated for. After the impression was taken, it was decided to produce the metal-framework RPD first and integrate the SFI-Anchors afterwards.

At the next appointment, the metal framework design was placed in occlusion using the occlusal rims to determine the jaw relationship (Fig 6).

The shade, material, and mold of the artificial teeth were specified. The next stage was a try-in of the trial denture (Fig 7). The wax was replaced by acrylic at the laboratory, and the denture was delivered at the next visit.

After 4 weeks, the healing caps were removed and the SFI-Anchor attachments were inserted into the Tissue Level implants. The abutments were torqued to 35 Ncm with the SFI-Anchor screwdriver and the Straumann ratchet with torque-control device.

The occlusal view of the mandible (Fig 8) demonstrates the modification of the Kennedy class I mandibular arch to a more favorable Kennedy class III arch with two implants and SFI-Anchor attachments.

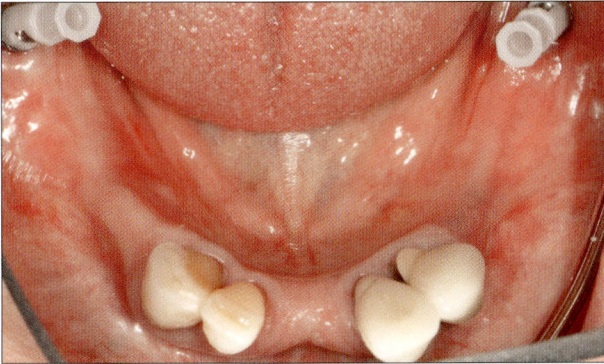

Fig 9   SFI-Anchor aligner positioned on the SFI abutments.

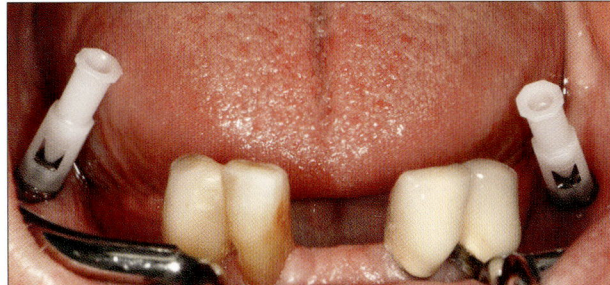

Fig 10   Frontal view: SFI-Anchor aligner on the SFI abutments.

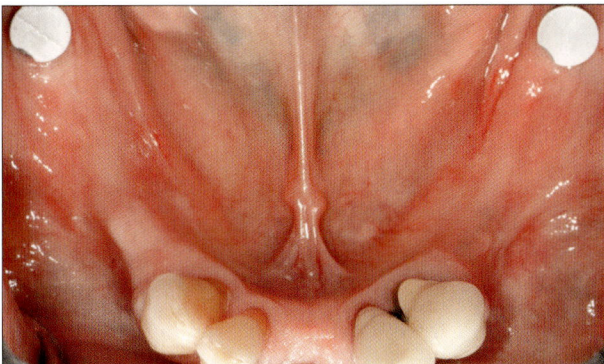

Fig 11   Occlusal view. SFI-Anchor impression post on the SFI-Anchor abutment.

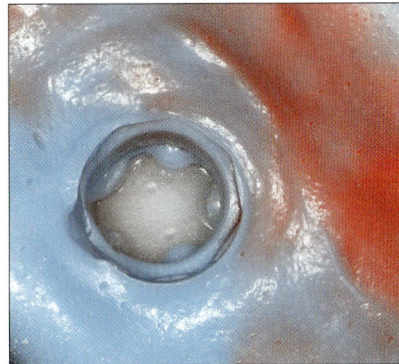

Fig 12   Impression with SFI-Anchor impression post.

The abutment aligners were placed on the Straumann SFI-Anchors (Figs 9 and 10). Self-adhesive dual-cure composite bonding cement (Multilink, Ivoclar Vivadent, Schaan, Liechtenstein) was inserted in the abutment aligner until excess cement came out of the vent holes. The two Straumann SFI-Anchor abutments were oriented with the help of the abutment aligner to achieve parallelism. Once the cement had completely cured, the aligners were removed.

The existing mandibular denture was relieved above the anchors. SFI-Anchor impression posts were placed on the SFI-Anchor abutments (Fig 11), and an impression was taken in silicone (Affinis; Coltene, Altstätten, Switzerland) (Fig 12). The denture was sent to the dental laboratory to polymerize the SFI-Anchor inserts into the relief areas of the denture.

Four color-coded polymer Pekkton (Cendres+Métaux, Biel, Switzerland) retention inserts (extra-low, low, medium, and strong) and the Elitor (highest retention strength; Institut Straumann AG, Basel, Switzerland) for different retention strength needs are available for the SFI-Anchor system. In this case, we opted for the red Pekkton insert (045.048) with low retention strength for both SFI-Anchors (Figs 13 to 15).

Once the maxillary complete denture was relined, the patient had enough retention and stability. The maxillary mucosa healed well after a vestibuloplasty (Fig 16). The insertion of the implant-supported metal-framework RPD proceeded uneventfully (Figs 17 and 18).

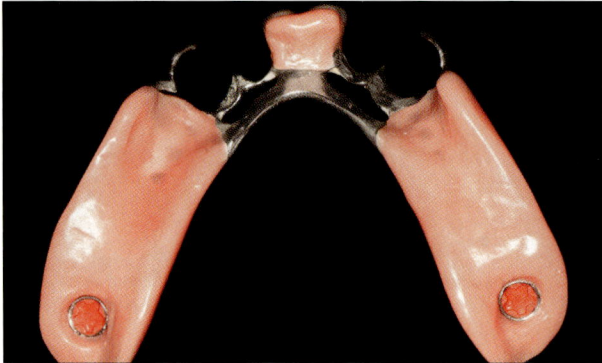

Fig 13   Removable metal-framework partial denture (RPD) with Pekkton inserts.

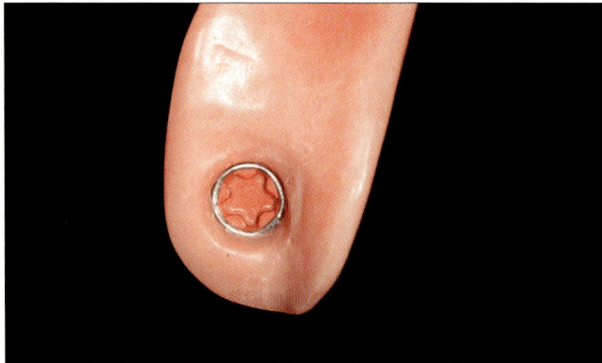

Fig 14   Polymerized five-star Pekkton insert in the mandibular denture (right side).

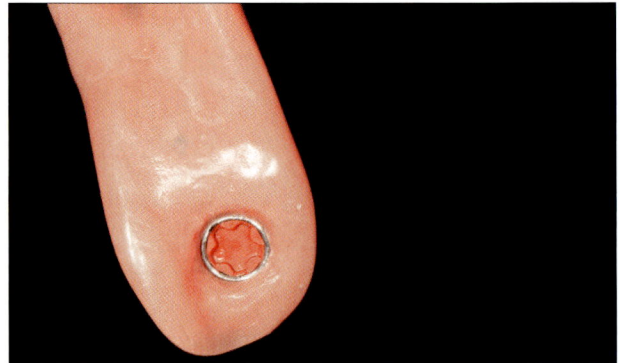

Fig 15   Polymerized five-star Pekkton insert in the mandibular denture (left side).

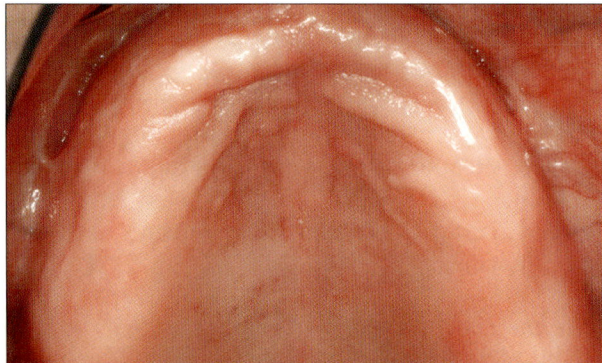

Fig 16   Occlusal view. Edentate maxilla 7 months after the vestibuloplasty.

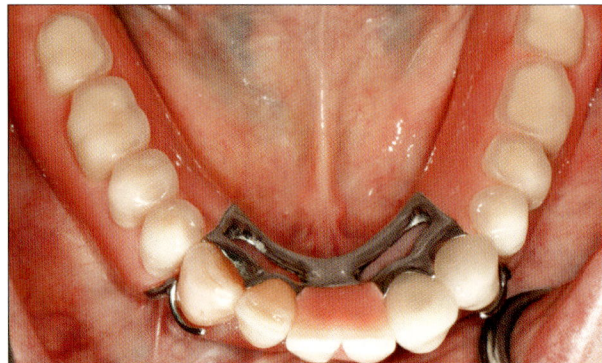

Fig 17   Occlusal view. Inserted implant-supported metal-framework RPD.

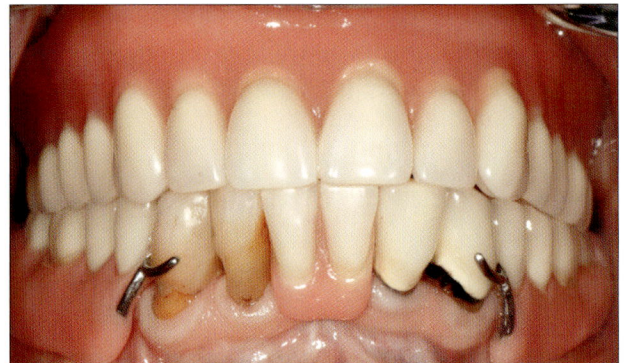

Fig 18   Frontal view after insertion of the denture.

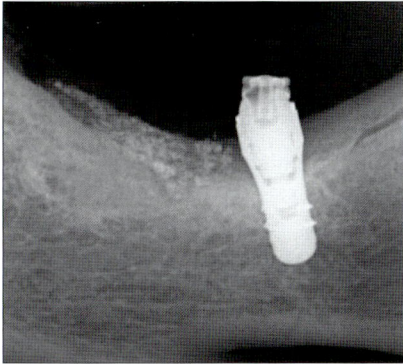

Fig 19   SFI-Anchor after insertion (left side).

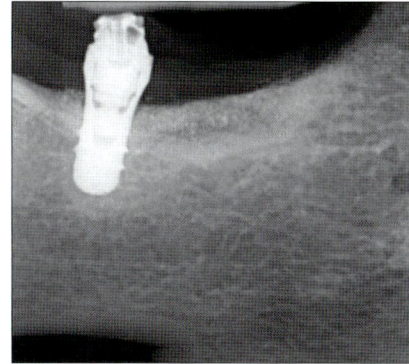

Fig 20   SFI-Anchor after insertion (right side).

The radiographs of the SFI-Anchors after insertion (Figs 19 and 20) impressively demonstrate the compensated angle of the two abutments.

The prosthetic design changed the Kennedy classification of the partially edentulous mandible from class I to class III. Additionally, the bilateral distal single implants changed the mandibular RPD from tooth/tissue-supported to tooth/implant-supported. The patient felt very comfortable wearing the new metal-framework RPD. After the initial assessment, the patient was seen every 6 months for a 2-year period. There were no complications.

At the dental appointment 2 years after insertion (Fig 21), the patient was still satisfied with the restoration, as she was able to perform routine oral functions and maintain good oral hygiene. A final panoramic radiograph was taken (Fig 22) that showed no change in crestal bone levels of the two distal mandibular implants after 2 years of loading.

Remark

With this abutment type, the retention cannot be easily restored when it diminishes by replacing a worn retentive five-star Pekkton insert, unlike the procedure when using Locator abutments. In the author's opinion, an intraoral pickup of the SFI-Anchor abutment will be necessary if the insert has to be replaced.

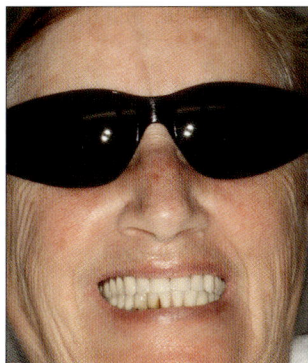

Fig 21   Happy patient 2 years after delivery of her RPD.

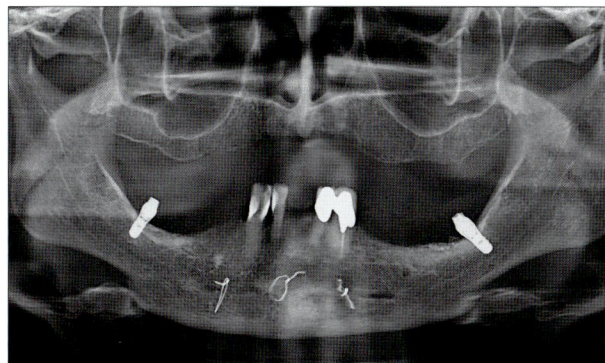

Fig 22   Panoramic radiograph 2 years after delivery.

13.9 Rehabilitation of a Mandibular Distal Extension Situation in a 89-year-old Patient with an Implant-supported Fixed Dental Prosthesis

D. Buser

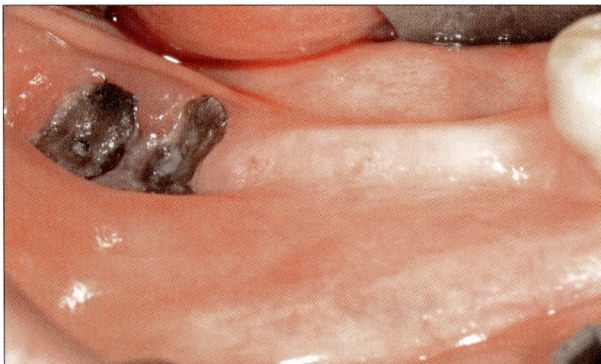

Fig 1   Distal extension situations due to the loss of retention of a three-unit FDP. Extraction site 45 showed complete soft-tissue healing, whereas the root of tooth 47 was still present. The ridge showed slight flattening at site 46.

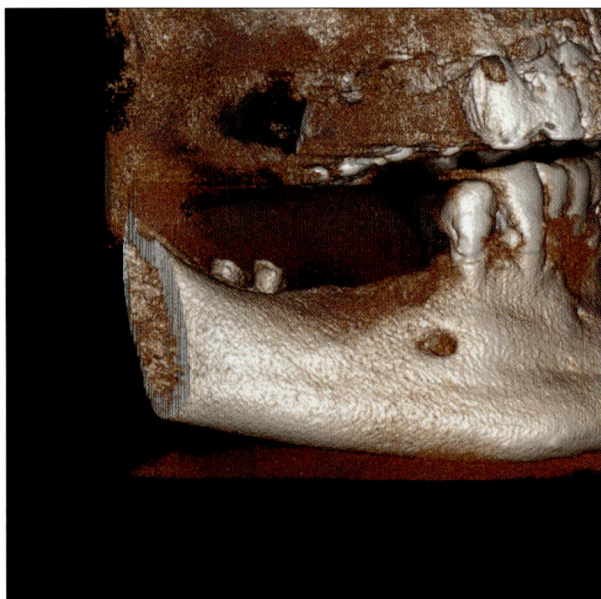

Fig 2   3D CBCT rendering. Distal extension situation, root 47, socket 45, and the buccal flattening at site 46. Note the position of the mental foramen.

A 89-year-old female patient had been referred to the Department of Oral Surgery and Stomatology at the University of Bern for consideration of implant therapy. A long-standing three-unit fixed dental prosthesis (FDP) supported by teeth 45 and 47 showed a loss of retention due to deep secondary caries at tooth 45. The referring dentist removed this tooth prior to referral. At that time, the patient had already undergone implant therapy at our department twice, at the age of 85, at which time hopeless maxillary premolars and molars had to be removed bilaterally. Implant-supported FDPs in both quadrants were provided by the referring dentist following implant surgery at our department, since the patient could not adapt to a removable dental prosthesis in the maxilla.

Preoperative examination
The preoperative examination clearly showed that the patient, despite her advanced age, was in very good physical shape and not mentally impaired at all; she reported taking Aspirin Cardio (Bayer Switzerland, Zürich, Switzerland) as her only medication. The patient insisted on an implant-supported FDP because she had been very pleased with the outcome of previous implant treatment in the maxilla. However, she also asked us to examine the option of a treatment without bone grafting.

The clinical examination showed a partially healed socket at site 45 and remnants of the roots of tooth 47 (Fig 1).

On palpation, the alveolar crest showed buccal flattening at site 46, where the former pontic has been located. Due to the local borderline anatomy, it was decided to analyze potential implant sites with a 3D radiographic examination using cone-beam computed tomography (CBCT). The 3D image—produced by a 3D Accuitomo 170 (Morita, Kyoto, Japan)—confirmed the buccal flattening in the right posterior mandible (Fig 2). The CBCT also showed that the bone height above the mandibular crest was sufficient for implant placement, even though it did not exceed 10 mm (Fig 3).

The axial cut confirmed slight buccal flattening in the mesial aspect of site 46 (Fig 4). Perpendicular orofacial cuts were made at all potential implant sites. The cut in site 45 (Fig 5) showed the extraction-socket defect with a typical reduction of the buccal bone wall. At this site, implant placement would have required a simultaneous GBR procedure to reestablish an intact buccal bone wall. At sites 46 (Figs 6 and 7), the images demonstrated that the alveolar crest was narrow at the top, but had a favorable shape with an increasing width in apical direction. In addition, there was no lingual undercut present. A favorable ridge anatomy allows the placement of a standard implant without bone grafting if the alveolar crest is reduced in height to yield a sufficient crest width of 5 mm for reduced-diameter implants, or 6 mm for standard-diameter implants. The sagittal cut on the mesial aspect of site 46 showed the need for a reduction of roughly 2 – 3 mm to allow the placement of a diameter-reduced implant (Fig 6). The bone height available following this crest reduction was more than 9 mm— sufficient for an 8-mm implant. On the distal aspect of site 46, the crest width was more favorable, requiring only minimal crest reduction for the placement of a standard-diameter 8-mm implant (Fig 7).

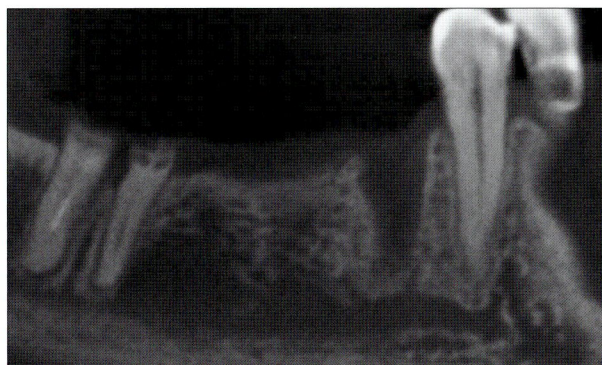

Fig 3 Panoramic cut of the CBCT. Root remnant 47, socket 45, and edentulous site 46. Bone height was limited by the mandibular canal and measures roughly 11 mm. 10-mm implants could not be utilized in this patient.

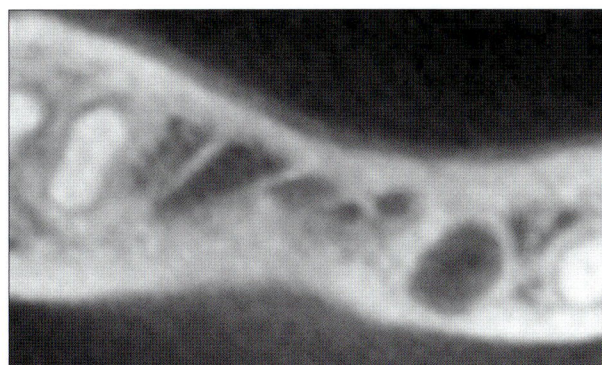

Fig 4 The axial cut confirms the buccal flattening of the crest on the mesial aspect of site 46.

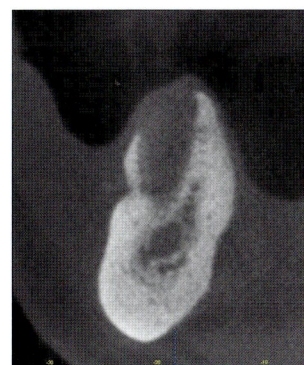

Fig 5 Sagittal cut of extraction socket 45. Typical buccal bone defect that would require contour augmentation in case of implant placement.

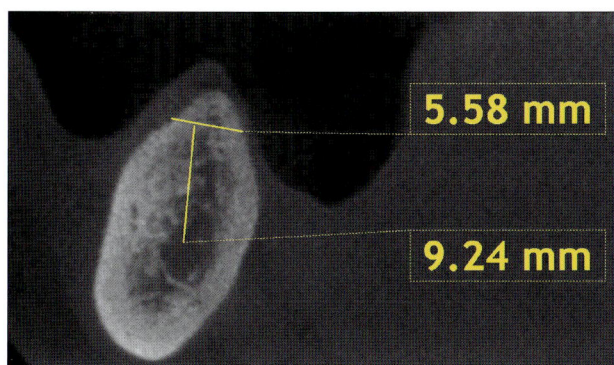

5.58 mm

9.24 mm

Fig 6 Sagittal cut at site 46 mesially. Narrow crest and a need for crest reduction to increase the crest width. The site was suitable for an 8-mm reduced-diameter NNC implant.

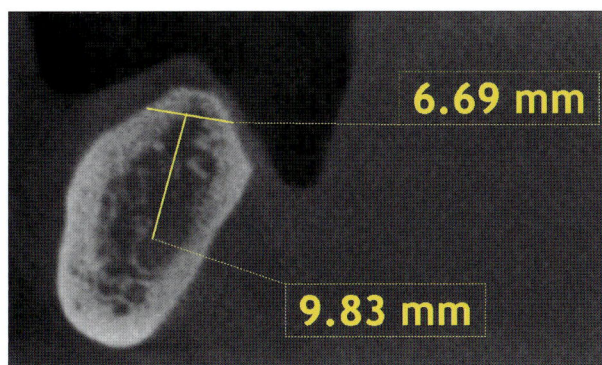

6.69 mm

9.83 mm

Fig 7 Sagittal cut at site 46 distally. Wider crest, allowing the placement of an 8-mm standard-diameter implant.

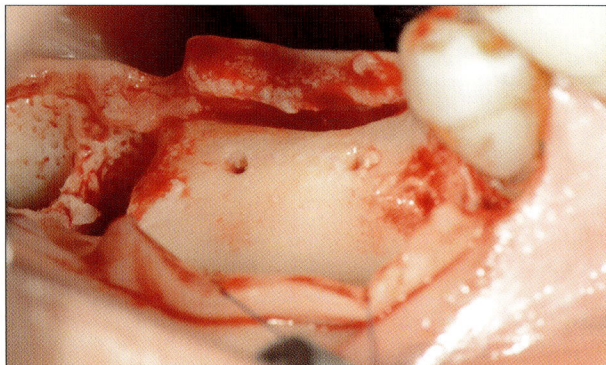

Fig 8   Flap elevated without relieving incision and root 47 extracted. The crest at site 46 was slightly shortened. The two implant sites were marked in the appropriate positions with a round bur.

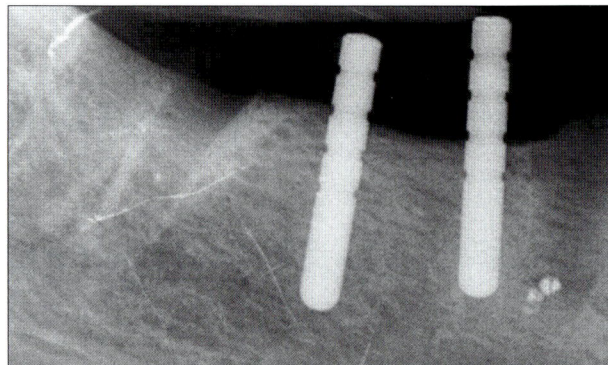

Fig 9   Intraoperative radiograph with two depth gauges in place following preparation with the first spiral drill. The mesial implant bed could be prepared 1 mm deeper without jeopardizing the alveolar nerve.

Based on this preoperative analysis, two treatment options were considered:

Option 1
- Implant placement at sites 45 and 46 with simultaneous GBR
- Both implants would be standard-diameter Tissue Level (TL) implants
- Submerged healing for 8 weeks
- Implant restoration with two single crowns

Option 2
- Implant placement at site 46 mesially with a reduced-diameter NNC (Narrow Neck CrossFit) implant
- Implant placement at site 46 distally with a standard-diameter TL implant
- Implant placement using a standard technique, no bone grafting
- Non-submerged healing for 8 weeks
- Implant restoration with two splinted single crowns and a mesial cantilever at site 45

The patient decided to go for option 2, since she wanted to avoid bone grafting.

Implant therapy
The surgery was undertaken in local anesthesia using an articaine 4% solution combined with a vasoconstrictor (Ubistesin forte; 3M ESPE, Seefeld, Germany), without sedative premedication. The medication with Aspirin Cardio was not interrupted. The flap was raised with a mid-crestal incision at sites 45 and 46 with the goal to obtain a band of keratinized mucosa on both flap margins. The incision was extended mesially into the distobuccal sulcus of tooth 44 without a releasing incision. Distally, the incision was extended through the sulcus of the root remnants 47, also without a releasing incision. The resulting full-thickness flap gave sufficient access to the alveolar crest.

The two root remnants of tooth 47 were removed. The crest was carefully flattened at site 46 and mesially of socket 47 to increase the crest width. The two implant positions were marked with a round bur: the first implant position roughly 10 mm distally of the contact point of tooth 44 and the second one 7 mm further distally (Fig 8).

The implant bed was prepared using a low-trauma technique and a protocol established more than 20 years ago, with a drilling speed of 500 to 800 rpm and copious irrigation with chilled sterile saline (Buser and von Arx 2000). Following the initial preparation of the implant bed with the first spiral drill, an intraoperative digital radiograph was taken with small depth gauges in place to examine the proximity to the mandibular canal. This first step of implant bed preparation often involves a reduced sink depth to eliminate the risk of nerve damage (Fig 9). In this case, it was obvious that the implant bed at site 46 could be prepared 1 to 1.5 mm deeper than planned. Implant-bed preparation continued for a reduced-diameter bed mesially (Figs 10 and 11) and for a standard-diameter implant bed distally, as outlined under option 2 (Fig 12).

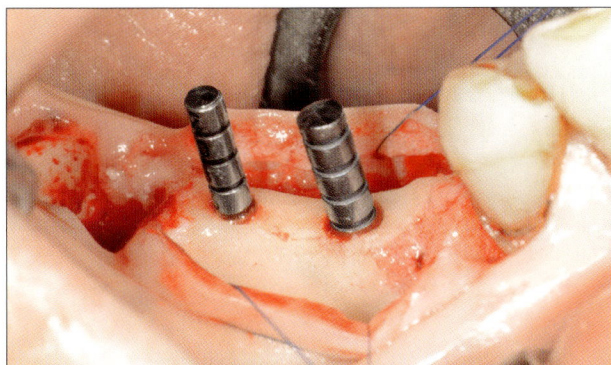

Fig 10 The preparation continued. It was decided to utilize a reduced-diameter NNC implant at the mesial site to maintain an intact buccal bone wall of sufficient thickness (1 mm or more).

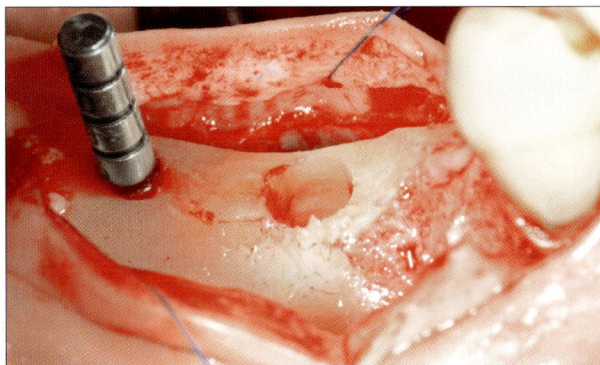

Fig 11 Implant bed prepared mesially, including the use of a profile drill for the NNC implant.

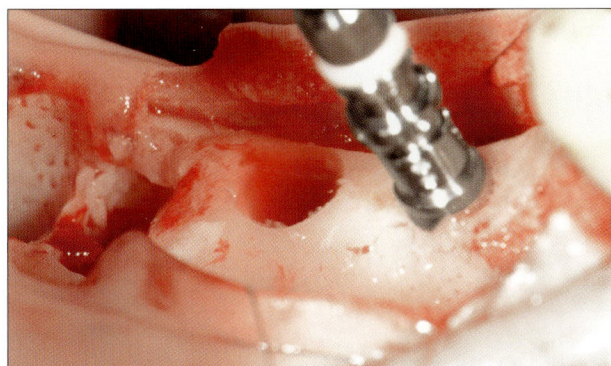

Fig 12 NNC implant inserted. The second implant bed was prepared for a standard-diameter TL implant (S 4.1).

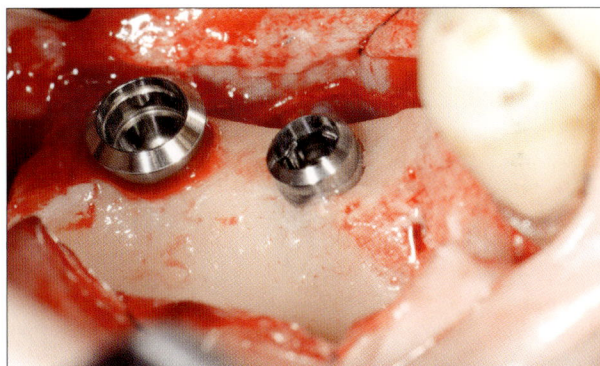

Fig 13 Both implants inserted. The border between the smooth and the SLA surface is located roughly 1 mm below the crest.

A sink depth of roughly 9 mm was chosen for both implant beds. It was important to maintain an intact lingual and buccal bone wall (1 mm or more) to avoid the need for bone grafting. The two 8-mm implants were inserted to a depth of roughly 8.5 to 9 mm. The mesial implant was a NNC Roxolid implant (Straumann, Basel, Switzerland), whereas the distal implant was a Standard Tissue Level (S 4.1) implant with a Regular Neck (RN) configuration (Straumann, Basel, Switzerland). With this insertion technique, the borderline between the ma-

chined surface of the implant neck, and the hydrophilic microrough surface of the implant body (SLActive) was located roughly 1 mm below the crest (Fig 13). Prior to flap closure, the extraction socket in site 47 was degranulated, rinsed with sterile saline, and filled with a collagen plug (TissueCone; Baxter AG, Volketswil, Switzerland) to stabilize the blood clot. The bone defect in the former extraction socket 45 was grafted with Bio-Oss Collagen (Geistlich Biomaterials, Wolhusen, Switzerland).

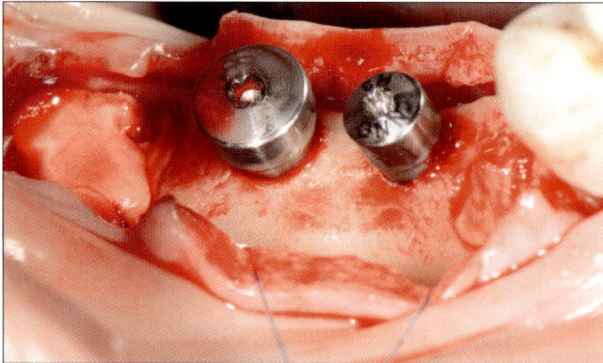

Fig 14 *3-mm healing caps inserted to facilitate easy adaptation of the wound margins for non-submerged healing. Extraction socket 47 is filled with a collagen plug.*

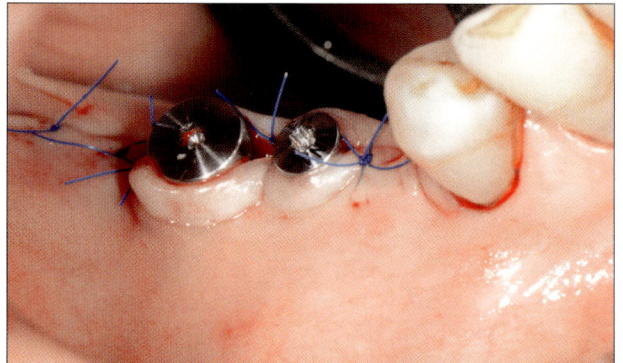

Fig 15 *Completed wound closure using 5-0 non-resorbable monofilament sutures.*

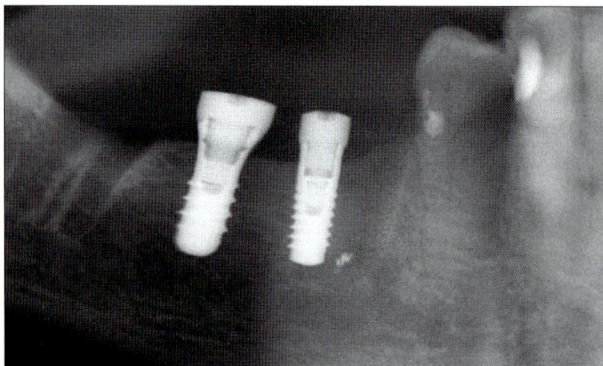

Fig 16 *Postsurgical panoramic radiograph. Correct position of both implants and a safe distance from the mandibular canal.*

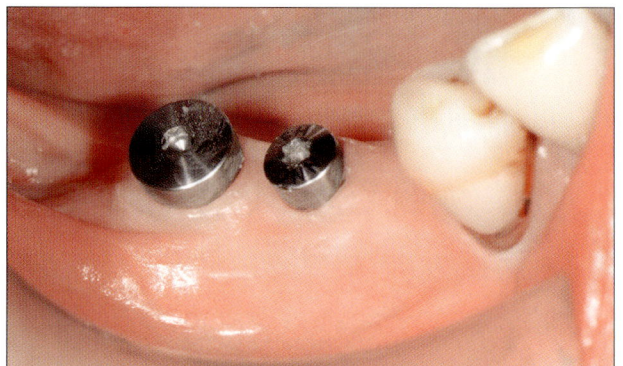

Fig 17 *Eight weeks later: The peri-implant soft tissues are well healed. The width of keratinized mucosa is sufficient.*

Prior to flap closure, 3-mm healing caps were inserted (Fig 14), and a thin layer of fibrin sealant (Tisseel; Baxter AG, Volketswil, Switzerland) was applied to immediately initiate blood coagulation underneath the flap. Then, the wound margins were carefully adapted to both healing caps and secured in place with interrupted single sutures utilizing 5-0 non-resorbable monofilament suture material (Fig 15). This facilitated non-submerged healing without a need for reopening. The postsurgical panoramic radiograph showed the two implants in their correct positions (Fig 16).

Following an uneventful healing period of 8 weeks, both implants were clinically well integrated. Both implants had a sufficient band of keratinized mucosa without visible signs of inflammation (Fig 17). The patient was referred back to the dentist. The two implants were restored with a screw-retained FDP supported by both implants including a mesial cantilever unit.

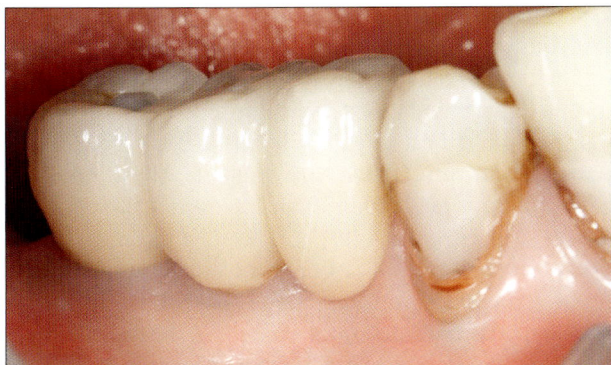

Fig 18 At the 1-year follow-up. The implants were restored with a FDP including a mesial cantilever unit. The peri-implant mucosa is healthy; the 90-year-old patient exercises good plaque control.

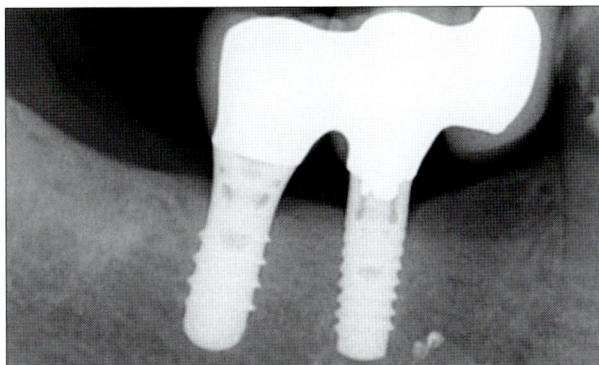

Fig 19 Periapical radiograph. Both implants were well integrated in the bone. The typical signs of slight bone remodeling in the crestal area are visible. The fit of the restoration is excellent.

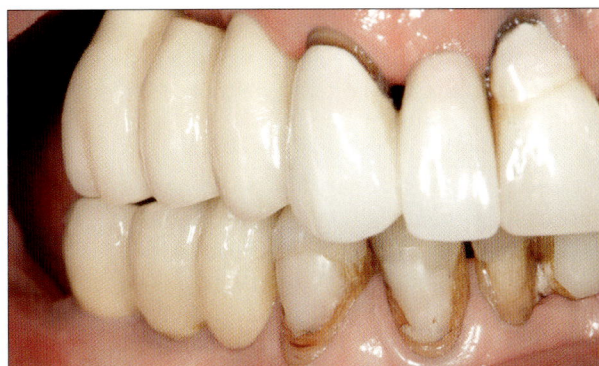

Fig 20 The two implant-supported FDP in the maxilla and mandible. Neighboring teeth show tooth-supported restorations and composite fillings with compromised esthetics, as often seen in patients of that age.

At the 1-year examination, the clinical status showed the two implants restored with a FDP including two splinted single crowns with a mesial cantilever crown. The peri-implant mucosa was clinically healthy and showed no signs of inflammation (Fig 18). The patient, now 90 years old, performed good oral hygiene, using interdental brushes every day. She was very satisfied with her chewing comfort in the right mandible. The periapical radiograph demonstrated some typical signs of bone remodeling at both implants (Fig 19). Overall, the radiograph showed two implants with direct bone apposition to the implant surface. The fit of the FDP on the implant shoulders was very good.

The elderly patient now has implant-supported FDP in the posterior mandible and in the maxilla, offering good chewing comfort (Fig 20). Neighboring teeth mesial to both FDPs show old composite fillings with compromised esthetics, as often seen in patients of that age category.

Discussion

In the present case, implant therapy had been performed in an 89-year-old patient. Such an age is not unusual today. Our department has witnessed an increase of the average age of our implant patients over the past 15 years. In a three-year patient pool treated with dental implants between 2002 and 2004, the percentage of patients aged over 80 years was 1.0% (Bornstein and coworkers 2008). In a later three-year period (2008–2010), representation of this age category had increased to 1.9% (Brügger and coworkers 2015). In 2014, another clear increase to 5.2% was noted (unpublished data). In 2014, the age group over 70 years made up 21.0% of all implant patients, which is quite remarkable. Of those 104 patients aged over 70 years, only 19 had been fully edentulous (18.2%), whereas the remaining patients were all partially edentulous (81.8%), presenting most often with distal extension situations, followed by single-tooth gaps and extended edentulous spaces. It is important to understand that patients of this age group in

Switzerland are no longer dominated by edentulism, as was the case 20 years ago. However, in both categories of patients—if fully or partially edentulous—the main objective of therapy is clearly to improve or maintain their chewing function. In the present patient, the alternative to implant therapy would have been a removable partial denture, which was no option for the female patient due to a non-satisfactory experience with a similar situation in the maxilla 4 years earlier.

During treatment planning, it is our strategy in elderly patients (age over 80 years) to limit the morbidity of therapy.

The most elegant treatment option is flapless implant placement, which requires an excellent bone volume and at least 7 mm of keratinized mucosa. This approach is very elegant in patients with anticoagulation therapy, since it limits the risk for postsurgical bleeding. In the present case, these conditions were not fulfilled due to the buccal flattening at site 46.

The second best treatment option is standard implant placement without the need for bone grafting and extended flap elevation. This approach was feasible in the present case, although a post-extraction bone defect was present at site 45. It was decided to avoid an implant placement in this area. The favorable shape of the mandible at site 46 allowed standard implant placement without bone grafting, as desired by the patient. The available bone height and the rather narrow crest at the top of the alveolar ridge required the shortening of the crest by 2-3 mm to a sufficient width. This shortening to optimize the crest width has been routine at our department for more than 15 years (Buser and von Arx 2000). In addition, the border between the smooth and the microrough SLA implant surface was positioned roughly 1 mm below the bone crest.

The main purpose of this insertion technique is to achieve an intact buccal and lingual bone wall of at least 1 mm thickness following the initial bone-healing phase, which always includes some physiologic bone remodeling caused by the surgical trauma. This helps avoid an exposed microrough SLA (sandblasted and acid-etched) surface in the supracrestal area. As consequence of this surgical technique, implant crowns are slightly longer, but this is no problem in the posterior segments of either jaw; the crown-to-implant ratio is slightly increased. This was acceptable as it is not a risk factor for the long-term performance of dental implants (Blanes and coworkers 2006; Schulte and coworkers 2007; Schneider and coworkers 2012).

Concerning the selection of implant types, Tissue Level implants with an SLA surface were utilized, since these implant types have shown excellent long-term results in our department since their introduction in 1997. As demonstrated in a large study on partially edentulous patients with more than 500 implants, these implants offer a failure rate of less than 2% for a 10-year period (Buser and coworkers 2012). This favorable long-term prognosis, however, is not applicable for heavy smokers (more than 10 cigarettes per day). The distal implant was an 8-mm standard-diameter implant (S 4.1) with a regular neck (RN) design and a machined surface 2.8 mm in height. The mesial implant was diameter-reduced, since the crest was slightly reduced in width as demonstrated by the CBCTs. The implant was an 8-mm NNC implant made of a titanium-zirconium alloy (Roxolid), which offers an increased mechanical strength when compared with commercially pure titanium. This implant type was introduced in our department in 2012 and is primarily utilized in implant sites with borderline crest width. So far, evidence for this implant is only short-term, but it has great potential for more widespread use (Chiapasco and coworkers 2012).

With the two 8-mm implants, the rehabilitation was achieved following an 8-week healing period with two splinted crowns and a mesial cantilever unit. This prosthesis, delivered by the referring dentist in private office, was screw-retained, as most of our implant restorations are these days. A cantilever unit attached to an implant-supported crown has been the standard of care at the University of Bern for roughly 15 years and has been documented by other groups as a valid treatment option in special situations. In the present case, the utilization of only one implant with a cantilever unit was no option, since the mesial implant had a reduced diameter and was only 8 mm long.

In summary, this 89-year-old woman could be treated with a low-morbidity approach using standard implant placement and no simultaneous bone augmentation at either implants. At the 1-year follow-up examination, the patient, now 90 years old, was highly satisfied with her implant-supported FDP, since it offered her the excellent chewing comfort she had hoped for.

13.10 Minimally Invasive Treatment of a Patient in Her Nineties After Removing Implants Affected by Severe Peri-implantitis

M. Roccuzzo

A 93-year-old female patient presented in September 2010 with an enlarged swelling on the lingual side of her lower incisors. At the time, she was essentially healthy, except for reduced vision due to bilateral age-related macular degeneration. She had been a heavy smoker (about 30 cigarettes a day) for the past 20 years after becoming a widow. The patient lived at home by herself, with full-time domestic support.

An extraoral examination revealed nothing adverse. Intraoral plaque control was anything but ideal, and a soft-tissue tumescence was visible around the lingual aspect of 41 – 42 (Fig 1). Because the nature of the lesion was not clear, a biopsy was carried out that revealed the inflammatory nature of the lesion. The panoramic radiograph (Fig 2) showed six irregularly distributed mandibular implants supporting a full-arch prosthesis, with various degrees of interproximal peri-implant resorption. The periapical radiograph (Fig 3) revealed interproximal bone resorption mesially and distally to implant 41.

Different therapeutic options were presented to the patient and her immediate family, explaining the risks and the benefits of each solution. Emphasis was placed on consulting her medical doctor. Even though a minimally invasive treatment was proposed, the patient refused further treatment because of her "old age" and reported that she was still pleased with her chewing capabilities. She accepted only to be seen by the dental hygienist for a session of "light" scaling and cleaning.

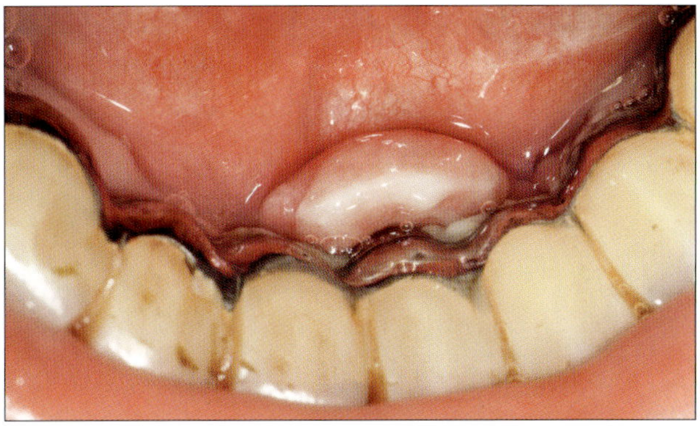

Fig 1   Soft-tissue tumescence lingually at site 41 – 42.

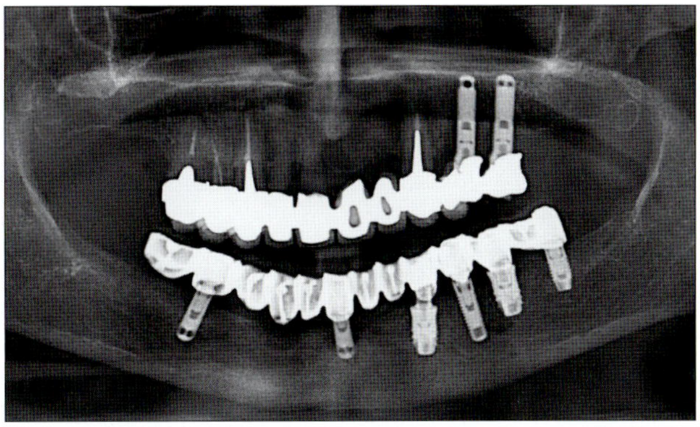

Fig 2   Panoramic radiograph. Six unevenly distributed mandibular implants supporting a full arch dental prosthesis.

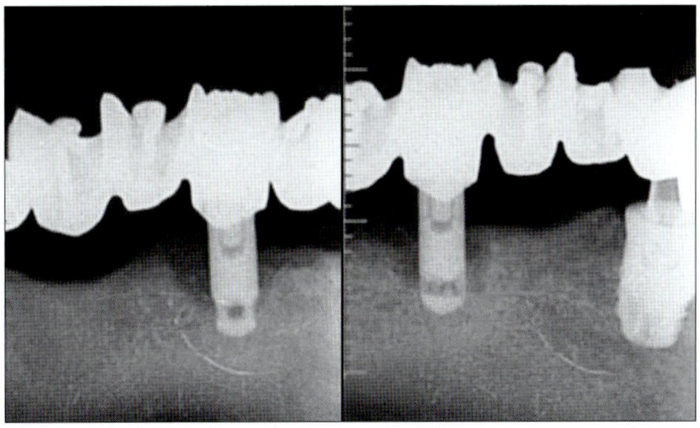

Fig 3   Periapical radiograph. Interproximal bone resorption mesial and distal to the implant at site 41.

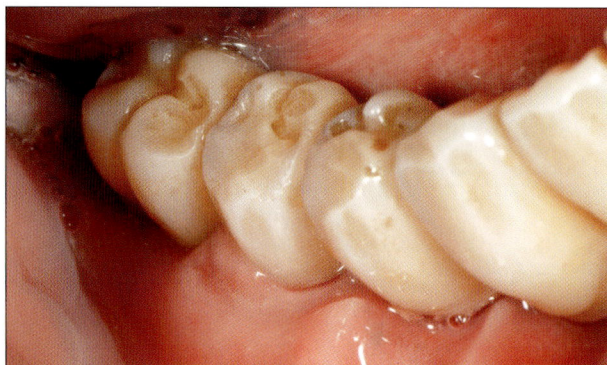

Fig 4   Swelling due to abscess in the lower right mandibular area. Accumulation of soft deposits on the gingival margin and on the adjacent tooth surfaces. The patient had experienced pain and tenderness of the area for several weeks.

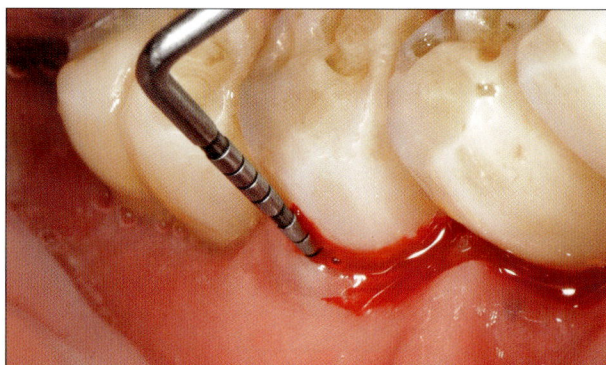

Fig 5   Probing at site 45 reveals deep pockets with severe inflammation of the gingival margin and abundant bleeding on probing.

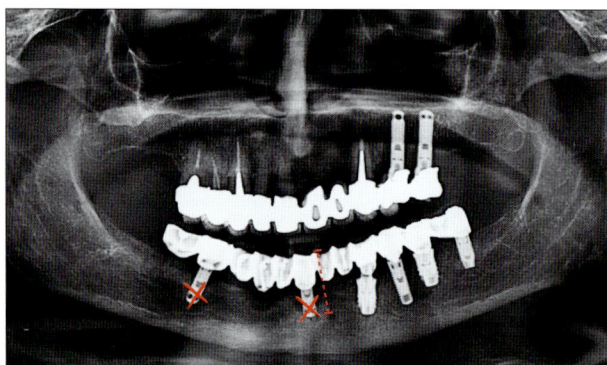

Fig 6   The minimally invasive treatment plan included segmentation of the existing full-arch reconstruction and removal of the two implants affected by peri-implantitis.

Seven months later, in April 2011, the patient returned because of a major abscess in the lower right mandible (Fig 4). It seemed related to implant 45 and presented with pocket depths of 8–9 mm, severe inflammation of the gingival margin, and abundant bleeding on probing (Fig 5). Soft deposits on the gingival margin and the adjacent tooth surfaces were visible to the naked eye.

The patient initially did not want to have the situation remedied, but she and her accompanying person were informed that this could hazardous. They finally accepted the treatment on condition that it be minimally invasive.

It was decided to segment the full-arch mandibular prosthesis, leaving the left half in situ (as the tissue was judged sufficiently healthy) while removing the right half (Fig 6).

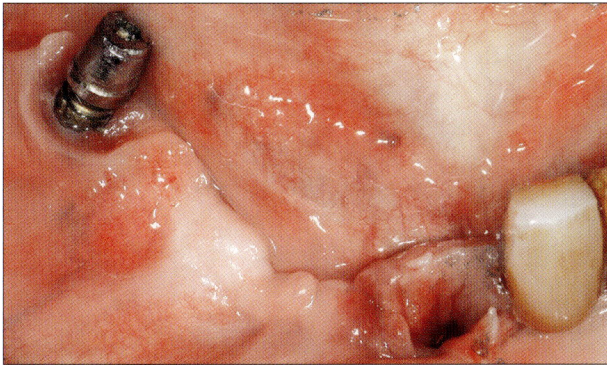

Fig 7   When the bridge was segmented, the implant at the incisor site came off spontaneously.

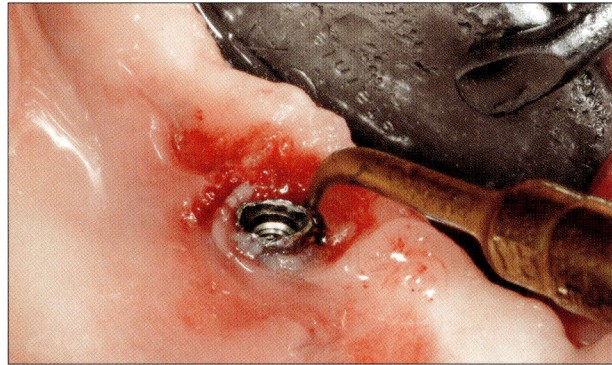

Fig 8   The removal of the implant is facilitated by piezosurgery.

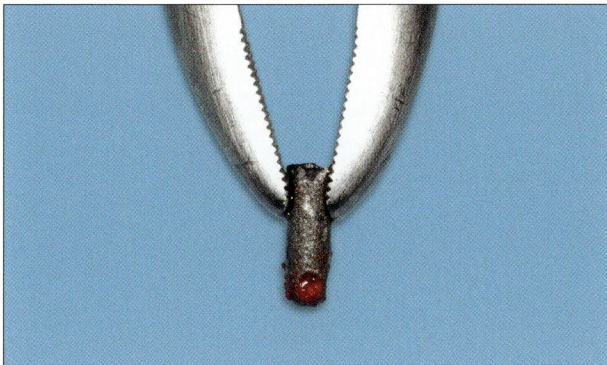

Fig 9   Extraction of the compromised implant at the molar site.

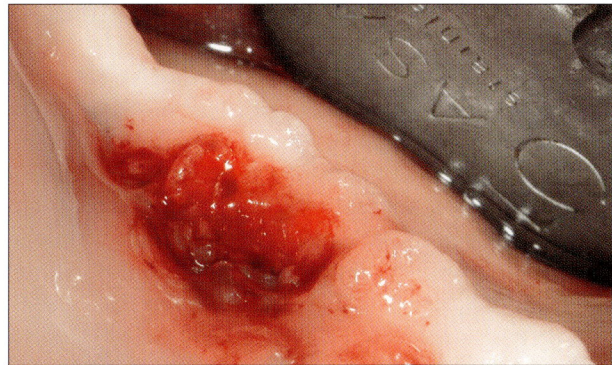

Fig 10   The mandibular left side immediately after implant removal.

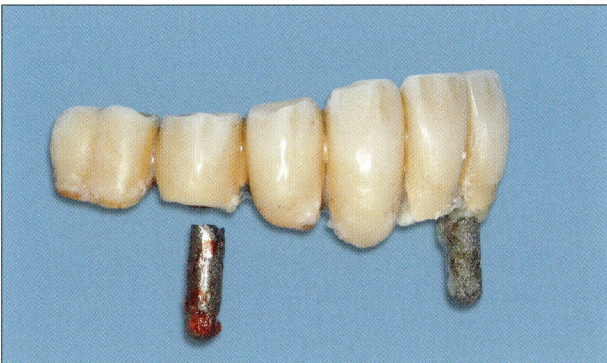

Fig 11   The old restoration after removal of the two implants.

When the bridge was cut between crowns 41 and 31 with a tungsten carbide bur, the implant at the incisor site came off spontaneously (Fig 7). The implant at the molar position, which has caused the abscess, was removed by piezosurgery (Figs 8 to 11).

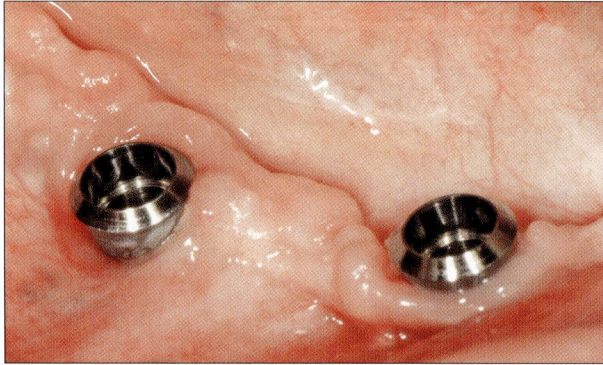

Fig 12   Five weeks after implant placement. Uneventful soft-tissue healing. The cover screws had been removed to connect the provisional fixed restoration.

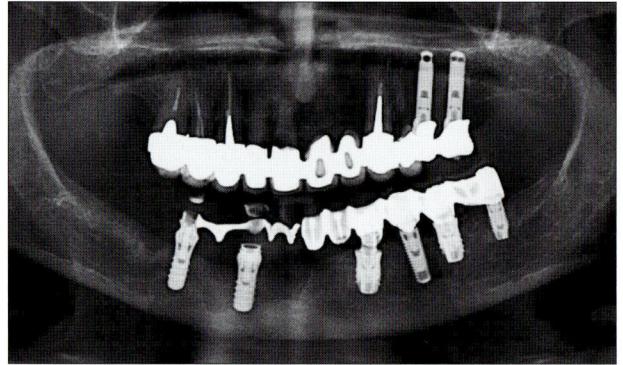

Fig 13   Panoramic radiograph at 4 months. Two new Tissue Level implants in the lower right mandible, with regular peri-implant bone levels. The two implants supported a provisional resin restoration with a double mesial cantilever.

The reconstructive procedure was based on the assumption that the primary objective was a functional outcome with a low risk of complications during healing, a minimum number of surgical interventions, and minimum pain and morbidity. In May 2011, two chemically modified titanium implants (Straumann SLActive, RN, diameter 4.1 mm, length 8 mm; Institut Straumann AG, Basel, Switzerland) were placed at sites 43 and 45. Interrupted Vicryl sutures were put in place for non-submerged healing. An impression was taken for a screw-retained provisional fixed restoration. As soon as the two implants could predictably support it (at 5 weeks), a provisional five-unit fixed restoration with a double mesial cantilever, was screwed onto implants 43 and 45 (Fig 12).

The original idea had been to keep the provisional restoration for several weeks to allow for sufficient tissue maturation and to make sure the patient was satisfied with the results. The patient was not willing to come back for the final restoration, as she was able to use her right side for chewing. She did accept a panoramic radiograph to be taken in September 2011, which confirmed stable peri-implant bone levels around the two new implants (Fig 13).

In June 2012, the definitive six-unit fixed prosthesis screw-retained on two implants was delivered and tightened to 35 Ncm (Figs 14a-b).

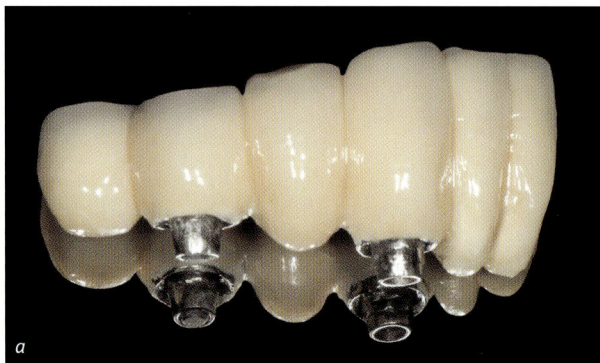

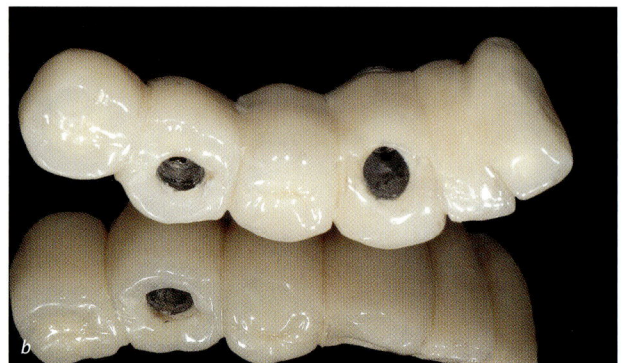

Fig 14a-b   The definitive six-unit fixed prosthesis with ceramic crowns on two implants, ready for delivery. (a) Lateral view. (b) Occlusal view.

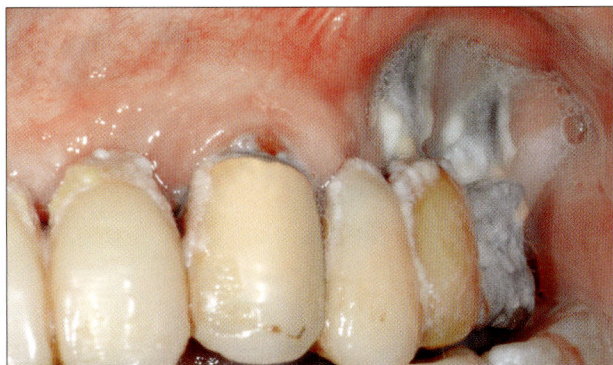

Fig 15 Painful condition with swelling in the left maxilla.

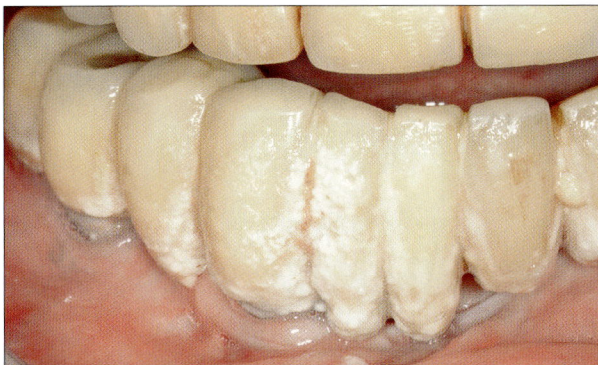

Fig 16 Very poor plaque control.

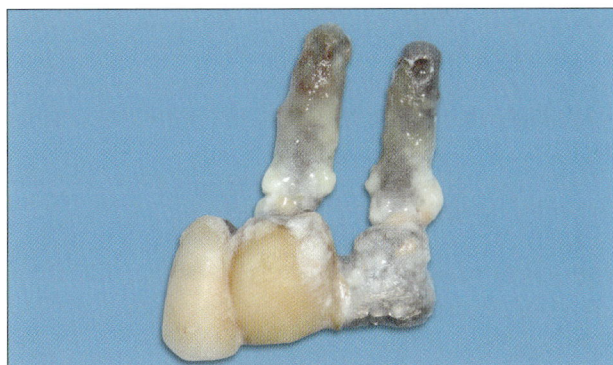

Fig 17 Removed three-unit bridge 24–26 and its two supporting implants.

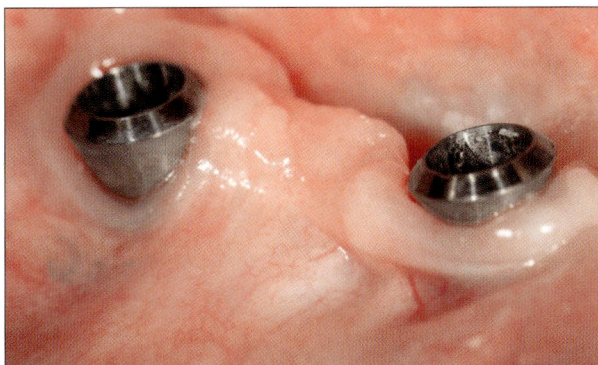

Fig 18 Lower right quadrant. The screw-retained bridge was removed and cleaned by the dental hygienist. Implant shoulders and peri-implant soft tissue were cleaned and gently treated.

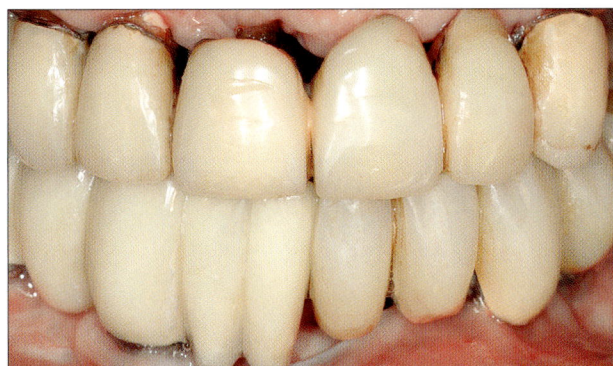

Fig 19 Scaling and root planning was performed on the natural dentition.

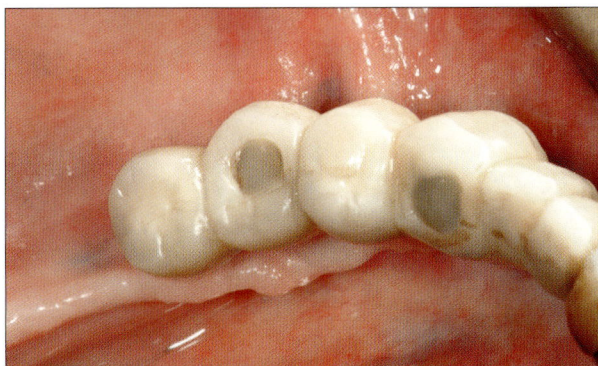

Fig 20 The fixed dental prosthesis was reconnected and the access holes were sealed with composite.

In June 2014, the patient came back reporting pain in the left maxilla (Fig 15), which exhibited very poor plaque control (Fig 16).

A three-unit bridge (24–26) and its two supporting implants were removed (Fig 17). After a few days, the patient was treated by the dental hygienist. The screw-retained bridge was removed and cleaned. The shoulders of the implants were carefully cleaned by the dental hygienist (Fig 18), and the peri-implant soft tissue was gently treated. Scaling and root planning was performed on the natural dentition, to the extent possible (Fig 19). The bridge was reconnected and the access holes were sealed with composite (Fig 20).

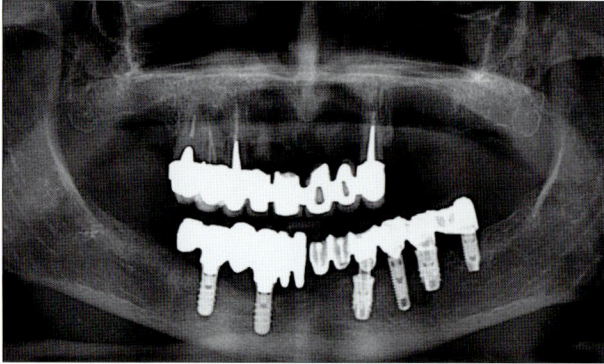

Fig 21   Panoramic radiographs of July 2014. Stable peri-implant levels around the two new implants.

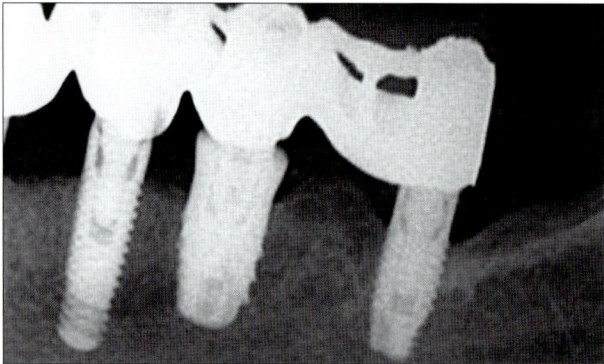

Fig 22   Intraoral radiograph of the left mandible. Limited peri-implant bone resorption around the four older implants.

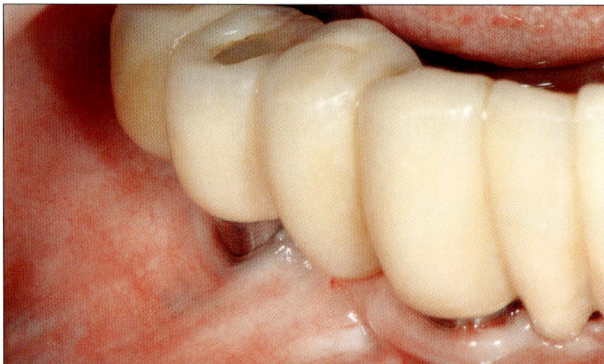

Fig 23   The last clinical view. Stable soft-tissue contours. No significant signs of inflammation and minimal soft-tissue recession.

The panoramic and intraoral radiographs of July 2014, confirmed stable peri-implant bone levels around the two newly placed implants and limited peri-implant bone resorption around the four older implants in the left mandible (Figs 21 and 22).

The last clinical picture, taken in October 2014 when the patient was almost 97 years old, more than 4 years after the first visit, revealed stable soft-tissue contours and no significant signs of inflammation or recession (Fig 23).

With this patient's history in mind, it is advisable to place implants with a long-term vision, so that maintenance is easy for the patient and the dentist. Moreover, given that peri-implantitis occurs not infrequently in partially and completely edentulous patients, the treatment plan should take possible complications into consideration and anticipate ways to resolve them, especially in older patients.

Acknowledgments

Laboratory Procedures
Francesco Cataldi – Master Dental Technician, Torino, Italy.

Periodontal Maintenance
Silvia Gherlone – Registered Dental Hygienist, Torino, Italy.

13.11 Implant-retained Rehabilitation after Mandibular Rim Resection

S. Shahdad

A 77-year-old woman was referred to our department by an oral and maxillofacial surgeon for rehabilitation of her dentition. She had been diagnosed with squamous cell carcinoma 6 months earlier and was treated surgically by right mandibular rim resection and local floor-of-mouth resection extending to tooth 33. No radiotherapy or chemotherapy had been considered necessary.

The patient complained that she was unable to eat and that her face was disfigured due to a lack of lip support on the resection side.

She reported a history of well-controlled asthma and angina, in addition to cardiac arrhythmia and an allergy to penicillin. Her medication included acetylsalicylic acid and diltiazem.

Clinical examination revealed an edentulous maxilla and only teeth 33 and 34 remaining in the mandible. Multiple extractions in the mandible had been carried out at the time of the mandibular rim resection. Due to the extent of resection, the buccal and lingual sulci were level with the floor of the mouth, with a complete lack of attached, keratinized mucosa (Fig 1). The mental foramen had been surgically relocated approximately to site 46. The patient reported reduced mental nerve sensation, which was confirmed during the clinical examination.

The radiographs showed less than 25% alveolar bone loss at teeth 33 and 34 (Fig 2). The distalized mental foramen was visible on the radiograph and showed the extent of the mandibular resection (Fig 3).

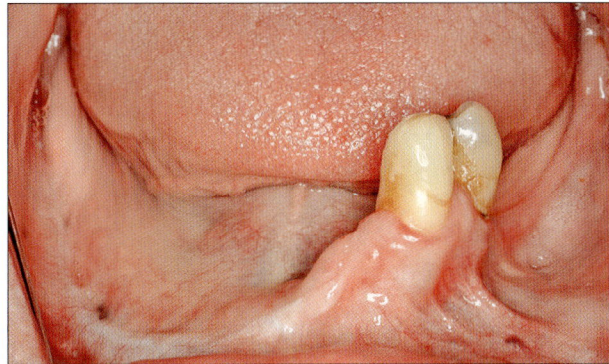

Fig 1   Initial mandibular clinical status after rim and floor-of-mouth resection on the right side. Completely absent sulcus, continuation of the lingual and buccal sulcus, and lack of keratinized mucosa.

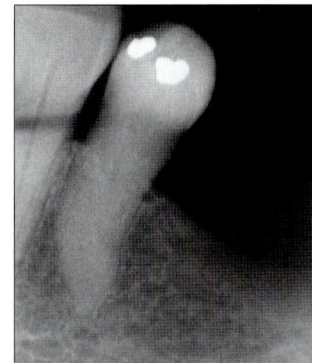

Fig 2   Periapical radiograph of teeth 33 and 34. Less than 25% alveolar bone loss.

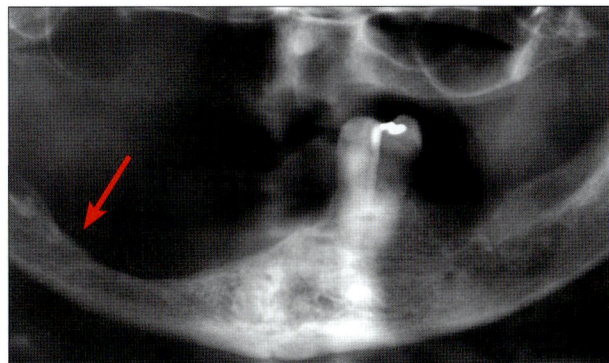

Fig 3   Panoramic radiograph. Mandibular rim resection and position of the relocated mental foramen (arrow).

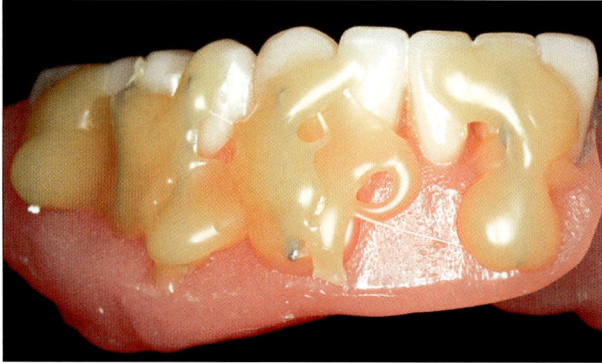

Fig 4   *Orthodontic wires of known dimensions attached to the denture with sticky wax for the radiographic template.*

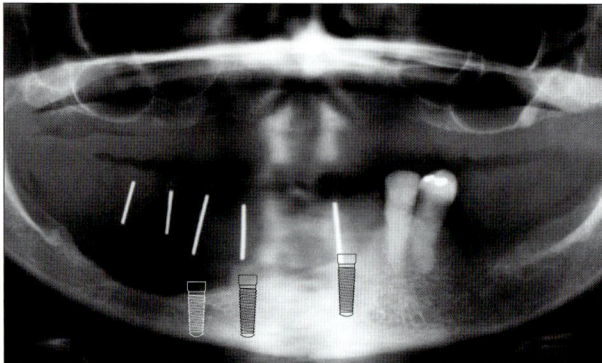

Fig 5   *Panoramic radiograph with wire bits used for implant planning.*

Taking into consideration the patient's medical history and the clinical and radiographic findings, the following treatment options were discussed with the patient:

Option 1
- Maxillary removable conventional acrylic denture.
- Mandibular removable conventional acrylic denture with retentive clasp and rest on teeth 33 and 34.

Option 2
- Maxillary removable conventional acrylic denture.
- Implant-retained fixed dental prosthesis (FDP) extending from site 32 to 45 or 46.

The patient requested option 1, as she was keen to avoid surgery and willing to try a removable partial denture. The challenges of achieving adequate stability and retention in the lower denture were discussed, and the patient was warned about the anticipated poor prognosis. Nonetheless, even for the implant option, determining an idealized tooth position was imperative, and at the least, the denture would be useful for finalizing the positions of the implants.

Treatment stage 1
In January 2006, treatment commenced with the fabrication of a maxillary conventional complete denture and a mandibular removable partial denture. The dentures were delivered in April 2006. The patient returned for denture adjustments on a couple of occasions. However, she continued to report an inability to eat and an "electric shock"-like sensation while chewing with the mandibular denture. Clinically, tenderness to palpation was present on the right side.

During the following 18 months, repeated ulceration of the mandibular mucosa due to trauma from the denture prevented any effective functional benefit or improvement in the quality of life of the patient.

Therefore, a decision was made in discussions with the patient to provide an implant-stabilized fixed dental prosthesis to replace the missing teeth based on the "shortened dental arch" concept (Käyser 1981).

Implant planning
The mandibular removable denture was used for radiographic planning (Fig. 4). Orthodontic wires in 8- and 10-mm lengths were used to localize the planned implants in relation to the inferior dental nerve and relocated mental foramen (Fig. 5).

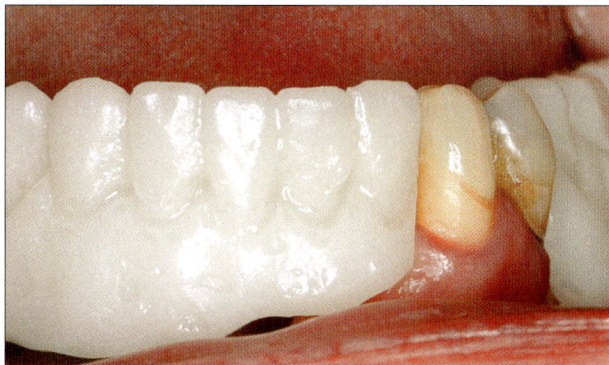
Fig 6   Copied mandibular denture for use as a surgical guide.

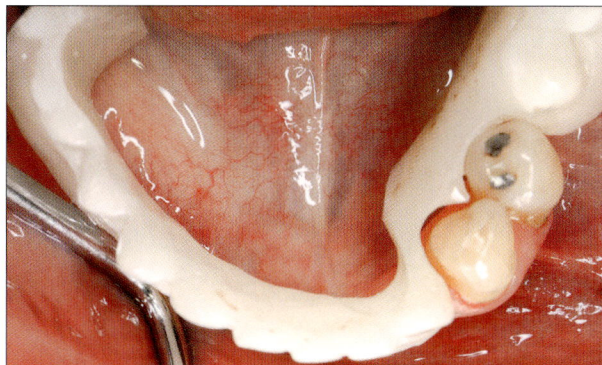
Fig 7   Surgical guide modified and adapted for access to implant drills.

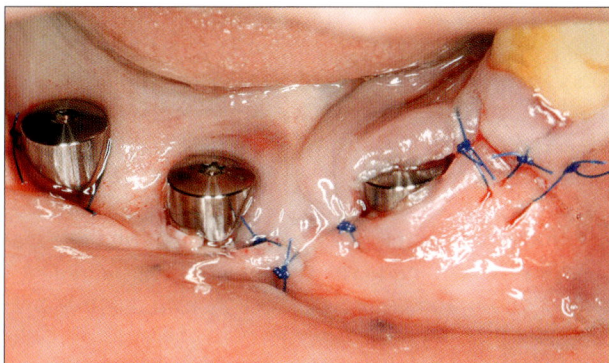
Fig 8   Immediately after implant placement with transmucosal closure. Specially ordered 6-mm healing abutments to aid healing and prevent submergence.

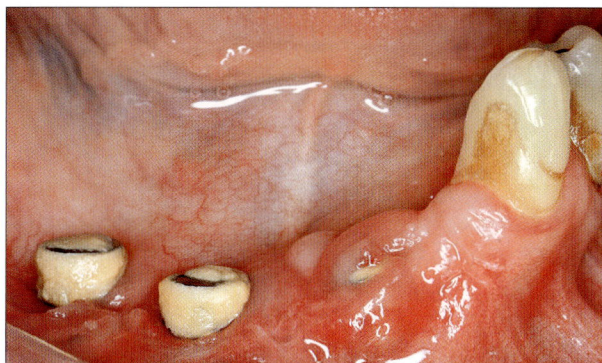
Fig 9   Calculus on healing abutments noted after 8 weeks of healing. Anterior implant 32 partially submerged.

No three-dimensional imaging was performed. At the time, no cone-beam CT scanning facility was available at the hospital. Conventional CT scans taken for mandibular resection were used to evaluate the shape of the mandible in cross-sections.

The mandibular removable prosthesis was duplicated and a surgical guide fabricated (Figs 6 and 7). The lingual flange was cut to aid the preparation of implant osteotomies.

In December 2007, three implants were placed:

- 31: Straumann S SLActive, RN, diameter 4.8 mm, length 10 mm
- 43: Straumann S SLActive, RN, diameter 4.8 mm, length 10 mm
- 45: Straumann S SLActive, RN, diameter 4.8 mm, length 8 mm
  (all Institut Straumann AG, Basel, Switzerland)

Customized healing abutments 6 mm in height were placed for transmucosal closure (Fig 8).

Implants were allowed to heal for 8 weeks before commencing prosthodontic treatment. The patient had a high propensity to accumulate calculus, as is evident on the healing abutments at the impression appointment (Fig 9). The healing abutment on implant 32 was partially submerged despite having used the highest available healing abutment.

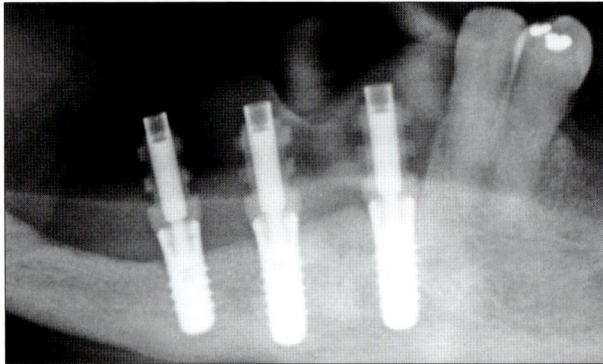

Fig 10   Radiograph to confirm accurate seating of the impression copings.

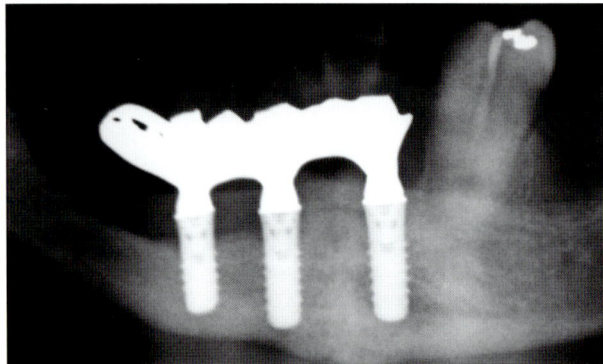

Fig 11   Radiograph confirming complete seating of the gold superstructure on the implants.

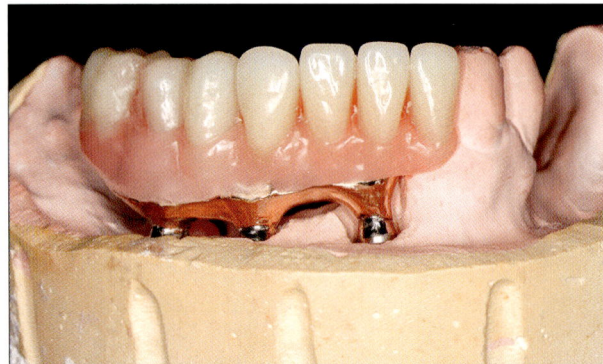

Fig 12   Working cast with wax tooth set-up on gold superstructure.

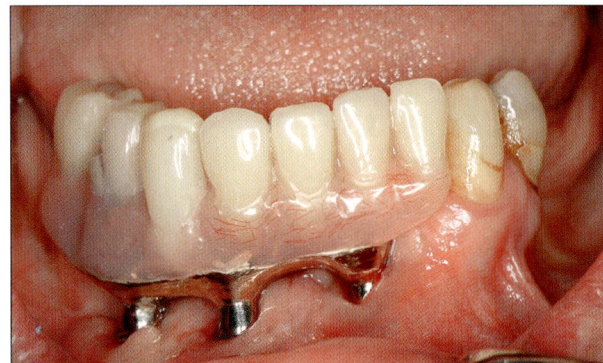

Fig 13   Intraoral try-in of the set-up.

The restorative plan was to use 1.5-mm synOcta abutments (Institut Straumann AG, Basel, Switzerland) with a screw-retained gold/acrylic hybrid superstructure. A definitive implant impression was taken after verifying the seating of the impression copings radiologically (Fig 10).

The accuracy of the impression was confirmed using a verification jig made from temporary abutments joined together with Pattern Resin (GC Corporation, Tokyo, Japan). A cast-gold framework was fabricated and its fit verified in situ with a radiograph (Fig 11).

The teeth were set up in wax on the framework (Fig 12), and the set-up was tried in to confirm the teeth's position, shape, shade, and occlusion. The definitive prosthesis was delivered in December 2008 (Fig 13). The synOcta abutments were torqued to 35 Ncm and the SCS occlusal screws to 15 Ncm. The screw-access holes were sealed with polytetrafluoroethylene (PTFE) tape followed by composite resin.

A control radiograph was taken (Fig 14), and the patient was reexamined after one month. The patient was placed on an annual recall, and a 4- to 6-monthly professional maintenance program was initiated. Regular radiographs were taken to assess the peri-implant bone levels.

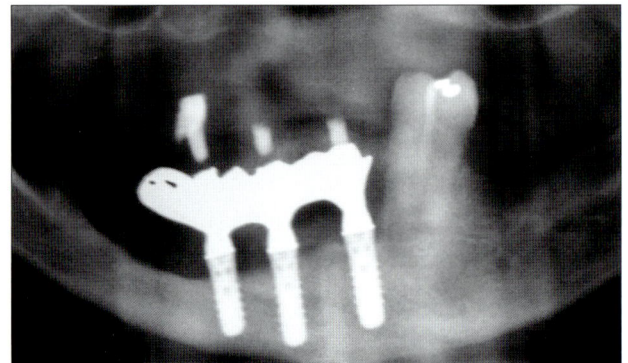

Fig 14   Control radiograph after delivery of the definitive prosthesis.

In July 2012, during one of the follow-up appointments, peri-implant mucositis was noted, particularly on the lingual aspect (Fig 15). It seemed the patient's manual dexterity was diminishing with age. She reported difficulty in effectively brushing the prosthesis and the peri-implant mucosa, especially lingually (Fig 16). She also found the peri-implant mucosa sensitive, which was affecting her ability to brush firmly. As a result, the decision was made to modify the intaglio surface of the prosthesis to provide additional space and allow easier access by interdental brushes (Figs 17a-b).

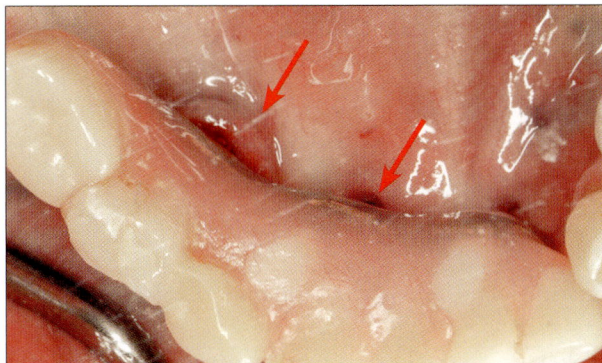

Fig 15   Peri-implant mucositis (arrows) on the lingual aspect.

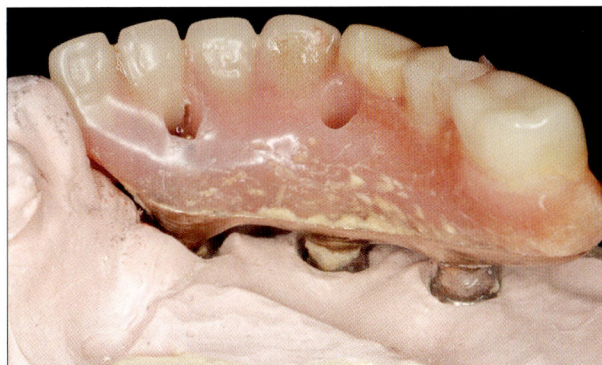

Fig 16   Prosthesis returned to the laboratory for modification of the lingual and intaglio surfaces.

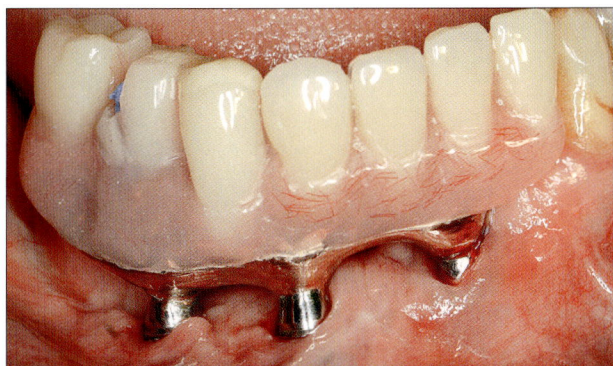

Fig 17a   Before adjustment.

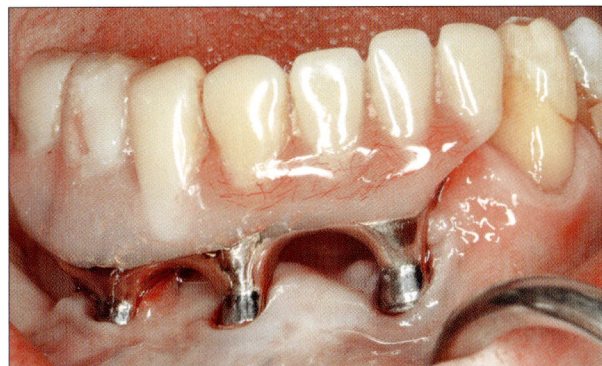

Fig 17b   After adjustment and trimming of the surface. More space to aid in oral hygiene.

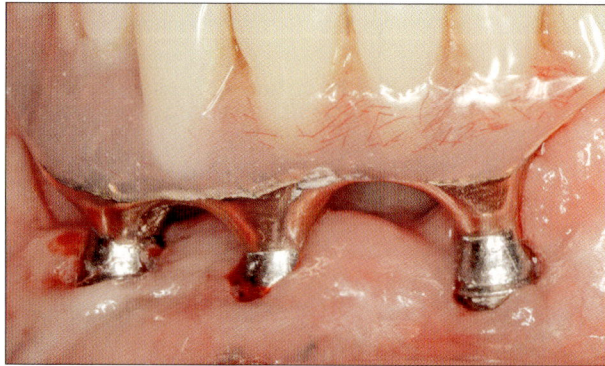

Fig 18   Signs of peri-mucositis persist with edematous tissues and bleeding on probing.

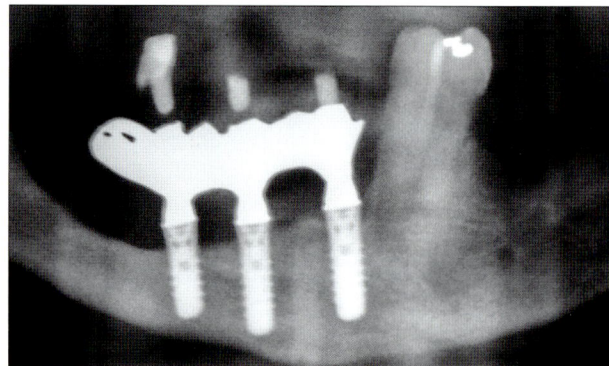

Fig 19   Follow-up radiograph after six years. Stable bone levels compared to the control radiograph.

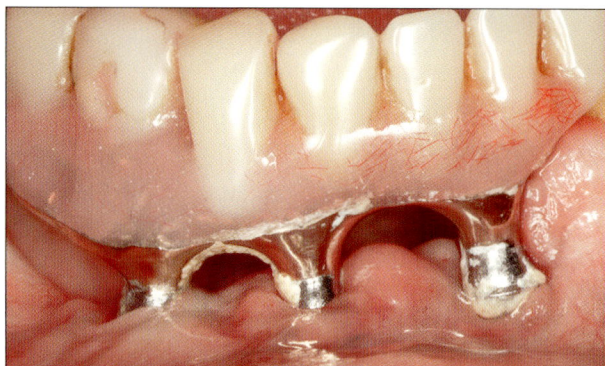

Fig 20   After seven years. Persistent peri-implant mucositis with calculus.

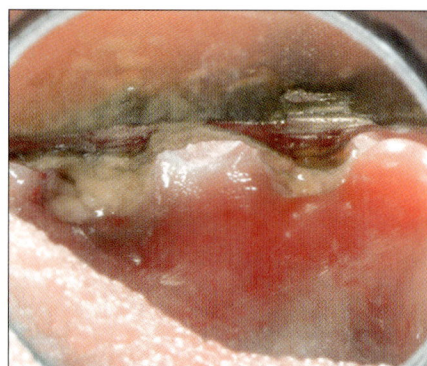

Fig 21   Lingual view. Deteriorated peri-implant mucosa and inability to maintain optimal oral hygiene.

The hospital then lost contact with the patient until January 2014, when she requested an appointment. It transpired that she had moved into a care home facility. During this time, the patient had not seen a dentist or a hygienist. Despite the previous adjustments to the prosthesis, the clinical examination showed persistent mucositis (Fig 18) with bleeding on probing and an edematous peri-implant mucosa, but with probing depths under 5 mm and stable bone levels (Fig 19).

The patient requested future implant maintenance to be carried out by a dentist nearer to her care home, as she was now finding it difficult and expensive to travel for her hospital appointments.

However, due to difficulty in accessing appropriate expertise for implant maintenance, the patient returned for help in March 2015. A local general dentist, instead of providing implant maintenance, had advised and persuaded her to reline the maxillary denture. The intervention has resulted in a complete loss of retention, incorrect occlusion, and a very bulky denture. A new maxillary denture was now indicated. Clinical examination again showed bleeding on probing, and supra- and submucosal calculus (Fig 20) on three implants and on the lingual and intaglio surfaces of the prosthesis (Fig 21). Nonetheless, after seven years, peri-implant bone levels remained stable despite persistent mucositis (Fig 22). Figures 23a-b show frontal and lateral views of the patient.

Discussion

This case demonstrates a multitude of challenges encountered by clinicians when rehabilitating a patient with mandibular rim and floor-of-mouth resection who has difficulty in tolerating a conventional removable denture, with implants in an unfavorable soft- and hard-tissue environment and persistent peri-implant mucositis due to the patient's inability to maintain adequate oral hygiene in old age.

The resective surgery resulted in the removal of the alveolus and part of the floor of mouth with a subsequent lack of sulcus depth. As the mental foramen had been distalized, the mandibular bone height was sufficient to accommodate implants in the basal bone. However, there was a complete lack of keratinized mucosa, and the peri-implant tissue comprising of the lining mucosa was sensitive in that area, with patient-reported pain and discomfort during brushing. The hyperesthesia could be attributed to the lining mucosa, or more plausibly to an inferior dental nerve injured during the resection. As a result, the patient struggled to maintain a clean peri-implant mucosal cuff.

There seems to be no conclusive evidence that the lack of adequate keratinized mucosa impairs oral hygiene, although pain and discomfort during brushing at sites with a bordering lining mucosa may hamper adequate cleaning (Wennström and Derks 2012).

There was a persistent insult to the peri-implant mucosa for more than seven years due to plaque and calculus accumulation with resultant peri-implant mucositis. Nonetheless, until most recent examination, there was no radiographic evidence of progression to peri-implantitis. While animal experiments have demonstrated a link and a progression of peri-mucositis to peri-implantitis (Lang and coworkers 2011b; Berglundh and coworkers 2011), longitudinal studies in humans have failed to corroborate the progression (Lang and Berglundh 2011a). Animal experiments also failed to demonstrate any significant difference in peri-implant bone loss around implants with keratinized or non-keratinized mucosa, although more pronounced recession was noted in the latter group (Warrer and coworkers 1995).

Despite a modified prosthesis, oral hygiene further deteriorated with the age of the patient, which demonstrates the challenges in maintaining implant-supported prostheses in geriatric patients as they experience diminishing manual dexterity. The patient now resides in a care home further away from access to specialist care. This raises further concerns about her ability to maintain an optimal level of oral hygiene in the coming years, with a detrimental effect on the implants.

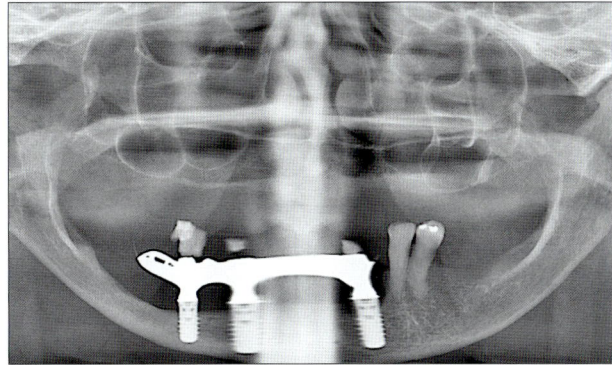

Fig 22   Panoramic radiograph after seven years. Stable bone levels despite persistent peri-implant mucositis.

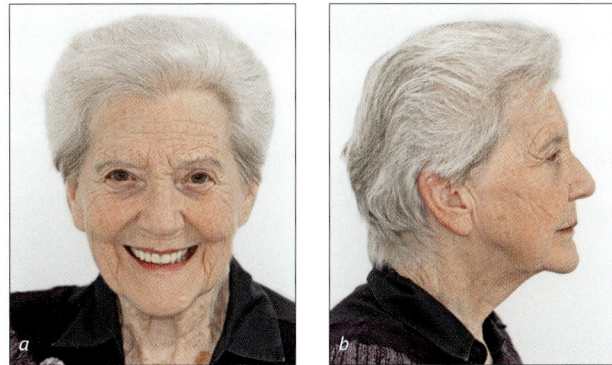

Figs 23a-b   The patient's facial and dental esthetics were restored once the replacement maxillary conventional denture was delivered.

13.12   Four Immediately Loaded Mini-implants Supporting a Mandibular Overdenture

S. Esfandiari

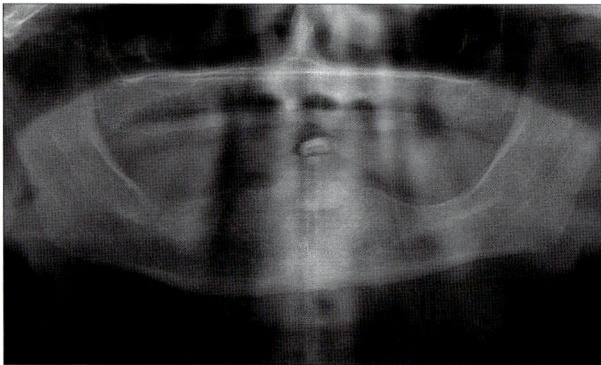

Fig 1   Preoperative radiograph showing favorable vertical bone height in the interforaminal region.

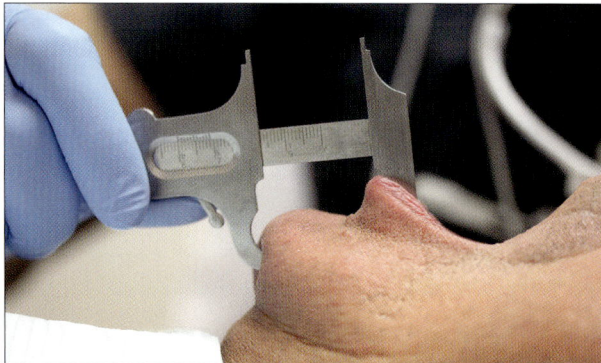

Fig 2   Approximate height measurement using a dental caliper.

A 74-year-old male patient, a non-smoker, who had been wearing complete dentures for more than 30 years, presented to our clinic complaining about discomfort in connection with his lower denture. The patient suffered from asthma and had a history of cardiac disease and blood pressure disorders. All conditions were medically controlled and stable.

The clinical inspection of the oral cavity revealed an ill-fitting complete mandibular denture. The patient expressed the wish for his lower denture to "stop moving when chewing, swallowing, and speaking." He reported having heard about dental implants and asked whether these could help in "fixing" his lower denture, but also requested non-invasive treatment. The mucosa presented healthy and was free of defects such as pressure sores. An band of keratinized mucosa approximately 2 mm wide was visible. The patient's mucosal biotype was medium thick to thin.

The panoramic radiograph (Fig 1) exhibited no anatomical abnormality that would have precluded implant placement. The height of the anterior mandibular region was screened by means of dental calipers (Fig 2), from the tip of the edentulous ridge to the outer lower part of the chin. A minimum height of approximate 27 mm is needed for the placement of a 10-mm implant. Any desired variations in implant length can be calculated based on this minimum required height.

Due to the reduced alveolar bone width and to respond to the patient's wish for a treatment approach that is as minimally invasive as possible, the placement of mini-implants was considered. The patient was asked if he would be willing to participate in a clinical trial at McGill University, whose treatment schedule called for the placement of four mini-implants in the edentulous anterior mandibular ridge, which he agreed to.

The study setup and treatment approach as defined in the clinical trial's protocol (flapless placement of four mini-implants (DMD; 3M ESPE, MN, USA) in the interforaminal region of the mandible and immediate loading with a transitional complete mandibular denture) were discussed with the patient. This included the risk of perforation of the cortical plates during surgery as a result of the flapless approach as outlined in the study protocol. The patient gave his informed consent.

Surgical procedure

Following the screening, the patient was scheduled for implant placement. He first received a chlorhexidine digluconate 0.12% rinse. The juxtaposed distal point of the canines and the mandibular midline on the inside of the mandibular denture were marked with an indelible marker (two equidistant points on each side of the midline and the canine line) (Fig 3).

The edentulous ridge was dried and the marked denture inserted, after which the marks were transferred to the patient's tissue—three lines and four points, each representing the future implant sites. This step may have to be repeated until all points are clearly visible (Fig 4).

The anterior mandibular region was anesthetized, first applying the topical anesthetic followed by the buccal mucosa infiltration. Block anesthetics was not required. The crest of the mandibular ridge was perforated with a 15c blade at each of the indicated points, not to elevate a flap but simply to confirm the width of the ridge (Fig 5).

For the first implant (MDI Collared Standard O-Ball, diameter 2.1 mm, length 13 mm; 3M ESPE), the pilot drill (1.1-mm Pilot Drill; 3M ESPE) was carefully placed on the initial entry point and moved up and down ever so lightly at the recommended drill speed of 1,200 to 1,500 rpm until the cortical plate was penetrated (Fig 6). Irrigation with sterile saline solution to avoid overheating the bone was mandatory throughout the drilling process. The drill hole created was as deep as one-third to one-half of the implant height.

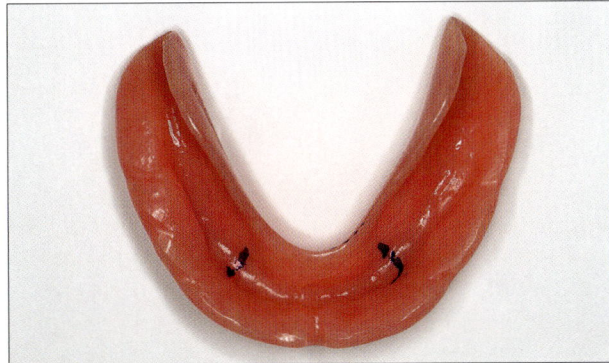

Fig 3   Juxtaposed canine marks.

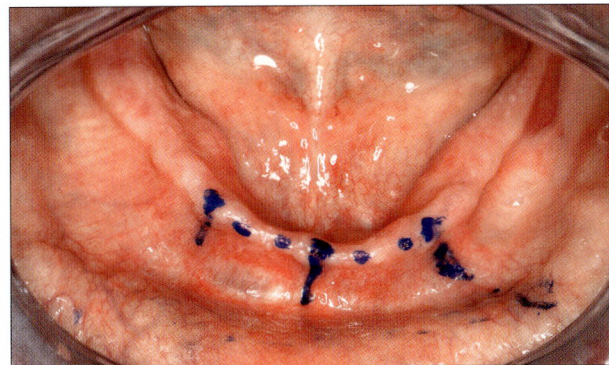

Fig 4   Equidistant implant positions.

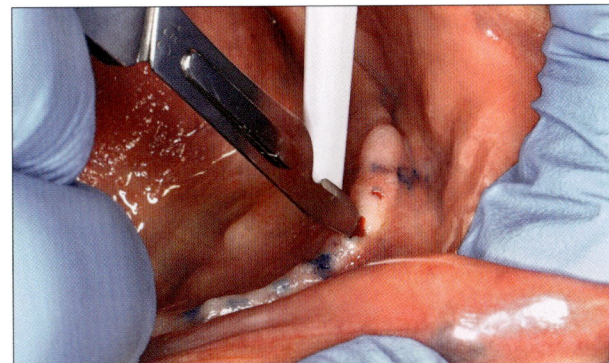

Fig 5   Locating the crest of the ridge.

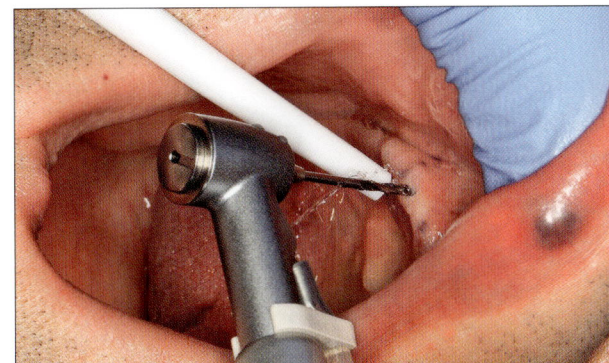

Fig 6   Initial perforation.

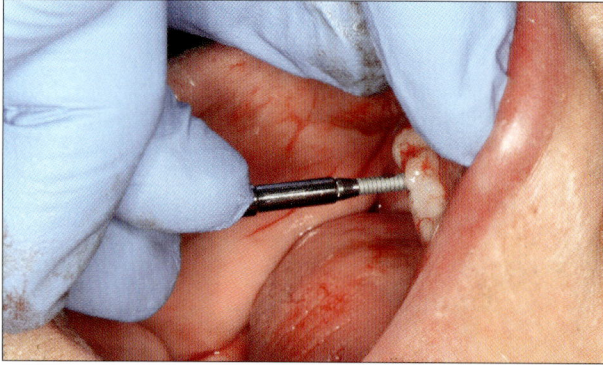

Fig 7   Implant placement.

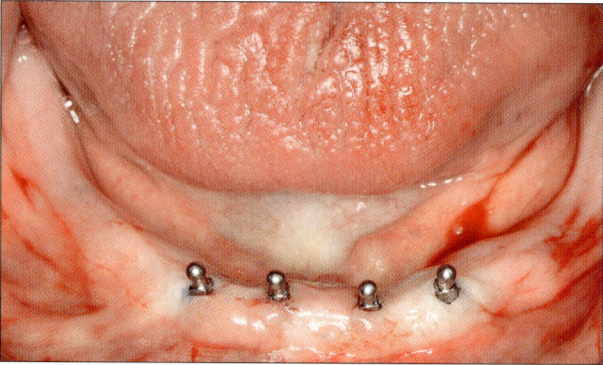

Fig 8   Verifying implant height and neck position.

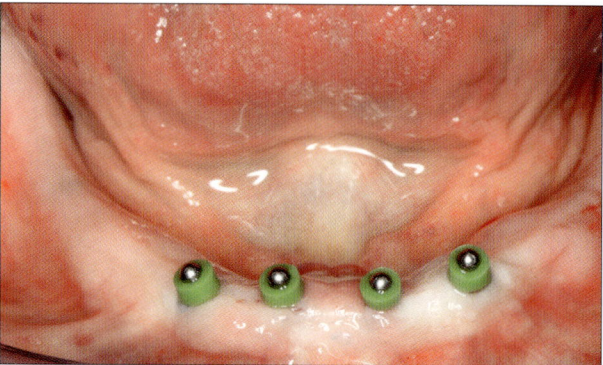

Fig 9   Rubber spacer tubing in place.

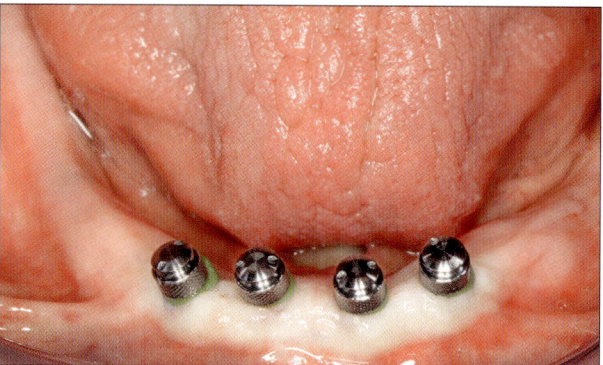

Fig 10   Metal housings in place.

The implant was then placed in the drill hole and the implant driver (Winged Thumb Wrench; 3M ESPE) attached to the head of the implant. After inserting the implant into the prepared bed, it was rotated clockwise to allow it to self-tap while exerting downward pressure until the wrench became more difficult to turn by hand, i.e. until noticeable resistance in the bone was encountered (Fig 7).

Next, the torque wrench (Adjustable Torque Wrench; 3M ESPE) was used to finalize the insertion of the implant, which was placed such that the abutment head was allowed to protrude from the gingival soft tissue at its full length but with no aspects of the neck or thread portions visible (Fig 8).

A minimum of 15 Ncm of resistance upon final insertion was sufficient for immediate loading of 4 mini-implants. Excessive torque (> 45 Ncm) may fracture the body of narrow-diameter implants (NDI).

Subsequent implants (all of the same endosteal diameter and length) were introduced following the same procedure. All implants axes should parallel to the maximum extent possible.

Prosthetic procedure
Prosthetic treatment was initially assisted by the patient's existing conventional complete dentures.

Segments of green rubber spacer tubing 2 to 2.5 mm in length (Blockout Shim; 3M ESPE) were cut and placed on each implant to block out undercuts (Fig 9), followed by the metal housings with O-rings (Metal Housing; 3M ESPE) (Fig 10).

Next, the existing mandibular denture was inserted in the mouth to inspect the locations of the implants in relation to the denture. The tissue side of the denture was relieved with a round acrylic bur, making sure not to extend trimming beyond the premolar regions. Posterior soft-tissue support is needed to make sure that patient occludes in a correct and comfortable position (Fig 11).

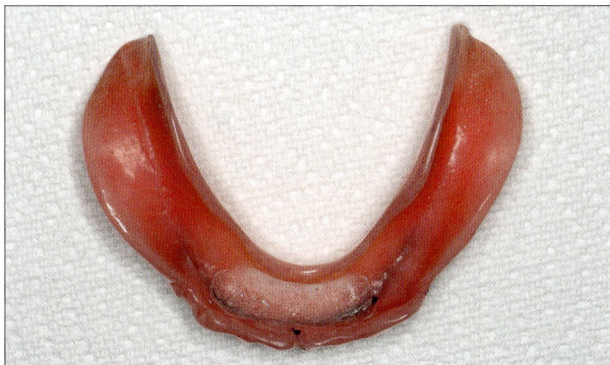

Fig 11   Relieved denture.

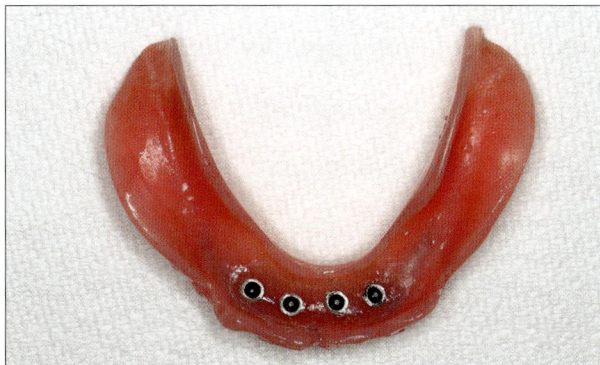

Fig 12   Polished overdenture with metal housings.

The denture was then returned to the patient's mouth and checked for a passive fit over the implants and housings, making sure the posterior region was in contact with the soft tissue. The relief area was roughened with an acrylic bur, then cleaned and dried. Petroleum jelly was applied to all areas not coming in touch with the autopolymerizing material during the following pick-up step, while a thin layer of adhesive was applied to the relief area of the denture. The pick-up acrylic resin (Secure Hard Pick-Up; 3M ESPE) was then extruded directly onto the metal housings and into the relief area of the denture.

Having slowly and carefully returned the denture to the patient's mouth, the patient was asked to close and apply normal bite pressure to confirm centric occlusion. The resin can take about 5 to 8 minutes to set. Excess resin was removed and the denture trimmed; all rubber tubes were removed, and the surfaces of the picked-up housings were polished (Fig 12).

The patient was instructed to keep the denture in place for the first 48 hours after placement to prevent tissue overgrowth and to stick to a soft diet for 2 weeks. He was prescribed chlorhexidine digluconate 0.12% for mouth rinses and ibuprofen 600 mg if needed for pain relief; antibiotics are not required with this procedure.

The overall chairside time for this procedure was 100 minutes.

Follow-up appointments were scheduled at 6, 12, and 24 months. The O-rings needed to be replaced three times during the last 2 years as part of regular maintenance.

The 2-year panoramic radiograph (Fig 13) showed stable implant and bone conditions. The patient was extremely satisfied with the outcome.

Conclusion
Reduced-diameter implants and mini dental implants are a good way to reduce the need for augmentation procedures prior to implant insertion. Implant treatment that is less invasive particularly benefits elderly patients or patients with systemic risk factors.

With flapless approaches, as in the present case, there is always the risk that the sharp and thin drills required might perforate the cortical plate of the mandible. These procedures should therefore be performed only by experienced surgeons, and pre-treatment assessment should include CBCT scans.

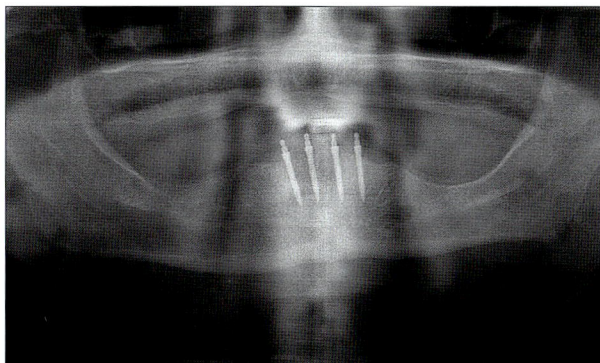

Fig 13   Panoramic radiograph at 2 years showing stable bone levels.

14 <u>Conclusions</u>

S. Barter, F. Müller

A real-life anecdote:

Today I was late for my first patient after lunch, who was due to have implant surgery. This patient was a fit and well 80-year-old lady who had only one missing tooth, the upper left second premolar (25). She did not want to wear a denture, feeling that she was "not old enough for that." She had the demeanor and appearance of someone in her mid-sixties. The adjacent teeth were healthy and unprepared, and an implant was the ideal solution.

We placed a tissue-level implant and performed some guided bone regeneration in a very short time, under local anesthesia, with no problems, and we had some cheerful conversation while the procedure was under way. The procedure was exactly as it would have been had the patient been eighteen rather than eighty. She could understand the postoperative instructions perfectly and will undoubtedly comply with them.

I was late because immediately before my lunch break, a 79-year-old patient, whom I had last seen in 2004, turned up unannounced at the clinic. She had been fit and well at the time and had undergone complex bone-grafting procedures using bone from iliac crest under general anesthesia. She had later had five maxillary and four mandibular implants placed, which had been restored with bar-retained overdentures. At that time, she had been delighted and it had changed her life. She had moved away after a year or so, and we did not see her again.

Today, she was confused, disorientated, disheveled, and very alone. She appeared 99 years old, not 79. She thought that she had lost her lower denture approximately a year previously and had since been chewing on the upper denture with the lower bar. Not only did she have significant deposits of plaque and calculus on the remaining maxillary denture and the bars, she also had rotting food in her mouth stuck under the denture and bars. Her clothes were dirty; she had obviously not washed properly in a long time, and she could not even remember how she got to us. In fact she was in such a state, I did not know how she had managed to get to us.

She claimed to live at home with her son, but when we made some enquiries, the address that she had given was not one she had lived at for some time. She could barely stand because she was so weak, and although not obviously suffering from Alzheimer's, she was clearly confused and disoriented, whether due to a form of dementia or possibly malnutrition, dehydration, infection, or illness.

We had to contact Adult Social Care Services and arrange for her to be taken for appropriate medical care. They would also assess her home living conditions and wider care needs. We then needed to liaise with her caregivers and medical attendants on appropriate dental care and on how it would be provided.

The difference between these two patients was less than a year in age. The older patient had a simple implant treatment, the other patient had had a more complex treatment carried out some eleven years previously. She had probably not had any care for that complex reconstruction in the last three years.

I found this experience very poignant and a perfect representation of the issues outlined in this volume. We are all going to encounter such cases more frequently, and we must know how to deal with them in the best interest of the patient.

For the first patient, an implant was the best option, being the simplest way to restore her appearance, self-esteem, and function. She spent less time in the chair than she might have for other restorative procedures, the economics were favorable, and that treatment option suited her personal circumstances.

Implants are a safe and predictable treatment option in elderly people. This is not new knowledge. As always, success depends on appropriate diagnosis and meticulous treatment planning. Nevertheless, failures and complications are inevitable, and now it seems we must also be able to see into the future!

For the second patient, her initially life-changing implant treatment had exactly the same advantages as for the first patient at the time the treatment was provided. However, it was now life-changing for a second time, but in the opposite sense. She was in pain, with a loss of function and appearance, and now had peri-implant disease. Treatment planning will be difficult, with issues of comprehension, consent, competence, access, affordability, and ongoing oral healthcare. If we roll back the rehabilitation to simple dentures, will she cope, having been used to a very retentive and resilient set of prostheses? How will her increasing cognitive impairment affect the treatment plan? What medical diagnoses exist, and how will these affect our decisions? What supporting services will she need? To whom can the dentist turn for advice and assistance?

There is clear evidence that we have an expanding aged population, with increasing rates of general multimorbidity, polypharmacy, and mental-health problems. The goals of treatment from the patients' perspective may progressively become more removed from the reality of the needs of those patients as they age. The patients, or their caregivers, may need to be carefully guided to an understanding of both the present and future implications of treatment.

Much of the content of previous volumes in this Treatment Guide series deals with the technical aspects of providing dental implant treatment and in dealing with the inevitable biological and technical complications that will occur. These excellent volumes have all highlighted in their conclusions the need for individualized treatment plans and ongoing supportive care programs. They have also stressed the importance of clinicians being aware of their own experience levels and skills.

There is a need for dental practitioners to have an increased level of knowledge regarding the medical status of their patients, and particularly the effect of aging on that status. Along with this knowledge, practitioners need to be prepared to accept the professional ethics of following up of their patients and to assure that, once frail and dependent, they are not left alone with their implant-supported restorations, often without access to dental care and in a institutionalized context, with limited knowledge and strong apprehensions in those caring for them. As a profession, we need to ensure that our patients receive lifelong oral health care and that oral comfort, infection control, and quality of life are provided until the last moments of life.

The term "team approach" is widely used when considering implant treatment – as you can see, the "team" comprises more than just the dental experts. We have an important role to play in the wider health care team, including geriatricians, social workers, care-home workers, and general medical practitioners.

It is not just about implants; it is about patients, about caring, and it is about you and me.

15 References

References have been listed in the order of (1) the first or only author's last name and (2) the year of publication. Identical short references are distinguished in the text by lowercase letters, which if used are given in parentheses at the end of the respective entry in this list of references.

AAOS/ADA (American Academy of Orthopaedic Surgeons/American Dental Association). Prevention of orthopaedic implant infection in patients undergoing dental procedures. **2014**. http://ebd.ada.org/~/media/EBD/Files/PUDP_guideline.ashx. Last accessed 20 December 2014.

Abate M, Vanni D, Pantalone A, Salini V. Cigarette smoking and musculoskeletal disorders. Muscles Ligaments Tendons J. **2013** Jul 9; 3(2): 63 – 69.

Abduo J. Occlusal schemes for complete dentures: a systematic review. Int J Prosthodont. **2013** Jan – Feb; 26(1): 26 – 33.

Abe S, Ishihara K, Adachi M, Okuda K. Tongue-coating as risk indicator for aspiration pneumonia in edentate elderly. Arch Gerontol Geriatr. **2008** Sep – Oct; 47(2): 267 – 275.

Abete P, Della-Morte D, Gargiulo G, Basile C, Langellott A, Galizia G, Testa G, Vincenzo C, Bonaduce D, Cacciatore F. Cognitive impairment and cardiovascular diseases in the elderly. A heart-brain continuum hypothesis. Ageing Res Rev. **2014** Nov; 18: 41 – 52.

Adamson JW, Eschbach J, Finch CA. The kidney and erythropoiesis. Am J Med. **1968** May; 44(5): 725 – 733.

Aghaloo TL, Felsenfeld AL, Tetradis S: Osteonecrosis of the jaw in a patient on denosumab. J Oral Maxillofac Surg. **2010** May; 68(5): 959 – 963.

Aghaloo TL, Kang B, Sung EC, Shoff M, Ronconi M, Gotcher JE, Bezouglaia O, Dry SM, Tetradis S. Periodontal disease and bisphosphonates induce osteonecrosis of the jaws in the rat. J Bone Miner Res. **2011** Aug; 26(8): 1871 – 1882.

Aglietta M, Siciliano VI, Zwahlen M, Brägger U, Pjetursson BE, Lang NP, Salvi GE. A systematic review of the survival and complication rates of implant supported fixed dental prostheses with cantilever extensions after an observation period of at least 5 years. Clin Oral Implants Res. **2009** May; 20(5): 441 – 451.

Aguirre JI, Akhter MP, Kimmel DB, Pingel JE, Williams A, Jorgensen M, Kesavalu L, Wronski TJ. Oncologic doses of zoledronic acid induce osteonecrosis of the jaw-like lesions in rice rats (Oryzomys palustris) with periodontitis. J Bone Miner Res. **2012** Oct; 27(10): 2130 – 2043.

Agustí A. Systemic effects of chronic obstructive pulmonary disease: what we know and what we don't know (but should). Proc Am Thorac Soc. **2007** Oct 1; 4(7): 522 – 525.

Ahmed T, Haboubi N. Assessment and management of nutrition in older people and its importance to health. Clin Interv Aging. **2010** Aug 9; 5: 207 – 216.

Akin H, Coskun ME, Akin EG, Ozdemir AK. Evaluation of the attractive force of different types of new-generation magnetic attachment systems. J Prosthet Dent. **2011** Mar; 105(3): 203 – 207.

Albrektsson T, Donos N, Working G. Implant survival and complications. The Third EAO Consensus Conference 2012. Clin Oral Implants Res. **2012** Oct; 23(Suppl 6): 63 – 65.

Ali A, Patton DW, El-Sharkawi AM, Davies J. Implant rehabilitation of irradiated jaws: a preliminary report. Int J Oral Maxillofac Implants. **1997** Jul – Aug; 12(4): 523 – 526.

Ali-Erdem M, Burak-Cankaya A, Cemil-Isler S, Demircan S, Soluk M, Kasapoglu C, Korhan-Oral C. Extraction socket healing in rats treated with bisphosphonate: Animal model for bisphosphonate related osteonecrosis of jaws in multiple myeloma patients. Med Oral Patol Oral Cir Bucal. **2011** Nov 1; 16(7): e879 – e883.

Al-Johany SS, Andres C. ICK classification system for partially edentulous arches. J Prosthodont. **2008** Aug; 17(6): 502 – 507.

Allen PF, McMillan AS, Walshaw D. A patient-based assessment of implant-stabilized and conventional complete dentures. J Prosthet Dent. **2001** Feb; 85(2): 141 – 147.

Allen F, Locker D. A modified short version of the oral health impact profile for assessing health-related quality of life in edentulous adults. **2002** Sep – Oct; 15(5): 446 – 450.

Allen PF, McMillan AS. A longitudinal study of quality of life outcomes in older adults requesting implant prostheses and complete removable dentures. Clin Oral Implants Res. **2003** Apr; 14(2): 173 – 179.

Allum SR, Tomlinson RA, Joshi R. The impact of loads on standard diameter, small diameter and mini implants: a comparative laboratory study. Clin Oral Implants Res. **2008** Jun; 19(6): 553–559.

Almirall J, Rofes L, Serra-Prat M, Icart R, Palomera E, Arreola V, Clavé P. Oropharyngeal dysphagia is a risk factor for community-acquired pneumonia in the elderly. Eur Respir J. **2013** Apr; 41(4): 923–928.

Alsaadi G, Quirynen M, Komárek A, van Steenberghe D. Impact of local and systemic factors on the incidence of oral implant failures, up to abutment connection. J Clin Periodontol. **2007** Jul; 34(7): 610–617.

Alsaadi G, Quirynen M, Komárek A, van Steenberghe D. Impact of local and systemic factors on the incidence of late oral implant loss. Clin Oral Implants Res. **2008** Jul; 19(7): 670–676.

AlSabeeha N, Payne AG, De Silva RK, Swain MV. Mandibular single-implant overdentures: a review with surgical and prosthodontic perspectives of a novel approach. Clin Oral Implants Res. **2009** Apr; 20(4): 356–365.

Alzheimer's Society. Dementia UK: Update. London: Alzheimer's Society; **2014**.

Amam A, Rustom J. Assessment of mandibular alveolar bone density in osteoporotic adults in Syria. Open Journal of Dentistry and Oral Medicine. **2014**; 2(2): 26–32.

Andersohn F, Konzen C, Garbe E. Systematic review: agranulocytosis induced by nonchemotherapy drugs. Ann Intern Med. **2007** May 1; 146(9): 657–665.

Andreiotelli M, Att W, Strub JR. Prosthodontic complications with implant overdentures: a systematic literature review. Int J Prosthodont. **2010** May–Jun; 23(3): 195–203.

Andres R, Bierman EL, Hazzard WR. Principles of geriatric medicine. New York: McGraw-Hill; **1990**.

American Psychiatric Association (APA). Diagnostic and statistical manual of mental disorders 4th ed. Washington: APA Publishing; **1994**.

Aparicio C, Ouazzani W, Garcia R, Arevalo X, Muela R, Fortes V. A prospective clinical study on titanium implants in the zygomatic arch for prosthetic rehabilitation of the atrophic edentulous maxilla with a

follow-up of 6 months to 5 years. Clin Implant Dent Relat Res. **2006**; 8(3): 114–122.

Araújo M, Lindhe J. Dimensional ridge alterations following tooth extraction. An experimental study in the dog. J Clin Periodontol. **2005** Feb; 32(2): 212–218.

Ardekian L, Oved-Peleg E, Mactei EE, Peled M. The clinical significance of sinus membrane perforation during augmentation of the maxillary sinus. J Oral Maxillofac Surg. **2006** Feb; 64(2): 277–282.

Aronow WS. Management of the older person with atrial fibrillation. J Gerontol A Biol Sci Med Sci. **2002** Jun; 57(6): M352-63.

Arora A, Arora M, Roffe C. Mystery of the missing denture: an unusual cause of respiratory arrest in a nonagenarian. Age Ageing. **2002** Sep; 34(5): 519–520.

ASA (American Society of Anesthesiologists). ASA physical status classification system. **2014**. https://www.asahq.org/resources/clinical-information/asa-physical-status-classification-system. Last accessed April 29, 2015.

Aslam M, Vaezi MF. Dysphagia in the elderly. Gastroenterol Hepatol. **2013** Dec; 9(12): 784–795.

Atchison KA, Dolan TA. Development of the Geriatric Oral Health Assessment Index. J Dent Educ. **1990** Nov; 54(11): 680–687.

August M, Chung K, Chang Y, Glowacki J. Influence of estrogen status on endosseous implant osseointegration. J Oral Maxillofac Surg. **2001** Nov; 59(11): 1285–1289; discussion 1290–1291.

Awad MA, Lund JP, Dufresne E, Feine JS. Comparing the efficacy of mandibular implant-retained overdentures and conventional dentures among middle-aged edentulous patients: satisfaction and functional assessment. Int J Prosthodont. **2003** Mar–Apr; 16(2): 117–122.

Awad MA, Rashid F, Feine JS; Overdenture Effectiveness Study Team Consortium. The effect of mandibular 2-implant overdentures on oral health-related quality of life: an international multicentre study. Clin Oral Implants Res. **2014** Jan; 25(1): 46–51.

Bacci C, Berengo M, Favero L, Zanon E. Safety of dental implant surgery in patients undergoing anticoagulation therapy: a prospective case-control study. Clin Oral Implants Res. **2011** Feb; 22(2): 151–156.

Baggi L, Cappelloni I, Di Girolamo M, Maceri F, Vairo G. The influence of implant diameter and length on stress distribution of osseointegrated implants related to crestal bone geometry: a three-dimensional finite element analysis. J Prosthet Dent. **2008** Dec; 100(6): 422–431.

Bahat O. Brånemark system implants in the posterior maxilla: clinical study of 660 implants followed for 5 to 12 years. Int J Oral Maxillofac Implants. **2000** Sep–Oct; 15(5): 646–653.

Baker MA. The management of leukaemia in the elderly. Baillieres Clin Haematol. **1987** Jun; 1(2): 427–448.

Baldwin JG: Hematopoietic function in the elderly. Arch Intern Med. **1988** Dec; 148(12): 2544–2546.

Barat I, Andreasen F, Damsgaard EM. Drug therapy in the elderly: what doctors believe and patients actually do. Br J Clin Pharmacol. **2001** Jun; 51(6): 615–622.

Barnes PJ. Inhaled glucocorticoids for asthma. N Engl J Med. **1995** Mar 30; 332(13): 868–875.

Barnett KN, McMurdo ME, Ogston SA, Morris AD, Evans JM.. Mortality in people diagnosed with type 2 diabetes at an older age: a systematic review. Age Ageing. **2006** Sep; 35(5): 463–468.

Barnett K, Mercer S W, Norbury M, Watt G, Wyke S, Guthrie B. Epidemiology of multimorbidity and implications for health care, research, and medical education: a cross-sectional study. The Lancet. **2012** Jul 7; 380(9836): 37–43.

Barros SP, Suruki R, Loewy ZG, Beck JD, Offenbacher S. A cohort study of the impact of tooth loss and periodontal disease on respiratory events among COPD subjects: modulatory role of systemic biomarkers of inflammation. PLoS One. **2013** Aug 8; 8(8): e68592.

Barrowman RA, Wilson PR, Wiesenfeld D. Oral rehabilitation with dental implants after cancer treatment. Aust Dent J. **2011** May 30; 56(2): 160–165.

Barter S, Stone P, Brägger U. A pilot study to evaluate the success and survival rate of titanium-zirconium implants in partially edentulous patients: results after 24 months of follow-up. Clin Oral Implants Res. **2012** Jul; 23(7): 873–881.

Bartlett JG, Gorbach SL. The triple threat of aspiration pneumonia. Chest. **1975** Oct; 68(4): 560–566.

Bashutski JD, D'Silva NJ, Wang HL. Implant compression necrosis: current understanding and case report. J Periodontol. **2009** Apr; 80(4): 700–7ß4.

Basker RM, Watson CJ). Tongue control of upper complete dentures: a clinical hint. Br Dent K. **1991** Oct; 170(12): 449–450.

Bassett JH, Williams AJ, Murphy E, Boyde A, Howell PG, Swinhoe R, Archanco M, Flamant F, Samarut J, Costagliola S, Vassart G, Weiss RE, Refetoff S, Williams GR. A lack of thyroid hormones rather than excess thyrotropin causes abnormal skeletal development in hypothyroidism. Mol Endocrinol. **2008** Feb; 22(2): 501–512.

Batty GM, Oborne CA, Swift CG, Jackson SH. The use of over-the-counter medication by elderly medical in-patients. Postgrad Med J. **1997** Nov; 73(865): 720–722.

Bauer KA, Weiss LM, Sparrow D, Vokonas PS, Rosenberg RD. Aging associated changes in indices of thrombin generation and protein C activation in humans: normative aging study. J Clin Invest. **1987** Dec; 80(6): 1527–1534.

Beers MH, Ouslander JG, Rollingher I, Reuben DB, Brooks J, Beck JC. Explicit criteria for determining inappropriate medication use in nursing home residents. Arch Intern Med. **1991** Sep; 151(9): 1825–1832.

Beijer HJ, de Blaey CJ. Hospitalisations caused by adverse drug reactions (ADR): a meta-analysis of observational studies. Pharm World Sci. **2002** Apr; 24(2): 46–54.

Beikler T, Flemmig TF. Implants in the medically compromised patient. Crit Rev Oral Biol Med. **2003**; 14(4): 305–316.

Bello SA, Adeyemo WL, Bamgbose BO, Obi EV, Adeyinka AA. Effect of age, impaction types and operative time on inflammatory tissue reactions following lower third molar surgery. Head Face Med. **2011** Apr 28; 7: 8.

Bellomo F, de Preux F, Chung JP, Julien N, Budtz-Jørgensen E, Müller F. The advantages of occupational therapy in oral hygiene measures for institutionalised elderly adults. Gerodontology. **2005** Mar; 22(1): 24–31.

Bergendal B, Anderson JD, Müller F. Comprehensive treatment planning for the patient with complex treatment needs. In: Jokstad A (ed). Osseointegration and dental implants. **2008**. John Wiley & Sons. 43–62.

Berglundh T, Persson L, Klinge B. A systematic review of the incidence of biological and technical complications in implant dentistry reported in prospective longitudinal studies of at least 5 years. J Clin Periodontol. **2002**; 29(Suppl. 3): 197–212.

Berglundh T, Zitzmann NU, Donati M. Are peri-implantitis lesions different from periodontitis lesions? J Clin Periodontol. **2011** Mar; 38(Suppl 11): 188–202.

Berr C, Wancata J, Ritchie K. Prevalence of dementia in the elderly in Europe.C384 Eur Neuropsychopharmacol. **2005** Aug; 15(4): 463–471.

Bethel MA, Sloan FA, Belsky D, Feinglos MN. Longitudinal incidence and prevalence of adverse outcomes of diabetes mellitus in elderly patients. Arch Intern Med. **2007** May 14; 167(9): 921–927.

Bidra AS, Almas K. Mini implants for definitive prosthodontic treatment: a systematic review. J Prosthet Dent. **2013** Mar; 109(3): 156–164.

Bilhan H, Mumcu E, Arat S. The comparison of marginal bone loss around mandibular overdenture-supporting implants with two different attachment types in a loading period of 36 months. Gerodontology. **2011** Mar; 28(1): 49–57.

Binon PP. Thirteen-year follow-up of a mandibular implant-supported fixed complete denture in a patient with Sjögren's syndrome: a clinical report. J Prosthet Dent. **2005** Nov; 94(5): 409–413.

Black DM, Reid IR, Boonen S, Bucci-Rechtweg C, Cauley JA, Cosman F, Cummings SR, Hue TF, Lippuner K, Lakatos P, Leung PC, Man Z, Martinez RL, Tan M, Ruzycky ME, Su G, Eastell R. The effect of 3 versus 6 years of zoledronic acid treatment of osteoporosis: A randomized extension to the HORIZON-Pivotal Fracture Trial (PFT). J Bone Miner Res. **2012** Feb; 27(2): 243–254.

Blanes RJ, Bernard JP, Blanes ZM, Belser UC. A 10-year prospective study of ITI dental implants placed in the posterior region. II: Influence of the crown-to-implant ratio and different prosthetic treatment modalities on crestal bone loss. Clin Oral Implants Res. **2007** Dec; 18(6): 707–714.

Boerrigter EM, Stegenga B, Raghoebar GM, Boering G. Patient satisfaction and chewing ability with implant-retained mandibular overdentures: a comparison with new complete dentures with or without preprosthetic surgery. J Oral Maxillofac Surg. **1995** Oct; 53(10): 1167–1173. (**a**)

Boerrigter EM, Geertman ME, Van Oort RP, Bouma J, Raghoebar GM, van Waas MA, van't Hof MA, Boering G, Kalk W: Patient satisfaction with implant-retained mandibular overdentures. A comparison with new complete dentures not retained by implants—a multicentre randomized clinical trial. Br J Oral Maxillofac Surg. **1995** Oct; 33(5): 282–288. (**b**)

Bonewald L. The amazing osteocyte. J Bone Miner Res. **2011** Feb; 26(2): 229–238.

Bornstein MM, Halbritter S, Harnisch H, Weber HP, Buser D. A retrospective analysis of patients referred for implant placement to a specialty clinic: indications, surgical procedures, and early failures. Int J Oral Maxillofac Implants. **2008** Nov-Dec; 23(6): 1109–1116.

Bornstein MM, Cionca N, Mombelli A. Systemic conditions and treatments as risks for implant therapy. Int J Oral Maxillofac Implants. **2009**; 24(Suppl): 12–27.

Borromeo GL, Brand C, Clement JG, McCullough M, Crighton L, Hepworth G, Wark JD. A large case-control study reveals a positive association between bisphosphonate use and delayed dental healing and osteonecrosis of the jaw. J Bone Miner Res. **2014** May 19; 29(6): 1363–1368.

Bortolini S, Natali A, Franchi M, Coggiola A, Consolo U. Implant-retained removable partial dentures: an 8-year retrospective study. J Prosthodont. **2011** Apr; 20(3): 168–172.

Boscolo-Rizzo P, Stellin M, Muzzi E, Mantovani M, Fuson R, Lupato V, Trabalzini F, Da Mosto MC. Deep neck infections: a study of 365 cases highlighting recommendations for management and treatment. Eur Arch Otorhinolaryngol. **2012** Sep 14; 269(4): 1241–1249.

Boskey AL, Coleman R. Aging and bone. J Dent Res. **2010** Dec; 89(12): 1333–1448.

Bots CP, Poorterman JH, Brand HS, Kalsbeek H, van Amerongen BM, Veerman EC, Nieuw Amerongen AV. The oral health status of dentate patients with chronic renal failure undergoing dialysis therapy. Oral Dis. **2006** Mar; 12(2): 176–180.

Boult C, Green AF, Boult LB, Pacala JT, Snyder C, Leff B. Successful models of chronic care for older adults with chronic conditions: evidence for the Institute of Medicine's "Retooling for an aging America" report. J Am Geriatr Soc. **2009** Dec; 57(12): 2328 – 2337.

Boyd CM, Darer J, Boult C, Fried LP, Boult L, Wu AW. Clinical practice guidelines and quality of care for older patients with multiple comorbid diseases: implications for pay for performance. JAMA. **2005** Aug 10; 294(6): 716 – 724.

Boyle JP, Thompson TJ, Gregg EW, Barker LE, Williamson DF. Projection of the year 2050 burden of diabetes in the US adult population: dynamic modeling of incidence, mortality, and prediabetes prevalence. Popul Health Metr. **2010** Oct 22; 8: 29.

Bozini T, Petridis H, Tzanas K, Garefis P. A meta-analysis of prosthodontic complication rates of implant- supported fixed dental prostheses in edentulous patients after an observation period of at least 5 years. Int J Oral Maxillofac Implants. **2011**; 26: 304 – 318.

Bradbury J, Thomason JM, Jepson NJ, Walls AW, Allen PF, Moynihan PJ. Nutrition counseling increases fruit and vegetable intake in the edentulous. J Dent Res. **2006** May; 85(5): 463 – 468.

Bradley JC. A radiological investigation into the age changes of the inferior dental artery. Br J Oral Surg. **1975** Jul; 13(1): 82 – 90.

Bradley JC. The clinical significance of age changes in the vascular supply to the mandible. Int J Oral Surg. **1981**; 10(Suppl 1): 71 – 76.

Brägger U, Gerber C, Joss A, Haenni S, Meier A, Hashorva E, Lang NP. Patterns of tissue remodelling after placement of ITI dental implants using an osteotome technique: a longitudinal radiographic case cohort study. Clin Oral Implants Res. **2004** Apr; 15(2): 158 – 166.

Brägger U, Karoussis I, Persson R, Pjetursson B, Salvi G, Lang N. Technical and biological complications/failures with single crowns and fixed partial dentures on implants: a 10-year prospective cohort study. Clin Oral Implants Res. **2005** Jun; 16(3): 326 – 334.

Brägger U, Hirt-Steiner S, Schnell N, Schmidlin K, Salvi GE, Pjetursson B, Matuliene G, Zwahlen M, Lang NP. Complication and failure rates of fixed dental prostheses in patients treated for periodontal disease. Clin Oral Implants Res. **2011** Jan; 22(1): 70 – 77.

Braman SS, Hanania NA. Asthma in older adults. Clin Chest Med. **2007** Dec; 28(4): 685 – 702.

Brånemark PI, Adell R, Albrektsson T, Lekholm U, Lindström J, Rockler B. An experimental and clinical study of osseointegrated implants penetrating the nasal cavity and maxillary sinus. J Oral Maxillofac Surg. **1984** Aug; 42(8): 497 – 505.

Bras J, de Jonge HK, van Merkesteyn JP. Osteoradionecrosis of the mandible: pathogenesis. Am J Otolaryngol. **1990** Jul – Aug; 11(4): 244 – 250.

Brecx M, Holm-Pedersen P, Theilade J. Early plaque formation in young and elderly individuals. Gerodontics. **1985** Feb; 1(1): 8 – 13.

Brill N, Tryde G, Schübeler S. The role of exteroceptors in denture retention. J Prosthet Dent. **1959**; 9: 761 – 768.

Brodeur JM, Laurin D, Vallee R, Lachapelle D. Nutrient intake and gastrointestinal disorders related to masticatory performance in the edentulous elderly. J Prosthet Dent. **1993** Nov; 70(5): 468 – 473.

Bronskill SE, Gill SS, Paterson JM, Bell CM, Anderson GM, Rochon PA. Exploring variation in rates of polypharmacy across long term care homes. J Am Med Dir Assoc. **2012** Mar; 13(3): 309

Brook I, Frazier HE. Immune response to Fusobacterium nucleatum and Prevotella intermedia in the sputum of patients with acute exacerbations of chronic bronchitis. Chest. **2003** Sep; 124(3): 832 – 833.

Brown RS, Rhodus NL. Adrenaline and local anaesthesia revisited. Oral Surg Oral Med Oral Pathol Oral Radiol Endod. **2005** Oct; 100(4): 401 – 408.

Brügger OE, Bornstein MM, Kuchler U, Janner SF, Chappuis V, Buser D. Implant therapy in a surgical specialty clinic: An analysis of patients, indications, surgical procedures, risk factors and early failures. Int J Oral Maxillofac Implants. **2015** Jan – Feb; 30(1): 151 – 160

Bryant SR. The effects of age, jaw site, and bone condition on oral implant outcomes. Int J Prosthodont. **1998** Sep – Oct; 11(5): 470 – 490.

Bryant SR, Zarb GA. Crestal bone loss proximal to oral implants in older and younger adults. J Prosthet Dent. **2003** Jun; 89(6): 589 – 597.

Bryant SR, MacDonald-Jankowski D, Kim K. Does the type of implant prosthesis affect outcomes for the completely edentulous arch? Int J Oral Maxillofac Implants. **2007**; 22(Suppl): 117–139.

Bryant SR, Walton JN, MacEntee MI. A 5-year randomized trial to compare 1 or 2 implants for implant overdentures. J Dent Res. **2015** Jan; 94(1): 36–43.

Buckeridge D, Huang A, Hanley J, Kelome A, Reidel K, Verma A, Winslade N, Tamblyn R. Risk of injury associated with opioid use in older adults. J Am Geriatr Soc. **2010** Sep; 58(9): 1664–1670.

Budtz-Jørgensen E, Isidor F. A 5-year longitudinal study of cantilevered fixed partial dentures compared with removable partial dentures in a geriatric population. J Prosthet Dent. **1990** Jul; 64(1): 42–47.

Budtz-Jørgensen E, Bochet G. Alternate framework designs for removable partial dentures. J Prosthet Dent. **1998** Jul; 80(1): 58–66.

Budtz-Jørgensen E. Prosthodontics for the elderly: diagnosis and treatment. Chicago: Quintessence. **1999.**

Buser D, Weber HP, Lang NP. Tissue integration of non-submerged implants. 1-year results of a prospective study with 100 ITI hollow-cylinder and hollow-screw implants. Clin Oral Implants Res. **1990** Dec; 1(1): 33–40.

Buser D, von Arx T. Surgical procedures in partially edentulous patients with ITI implants. Clin Oral Implants Res. **2000**; 11(Suppl 1): 83–100.

Buser D, Janner SF, Wittneben JG, Brägger U, Ramseier CA, Salvi GE. 10-year survival and success rates of 511 titanium implants with a sandblasted and acid-etched surface: a retrospective study in 303 partially edentulous patients. Clin Implant Dent Relat Res. **2012** Dec; 14(6): 839–851.

Cabre M, Serra-Prat M, Palomera E, Almirall J, Pallares R, Clavé P. Prevalence and prognostic implications of dysphagia in elderly patients with pneumonia. Age Ageing. **2010** Jan; 39(1): 39–45.

Cancer Research UK. **2014**. http://www.cancerres earchuk.org/health-professional/cancer-statistics/ statistics-by-cancer-type/oral-cancer/incidence. Last accessed December 21, 2014.

Candel-Marti ME, Ata-Ali J, Peñarrocha-Oltra D, Peñarrocha-Diago M, Bagán JV. Dental implants in patients with oral mucosal alterations: an update. Med Oral Patol Oral Cir Bucal. **2011** Sep 1; 16(6): e787–793.

Cardaropoli G, Araújo M, Lindhe J. Dynamics of bone tissue formation in tooth extraction sites. An experimental study in dogs. J Clin Periodontol. **2003** Sep; 30(9): 809–818.

Carter RB, Keen EN. The intramandibular course of the inferior alveolar nerve. J Anat. **1971**; 108(Pt 3): 433–440.

Castle SC, Uyemura K, Rafi A, Akande O, Makinodan T. Comorbidity is a better predictor of impaired immunity than chronological age in older adults. J Am Geriatr Soc. **2005** Sep; 53(9): 1565–1569.

Cawood JI, Howell RA. A classification of the edentulous jaws. Int J Oral Maxillofac Surg. **1988** Aug; 17(4): 232–236.

Cawood JI, Howell RA. A classification of the edentulous jaws. Int J Oral Maxillofac Surg. **1988** Aug; 17(4): 232–236.

Challacombe SJ, Percival RS, Marsh PD. Age-related changes in immunoglobulin isotypes in whole and parotid saliva and serum in healthy individuals. Oral Microbiol Immunol. **1995** Aug; 10(4): 202–207.

Chambrone L, Mandia J Jr, Shibli JA, Romito GA, Abrahao M. Dental implants installed in irradiated jaws: a systematic review. J Dent Res. **2013** Dec; 92(12 Suppl): 119S–130S.

Chamizo Carmona E, Gallego Flores A, Loza Santamaría E, Herrero Olea A, Rosario Lozano MP. Systematic literature review of bisphosphonates and osteonecrosis of the jaw in patients with osteoporosis. Reumatol Clin. **2012** May–Jun; 9(3); 172–177.

Chapuy MC, Durr F, Chapuy P. Age-related changes in parathyroid hormone and 25 hydroxycholecalciferol levels. J Gerontol. **1983** Jan; 38(1): 19–22.

Charlson ME, Pompei P, Ales KL, MacKenzie CR. A new method of classifying prognostic comorbidity in longitudinal studies: development and validation. J Chronic Dis. **1987**; 40(5): 373–383.

Chen S, Buser D. Advantages and disadvantages of treatment options for implant placement in post-extraction sites. In: Buser D, Wismeijer D, Belser U (eds). ITI Treatment Guide, Vol 3: Implant placement in post-extraction sites. Berlin: Quintessence. **2008**: 29 – 35.

Chen S, Buser D, Cordaro L. Classification of surgical cases. In: Dawson A, Chen S (eds). The SAC classification in implant dentistry. Berlin: Quintessence. **2009**: 27 – 81.

Chiapasco M, De Cicco L, Marrone G. Side effects and complications associated with third molar surgery. Oral Surg Oral Med Oral Pathol. **1993** Oct; 76(4): 412 – 420.

Chiapasco M, Felisati G, Maccari A, Borloni R, Gatti F, Di Leo, F. The management of complications following displacement of oral implants in the paranasal sinuses: a multicenter clinical report and proposed treatment protocols. Int J Oral Maxillofac Surg. **2009** Dec; 38(12): 1273 – 1278.

Chiapasco M, Casentini P, Zaniboni M, Corsi E, Anello T. Titanium zirconium alloy narrow-diameter implants (Straumann Roxolid) for the rehabilitation of horizontally deficient edentulous ridges: prospective study on 18 consecutive patients. Clin Oral Implants Res. **2012** Oct; 23(10): 1136 – 1141.

Chiarella G, Leopardi G, De Fazio L, Chiarella R, Cassandro E. Benign paroxysmal positional vertigo after dental surgery. Eur Arch Otorhinolaryngol. **2008** Jan; 265(1): 119 – 122.

Chou KL, Evatt M, Hinson V, Kompoliti K. Sialorrhea in Parkinson's disease: a review. Mov Disord. **2007** Dec; 22(16): 2306 – 2313.

Chrcanovic BR, Custódio ALN. Mandibular fractures associated with endosteal implants. Oral Maxillofac Surg. **2009** Dec; 13(4): 231 – 238.

Chrcanovic BR, Albrektsson T, Wennerberg A. Diabetes and oral implant failure: a systematic review. J Dent Res. **2014** Sep; 93(9): 859 – 867.

Chuang SK, Wei LJ, Douglass CW, Dodson TB. Risk factors for dental implant failure: a strategy for the analysis of clustered failure-time observations. J Dent Res. **2002** Aug; 81(8): 572 – 577.

Chui MA, Stone JA, Martin BA, Croes KD, Thorpe JM. Safeguarding older adults from inappropriate over-the-counter medications: the role of community pharmacists. Gerontologist. **2013** Nov 6; 54(6): 980 – 1000.

Chung WE, Rubenstein JE, Phillips KM, Raigrodski AJ. Outcomes assessment of patients treated with osseointegrated dental implants at the University of Washington Graduate Prosthodontic Program, 1988 to 2000. Int J Oral Maxillofac Implants. **2009** Sep-Oct; 24(5): 927 – 935.

CKD-MBD Work Group. KDIGO clinical practice guideline for the diagnosis, evaluation, prevention, and treatment of Chronic Kidney Disease—Mineral and Bone Disorder (CKD-MBD). Kidney Int Suppl. **2009** Aug; (113): S1 – S130.

Claffey N, Clarke E, Polyzois I, Renvert S. Surgical treatment of peri-implantitis. J Clin Periodontol. **2008** Sep; 35(Suppl. 8): 316 – 332.

Claudy MP, Miguens SA Jr, Celeste RK, Camara Parente R, Hernandez PA, da Silva AN Jr. Time interval after radiotherapy and dental implant failure: systematic review of observational studies and meta-analysis. Clin Implant Dent Relat Res. **2015** Apr; 17(2): 401 – 411.

Claxton AJ, Cramer J, Pierce C. A systematic review of the associations between dose regimens and medication compliance. Clin Ther. **2001** Aug; 23(8): 1296 – 1310.

Cochran DL, Schou S, Heitz-Mayfield LJA, Bornstein MM, Salvi GE, Martin WC. Consensus statements and recommended clinical procedures regarding risk factors in implant therapy. Int J Oral Maxillofac Implants. **2009**; 24(Suppl): 86 – 89.

Colella G, Cannavale R, Pentenero M, Gandolfo S. Oral implants in radiated patients: A systematic review. Int J Oral Maxillofac Implants. **2007** Jul – Aug; 22(4): 616 – 622.

Cooper C, Livingston G. Mental health/psychiatric issues in elder abuse and neglect. Clin Geriatr Med. **2014** Nov; 30(4): 839 – 850.

Coresh J, Selvin E, Stevens LA, Manzi J, Kusek JW, Eggers P, Van Lente F, Levey AS: Prevalence of chronic kidney disease in the United States. JAMA. **2007** Nov 7: 298(17): 2038 – 2047.

Cosman F, de Beur SJ, LeBoff MS, Lewiecki EM, Tanner B, Randall S, Lindsay R; National Osteoporosis Foundation. Clinician's Guide to Prevention and Treatment of Osteoporosis. Osteoporos Int. **2014** Oct; 25(10): 2359 – 2381.

Costa FO, Takenaka-Martinez S, Cota LO, Ferreira SD, Silva GL, Costa JE. Peri-implant disease in subjects with and without preventive maintenance: a 5-year follow-up. J Clin Periodontol. **2012** Feb; 39(2): 173–181.

Czerninski R, Eliezer M, Wilensky A, Soskolne A. Oral lichen planus and dental implants—a retrospective study. Clin Implant Dent Relat Res. **2013** Apr; 15(2): 234–242.

Daubländer M, Müller R, Lipp MD. The incidence of complications associated with local anesthesia in dentistry. Anesth Prog. **1997** Fall; 44(4): 132–141.

David LA, Sandor GK, Evans AW, Brown DH. Hyperbaric oxygen therapy and mandibular osteoradionecrosis: a retrospective study and analysis of treatment outcomes. J Can Dent Assoc. **2001** Jul–Aug; 67(7): 384.

Davidovich E, Schwarz Z, Davidovitch M, Eidelman E, Bimstein E. Oral findings and periodontal status in children, adolescents and young adults suffering from renal failure. J Clin Periodontol. **2005** Oct; 32(10): 1076–1082.

Dawson A, Martin W, Belser U. Classification of restorative cases. In: Dawson A, Chen S (eds). The SAC classification in implant dentistry. Berlin: Quintessence. **2009**: 83–111.

Dayer R, Badoud I, Rizzoli R, Ammann P. Defective implant osseointegration under protein undernutrition: prevention by PTH or pamidronate. J Bone Miner Res. **2007** Oct; 22(10): 1526–1533.

de Albuquerque Júnior RF, Lund JP, Tang L, Larivée J, de Grandmont P, Gauthier G, Feine JS. Within-subject comparison of maxillary long-bar implant-retained prostheses with and without palatal coverage: patient-based outcomes. Clin Oral Implants Res. **2000** Dec; 11(6): 555-565.

de Baat C. Success of dental implants in elderly people—a literature review. Gerodontology. **2000** Jul; 17(1): 45–48.

de Groot V, Beckerman H, Lankhorst GJ, Bouter LM. How to measure comorbidity: a critical review of available methods. J Clin Epidemiol. **2003** Mar; 56(3): 221–229.

de Jong MH, Wright PS, Meijer HJ, Tymstra N. Posterior mandibular residual ridge resorption in patients with overdentures supported by two or four endos-seous implants in a 10-year prospective comparative study. Int J Oral Maxillofac Implants. **2010** Nov–Dec; 25(6): 1168–1174.

De Rossi SS, Glick M. Dental considerations for the patient with renal disease receiving hemodialysis. J Am Dent Assoc. **1996** Feb; 127(2): 211–219.

De Rossi SS, Slaughter YA. Oral changes in older patients: a clinician's guide. Quintessence Int. **2007** Oct; 38(9): 773–780.

de Souza RF, de Freitas Oliveira Paranhos H, Lovato da Silva CH, Abu-Naba'a L, Fedorowicz Z, Gurgan CA. Interventions for cleaning dentures in adults. Cochrane Database Syst Rev. **2009** Oct 7; (4): CD007395.

de Torres EM, Barbosa GAS, Bernardes SR, de Mattos Mda G, Ribeiro RF. Correlation between vertical misfits and stresses transmitted to implants from metal frameworks. J Biomech. **2011** Jun 3; 44(9): 1735–1739.

Degidi M, Piattelli A. Immediately loaded bar-connected implants with an anodized surface inserted in the anterior mandible in a patient treated with diphosphonates for osteoporosis: a case report with a 12-month follow-up. Clin Implant Dent Relat Res. **2003**; 5(4): 269–272.

Del Fiol G, Weber AI, Brunker CP, Weir CR. Clinical questions raised by providers in the care of older adults: a prospective observational study. BMJ Open. **2014** Jul 4; 4(7): e005315.

Deliberador TM, Marengo G, Scaratti R, Giovanni AF, Zielak JC, Baratto Filho F. Accidental aspiration in a patient with Parkinson's disease during implant-supported prosthesis construction: a case report. Special Care Dentist. **2011** Sep–Oct; 31(5): 156–161.

Dello Russo NM, Jeffcoat MK, Marx RE, Fugazzotto P. Osteonecrosis in the jaws of patients who are using oral bisphosphonates to treat osteoporosis. Int J Oral Maxillofac Implants. **2007** Jan–Feb; 22(1): 146–153.

Department of Health, United Kingdom. Long term conditions compendium of information: Third edition. **2012** May 12. https://www.gov.uk/government/uploads/system/uploads/attachment_data/file/216528/dh_134486.pdf. Last accessed October 29, 2015.

Devlin J. Patients with chronic obstructive pulmonary disease: management considerations for the dental team. Br Dent J. **2014** Sep; 217(5): 235–237.

Dhanuthai K, Rojanawatsirivej S, Somkotra T, Shin HI, Hong SP, Darling M, Ledderhof N, Khalili M, Thosaporn W, Rattana-Arpha P, Saku T. Geriatric oral lesions: A multicentric study. Geriatr Gerontol Int. **2016** Feb; 16(2): 237 – 243.

Di Girolamo M, Napolitano B, Arullani CA, Bruno E, Di Girolamo S. Paroxysmal positional vertigo as a complication of osteotome sinus floor elevation. Eur Arch Ootorhinolaryngol. **2005** Aug; 262(8): 631 – 633.

Dijakiewicz M, Wojtowicz A, Dijakiewicz J, Szycik V, Rutkowski P, Rutkowski B. Is implanto-prosthodontic treatment available for haemodialysis patients? Nephrol Dial Transplant. **2007** Sep; 22(9): 2722 – 2724.

Dimopoulos MA, Kastritis E, Bamia C, Melakopoulos I, Gika D, Roussou M, Migkou M, Eleftherakis-Papaiakovou E, Christoulas D, Terpos E, Bamias A. Reduction of osteonecrosis of the jaw (ONJ) after implementation of preventive measures in patients with multiple myeloma treated with zoledronic acid. Ann Oncol. **2009** Jan; 20(1): 117 – 120.

Ding X, Zhu XH, Liao SH, Zhang XH, Chen H. Implant-bone interface stress distribution in immediately loaded implants of different diameters: a three-dimensional finite element analysis. J Prosthodont. **2009** Jul; 18(5): 393 – 402.

Diz P, Scully C, Sanz M. Dental implants in the medically compromised patient. J Dent. **2013** Mar 1; 41(3): 195 – 206.

Dodd MJ, Facione NC, Dibble SL, MacPhail L. Comparison of methods to determine the prevalence and nature of oral mucositis. Cancer Pract. **1996** Nov – Dec; 4(6): 312 – 318.

Donoff RB. Treatment of the irradiated patient with dental implants: The case against hyperbaric oxygen treatment. J Oral Maxillofac Surg. **2006** May; 64(5): 819 – 822.

Donos N, Laurell L, Mardas N. Hierarchical decisions on teeth vs. implants in the periodontitis-susceptible patient: the modern dilemma. Periodontol 2000. **2012** Jun; 59(1): 89 – 110.

Doud Galli SK, Lebowitz RA, Giacchi RJ, Glickman R, Jacobs JB. Chronic sinusitis complicating sinus lift surgery. Am J Rhinol. **2001** May – Jun; 15(3): 181 – 186.

Douglass CW, Shih A, Ostry L. Will there be a need for complete dentures in the United States in 2020? J Prosthet Dent. **2002** Jan; 87(1): 5 – 8.

Dubois L, de Lange J, Baas E, Van Ingen J. Excessive bleeding in the floor of the mouth after endosseous implant placement: a report of two cases. Int J Oral Maxillofac Surg **2010**; 39: 412 – 415.

Dudley J. Implants for the ageing population. Aust Dent J. **2015** Mar; 60(Suppl 1): 28 – 43.

Dvorak G, Arnhart C, Heuberer S, Huber CD, Watzek G, Gruber R. Peri-implantitis and late implant failures in postmenopausal women: a cross-sectional study. J Clin Periodontol. **2011** Oct; 38(10): 950 – 955.

Dwyer LL, Han B, Woodwell DA, Rechtsteiner EA. Polypharmacy in nursing home residents in the United States: results of the 2004 National Nursing Home Survey. Am J Geriatr Pharmacother. **2010** Feb; 8(1): 63 – 72.

Eder A, Watzek G. Treatment of a patient with severe osteoporosis and chronic polyarthritis with fixed implant-supported prosthesis: a case report. Int J Oral Maxillofac Implants. **1999** Jul – Aug; 14(4): 587 – 590.

Edwards LL, Pfeiffer RF, Quigley EM, Hofmann R, Balluff M. Gastrointestinal symptoms in Parkinson's disease. Mov Disord. **1991**; 6(2): 151 – 156.

Eiseman B, Johnson LR, Coll JR. Ultrasound measurement of mandibular arterial blood supply: techniques for defining ischemia in the pathogenesis of alveolar ridge atrophy and tooth loss in the elderly. Oral Maxillofac Surg. **2005**; 63: 28 – 35.

El Mekawy NH, El-Negoly SA, Grawish Mel A, El-Hawary YM. Intracoronal mandibular Kennedy Class I implant-tooth supported removable partial overdenture: a 2-year multicenter prospective study. Int J Oral Maxillofac Implants. **2012** May – Jun; 27(3): 677 – 683.

Emami E, Heydecke G, Rompré PH, de Grandmont P, Feine JS. Impact of implant support for mandibular dentures on satisfaction, oral and general health-related quality of life: a meta-analysis of randomized-controlled trials. Clin Oral Implants Res. **2009** Jun; 20(6): 533 – 544.

Engeland CG, Bosch JA, Cacioppo JT, Marucha PT. Mucosal wound healing: the roles of age and sex. Arch Surg. **2006** Dec; 141(12): 1193 – 1187; discussion 1198.

Engfors I, Ortorp Am Jemt T. Fixed implant-supported prostheses in elderly patients: a 5-year retrospective study of 133 edentulous patients older than 79 years. Clin Implant Dent Relat Res. **2004**; 6(4): 190–198.

Eom CS, Park SM, Myung SK, Yun JM, Ahn JS. Use of acid-suppressive drugs and risk of fracture: a meta-analysis of observational studies. Ann Fam Med. **2011** May–Jun; 9(3): 257–267.

Epstein JB, Lunn R, Le N, Stevenson-Moore P. Periodontal attachment loss in patients after head and neck radiation therapy. Oral Surg Oral Med Oral Pathol Oral Radiol Endod. **1998** Dec; 86(6): 673–677.

Ersanli S, Olgac V, Leblebicioglu B. Histologic analysis of alveolar bone following guided bone regeneration. J Periodontol. **2004** May; 75(5): 750–756.

Esposito SJ, Camisa C, Morgan M. Implant retained overdentures for two patients with severe lichen planus: a clinical report. J Prosthet Dent. **2003** Jan; 89(1): 6–10.

Esposito M, Worthington HV. Interventions for replacing missing teeth: hyperbaric oxygen therapy for irradiated patients who require dental implants. Cochrane Database Syst Rev. **2013** Sep 30; 9: CD003603.

Esser E, Wagner W. Dental implants following radical oral cancer surgery and adjuvant radiotherapy. Int J Oral Maxillofac Implants. **1997** Jul–Aug; 12(4): 552–557.

Ettinger RL, Pinkham JR. Dental care for the homebound—assessment and hygiene. Aust Dent J. **1977** Apr; 22(2): 77–82.

Evans WJ. Exercise, nutrition and aging. Clin Geriatr Med. **1995** Nov; 11(4): 725–734.

Fadaei Fathabady F, Norouzian M, Azizi F. Effect of hypothyroidism on bone repair in mature female rats. Int J Endocrinol Metab. **2005**; 1: 126–129.

Faggion CM Jr. Critical appraisal of evidence supporting the placement of dental implants in patients with neurodegenerative diseases. Gerodontology. **2013** Dec 10. [Epub ahead of print.]

Farrell B, Shamji S, Monahan A, French Merkley V. Reducing polypharmacy in the elderly: Cases to help you "rock the boat." Can Pharm J (Ott). **2013** Sep; 146(5): 243–244.

Faxen-Irving G, Basun H, Cederholm. Nutritional and cognitive relationships and long-term mortality in patients with various dementia disorders. Age Ageing. **2005** Mar; 34(2): 136–141.

FDA (United States Food and Drug Administration). Background document for meeting of advisory committee for reproductive health drugs and drug safety and risk management advisory committee. **2011**. http://www.fda.gov/downloads/AdvisoryCommittees/CommitteesMeetingMaterials/drugs/DrugSafetyandRiskManagementAdvisoryCommittee/ucm270958.pdf. Last accessed February 10, 2014.

FDA (United States Food and Drug Administration). Avastin (bevacizumab). Safety information. **2014**. http://www.fda.gov/safety/medwatch/safetyinformation/ucm275758.htm. Last accessed December 7, 2014. (**a**)

FDA (United States Food and Drug Administration). Sutent (sunitinib malate) capsules. Safety information. **2014**. http://www.fda.gov/safety/medwatch/safetyinformation/ucm224050.htm. Last accessed December 7, 2014. (**b**)

Feine JS, de Grandmont P, Boudrias P, Brien N, LaMarche C, Taché R, Lund JP. Within-subject comparisons of implant-supported mandibular prostheses: choice of prosthesis. J Dent Res. **1994** May; 73(5): 1105–1111.

Feine JS, Carlsson GE, Awad MA, Chehade A, Duncan WJ, Gizani S, Head T, Heydecke G, Lund JP, MacEntee M, Mericske-Stern R, Mojon P, Morais JA, Naert I, Payne AG, Penrod J, Stoker GT, Tawse-Smith A, Taylor TD, Thomason JM, Thomson WM, Wismeijer D. The McGill consensus statement on overdentures. Mandibular two-implant overdentures as first choice standard of care for edentulous patients. Gerodontology. **2002** Jul; 19(1): 3–4.

Feitosa Dda S, Bezerra Bde B, Ambrosano GM, Nociti FH, Casati MZ, Sallum EA, de Toledo S. Thyroid hormones may influence cortical bone healing around titanium implants: a histometric study in rats. J Periodontol. **2008** May; 79(5): 881–887.

Felsenberg D, Hoffmeister B: Kiefernekrosen nach hoch dosierter Bisphosphanattherapie. [Necrosis of the jaw after high-dose bisphosphonate therapy.] Dtsch Ärztebl. 2006; 103(46): A-3078/B-2681/C-2572.

Ferguson DB. The Aging Mouth. (Frontiers of Oral Biology, Vol. 6.) Basel: Karger AG; **1987**.

Ferreira SD, Silva GL, Cortelli JR, Costa JE, Costa FO. Prevalence and risk variables for peri-implant disease in Brazilian subjects. J Clin Periodontol. **2006** Dec; 33(12): 929 – 935.

Fialová D, Topinková E, Gambassi G, Finne-Soveri H, Jónsson PV, Carpenter I, Schroll M, Onder G, Sørbye LW, Wagner C, Reissigová J, Bernabei R; AdHOC Project Research Group. Potentially inappropriate medication use among elderly home care patients in Europe. JAMA. **2005** Mar 16; 293(11): 1348 – 1358.

Fich A, Camilleri M, Phillips SF. Effect of age on human gastric and small bowel motility. J Clin Gastroenterol. **1989** Aug; 11(4); 416 – 420.

Fick DM, Cooper JW, Wade WE, Waller JL, Maclean JR, Beers MH. Updating the Beers criteria for potentially inappropriate medication use in older adults: results of a US consensus panel of experts. Arch Intern Med. **2003** Dec 8 – 22; 63(22): 2716 – 2724.

Fillion M, Aubazac D, Bessadet M, Allegre M, Nicolas E. The impact of implant treatment on oral health related quality of life in a private dental practice: a prospective cohort study. Health Quality Life Outcomes. **2013** Nov; 11: 197.

Findler M, Galili D, Meidan Z, Yakirevitch V, Garfunkel AA. Dental treatment in very high-risk patients with active ischemic heart disease. Oral Surg Oral Med Oral Pathol. **1993** Sep; 76(3): 298 – 300.

Fiorellini JP, Nevins M. Dental implant considerations in the diabetic patient. Periodontology 2000. **2000** Jun; 23, 73 – 77.

Fiske J, Frenkel H, Griffiths J, Jones V. Guidelines for the development of local standards of oral health care for people with dementia. Gerodontology. **2006** Dec; 23 (Suppl 1): 5 – 32.

Folstein MF, Folstein SE, McHugh PR. "Mini-mental state." A practical method for grading the cognitive state of patients for the clinician. J Psychiatr Res. **1975** Nov; 12(3): 189 – 198.

Friberg B, Ekestubbe A, Mellström D, Sennerby L. Brånemark implants and osteoporosis: a clinical exploratory study. Clin Implant Dent Relat Res. **2001**; 3(1): 50 – 56.

Fried LP, Guralnik JM. Disability in older adults: evidence regarding significance, etiology, and risk. J Am Geriatr Soc. **1997** Jan; 45(1): 92 – 100.

Fried LP, Walston J. Frailty and failure to thrive. In: Hazzard WR, Blass JP, EW (eds). Principles of geriatric medicine and gerontology. New York: McGraw Hill; **1998**: 1387 – 1402.

Fried LP, Tangen CM, Walston J, Newman AB, Hirsch C, Gottdiener J, Seeman T, Tracy R, Kop WJ, Burke G, McBurnie MA; Cardiovascular Health Study Collaborative Research Group. Frailty in older adults: evidence for a phenotype. J Gerontol A Biol Sci Med Sci. **2001** Mar; 56(3): M146 – 156.

Fried LP, Hadley EC, Walston JD, Newman AB, Guralnik JM, Studenski S, Harris TB, Ershler WB, Ferrucci L. From bedside to bench: research agenda for frailty. Sci Aging Knowl Environ. **2005** Aug 3; 2005(31): pe24.

Fried TR, Tinetti ME, Iannone L. Primary care clinicians' experiences with treatment decision making for older persons with multiple conditions. Arch Int Med. **2011** Jan 10; 171(1): 75 – 80. (**a**)

Fried TR, Tinetti ME, Iannone L, O'Leary JR, Towle V, Van Ness PH. Health outcome prioritization as a tool for decision making among older persons with multiple chronic conditions. Arch Intern Med. **2011** Nov 14; 171(20): 1854 – 1856. (**b**)

Frith J, Jones D, Newton JL. Chronic liver disease in an ageing population. Age and Ageing. **2008** Nov 13; 38(1): 11 – 8.

Fujimoto T, Niimi A, Nakai H, Ueda M. Osseointegrated implants in a patient with osteoporosis: a case report. Int J Oral Maxillofac Implants. **1996** Jul – Aug; 11(4): 539 – 542.

Gallo JJ, Bogner HR, Morales KH, Post EP, Ten Have T, Bruce ML. Depression, cardiovascular disease, diabetes, and two-year mortality among older, primary-care patients. Am J Geriatr Psychiatry. **2005** Sep; 13(9): 748 – 755.

Gallucci GO, Bernard JP, Belser UC. Treatment of completely edentulous patients with fixed implant-supported restorations: three consecutive cases of simultaneous immediate loading in both maxilla and mandible. Int J Periodontics Restorative Dent. **2005** Feb; 25(1): 27 – 37.

Gallucci GO, Doughtie CB, Hwang JW, Fiorellini JP, Weber HP. Five-year results of fixed implant-supported rehabilitations with distal cantilevers for the edentulous mandible. Clin Oral Implants Res. **2009** Jun; 20(6): 601 – 607. (**a**)

Gallucci GO, Morton D, Weber HP. Loading protocols for dental implants in edentulous patients. Int J Oral Maxillofac Implants. **2009**; 24(Suppl): 132–146. (**b**)

Gallucci GO, Benic GI, Eckert SE, Papaspyridakos P, Schimmel M, Schrott A, Weber HP. Consensus statements and clinical recommendations for implant loading protocols. Int J Oral Maxillofac Implants. **2014**; 29(Suppl): 287–290.

Gandhi TK, Weingart SN, Borus J, Seger AC, Peterson J, Burdick E, Seger DL, Shu K, Federico F, Leape LL, Bates DW. Adverse drug events in ambulatory care. N Engl J Med. **2003** Apr 17; 348(16): 1556–1564.

Gavalda C, Bagan JV, Scully C, Silvestre F, Milian M, Jimenez V. Renal hemodialysis patients: oral, salivary, dental and periodontal findings in 105 adult cases. Oral Dis. **1999** Oct; 5(4): 299–302.

Gegauff AG, Laurell KA, Thavendrarajah A, Rosenstiel SF. A potential MRI hazard: forces on dental magnet keepers. J Oral Rehabil. **1990** Sep; 17(5): 403–410.

Gesing A, Lewiński A, Karbownik-Lewińska M. The thyroid gland and the process of ageing; what is new? Thyroid Res. **2012** Nov 24, 5(1): 16.

Gibson PG, McDonald VM, Marks GB. Asthma in older adults. Lancet. **2010** Sep 4; 376(9743): 803–813.

Gisbert JP, Chaparro M. Systematic review with meta-analysis: inflammatory bowel disease in the elderly. Aliment Pharmacol Ther. **2014** Jan 9; 39(5): 459–477.

Givol N, Chaushu G, Halamish-Shani T, Taicher S. Emergency tracheostomy following life-threatening hemorrhage in the floor of the mouth during immediate implant placement in the mandibular canine region. J Periodontol. **2000** Dec; 71(12): 1893–1895.

Glaser DL, Kaplan FS. Osteoporosis. Definition and clinical presentation. Spine. **1997** Dec 15; 22(24 Suppl): 12S-16S.

Gleissner C, Willershausen B, Kaesser U, Bolten WW. The role of risk factors for periodontal disease in patients with rheumatoid arthritis. Eur J Med Res. **1998** Aug 18; 3(8): 387–392.

Goiato MC, dos Santos DM, Santiago JF Jr, Moreno A, Pellizzer EP. Longevity of dental implants in type IV bone: a systematic review. Int J Oral Maxillofac Surg. **2014** Sep; 43(9): 1108–1116.

Goldman KE. Dental management of patients with bone marrow and solid organ transplantation. Dent Clin North Am. **2006** Oct; 50(4): 659–676.

Goodacre CJ, Kan JY, Rungcharassaeng K. Clinical complications of osseointegrated implants. J Prosthet Dent. **1999** May; 81(5): 537–552.

Gosain A, DiPietro LA. Aging and wound healing. World J Surg. **2004** Mar; 28(3): 321–326.

Gotfredsen K, Holm B. Implant-supported mandibular overdentures retained with ball or bar attachments: a randomized prospective 5-year study. Int J Prosthodont. **2000** Mar–Apr; 13(2): 125–130.

Gottrup F. Oxygen in wound healing and infection. World J Surg. **2004** Mar; 28(3): 312–315.

Granström G, Jacobsson M, Tjellström A. Titanium implants in irradiated tissue: benefits from hyperbaric oxygen. Int J Oral Maxillofac Implants. **1992** Spring; 7(1): 15–24.

Granström G, Tjellström A. Effects of irradiation on osseointegration before and after implant placement: a report of three cases. Int J Oral Maxillofac Implants. **1997** Jul–Aug; 12(4): 541–551.

Granström G. Radiotherapy, osseointegration and hyperbaric oxygen therapy. Periodontol 2000. **2003**; 33: 145–162.

Granström G. Osseointegration in irradiated cancer patients: An analysis with respect to implant failures. J Oral Maxillofac Surg. **2005** May; 63(5): 579–585.

Grant DJ, McMurdo ME, Mole PA, Paterson CR, Davies RR. Suppressed TSH levels secondary to thyroxine replacement therapy are not associated with osteoporosis. Clin Endocrinol (Oxford). **1993** Nov; 39(5): 529–533.

Grant BT, Amenedo C, Freeman K, Kraut RA. Outcomes of placing dental implants in patients taking oral bisphosphonates: a review of 115 cases. J Oral Maxillofac Surg. **2008** Feb; 66(2): 223–230.

Gravenstein S, Fillit HM, Ershler WB. Clinical immunology of aging. In: Tallis RC, Fillit HM (eds). Brocklehurst's textbook of geriatric medicine and gerontology. 6th edition. Churchill Livingstone; **2003**: 117–118.

Graves AB, Larson EB, Edland SD, Bowen JD, McCormick WC, McCurry SM, Rice MM, Wenzlow A, Uomoto JM.

Prevalence of dementia and its subtypes in the Japanese American population of King County, Washington state. The Kame Project. Am J Epidemiol. **1996** Oct; 144(8): 760–771.

Graziani F, Donos N, Needleman I, Gabriele M, Tonetti M. Comparison of implant survival following sinus floor augmentation procedures with implants placed in pristine posterior maxillary bone: a systematic review. Clin Oral Implants Res. **2004** Dec; 15(6): 677-682.

Grbic JT, Landesberg R, Lin SQ, Mesenbrink P, Reid IR, Leung PC, Casas N, Recknor CP, Hua Y, Delmas PD, Eriksen EF. Incidence of osteonecrosis of the jaw in women with postmenopausal osteoporosis in the health outcomes and reduced incidence with zoledronic acid once yearly pivotal fracture trial. J Am Dent Assoc. **2008** Jan; 139(1): 32–40.

Grbic JT, Black DM, Lyles KW, Reid DM, Orwoll E, McClung M, Bucci-Rechtweg C, Su G. The incidence of osteonecrosis of the jaw in patients receiving 5 milligrams of zoledronic acid: Data from the health outcomes and reduced incidence with zoledronic acid once yearly clinical trials program. J Am Dent Assoc. **2010** Nov; 141(11): 1365–1370.

Gross MD, Nissan J, Samuel R. Stress distribution around maxillary implants in anatomic photoelastic models of varying geometry. Part I. J Prosthet Dent. **2001** May; 85(5): 442–449. (**a**)

Gross MD, Nissan J. Stress distribution around maxillary implants in anatomic photoelastic models of varying geometry. Part II. J Prosthet Dent. **2001** May; 85(5): 450–454. (**b**)

Gross CP, Mallory R, Heiat A, Krumholz HM. Reporting the recruitment process in clinical trials: who are these patients and how did they get there? Ann Intern Med. **2002** Jul 2; 137(1): 10–16.

Grubbs V, Plantinga LC, Tuot DS, Powe NR. Chronic kidney disease and use of dental services in a United States public healthcare system: a retrospective cohort study. BMC Nephrol. **2012** Apr 2; 13(1): 16.

Gu L, Wang Q, Yu YC. Eleven dental implants placed in a liver transplantation patient: a case report and 5-year clinical evaluation. Chin Med J (Engl). **2011** Feb; 124(3): 472–475.

Gu L, Yu YC. Clinical outcome of dental implants placed in liver transplant recipients after 3 years: a case series. Transplant Proc. **2011** Sep; 43(7): 2678–2682.

Guarneri V, Miles D, Robert N, Diéras V, Glaspy J, Smith I, Thomssen C, Biganzoli L, Taran T, Conte P. Bevacizumab and osteonecrosis of the jaw: Incidence and association with bisphosphonate therapy in three large prospective trials in advanced breast cancer. Breast Cancer Res Treat. **2010** Jul; 122(1): 181–188.

Guigoz Y, Vellas B, Garry PJ. Mini nutritional assessment: a practical assessment tool for grading the nutritional state of elderly patients. In: The mini nutritional assessment. Facts and research in gerontology (suppl I). Paris: Serdi; **1994**.

Guo S, DiPietro LA. Factors affecting wound healing. J Dent Res. **2010** Mar; 89(3): 219–229.

Gupta A, Pansari K, Shett H. Post-stroke depression. Int J Clin Pract. **2002** Sep; 56(7): 531–537.

Guralnik JM, Eisenstaedt RS, Ferrucci L, Klein HG, Woodman RC. Prevalence of anemia in persons 65 years and older in the United States: evidence for a high rate of unexplained anemia. Blood. **2004** Oct; 104(8): 2263–2268.

Gurwitz JH, Avorn J, Ross-Degnan D, Choodnovskiy I, Ansell J. Aging and the anticoagulant response to warfarin therapy. Ann Intern Med. **1992** Jun 1; 116(11): 901–904.

Gurwitz JH, Field TS, Harrold LR, Rothschild J, Debellis K, Seger AC, Cadoret C, Fish LS, Garber L, Kelleher M, Bates DW. Incidence and preventability of adverse drug events among older persons in the ambulatory setting. JAMA. **2003** Mar; 289(9): 1107–1116.

Guyatt GH, Sackett DL, Cook DJ. Users' guides to the medical literature. II. How to use an article about therapy or prevention. B. What were the results and will they help me in caring for my patients? JAMA. **1994** Jan 5; 271(1): 59–63.

Haider R, Watzek G, Plenk H Jr. Histomorphometric analysis of bone healing after insertion of IMZ-1 implants independent of bone structure and drilling method (in German). Z Stomatol. **1991**; 88: 507–521.

Hajjar ER, Hanlon JT, Sloane RJ, Lindblad CI, Pieper CF, Ruby CM, Branch LC, Schmader KE. Unnecessary drug use in frail older people at hospital discharge. J Am Geriatr Soc. **2005** Sep; 53(9): 1518–1523.

Hajjar ER, Cafiero AC, Hanlon JT. Polypharmacy in elderly patients. Am J Geriatr Pharmacother. **2007** Dec; 5(4): 345–351.

Hakim FT, Gress RE. Immunosenescence: deficits in adaptive immunity in the elderly. Tissue antigens. **2007** Sep; 70(3): 179–189.

Halbert RJ, Natoli JL, Gano A, Badamgarav E, Buist AS, Mannino DM. Global burden of COPD: systematic review and meta-analysis. Eur Respir J. **2006** Sep; 28(3): 523–532.

Hamdan NM, Gray-Donald K, Awad MA, Johnson-Down L, Wollin S, Feine JS. Do implant overdentures improve dietary intake? A randomized clinical trial. J Dent Res. **2013** Dec; 92(12 Suppl): 146S-153S.

Han CH, Johansson CB, Wennerberg A, Albrektsson T. Quantitative and qualitative investigations of surface enlarged titanium and titanium alloy implants. Clin Oral Implants Res. **1998** Feb; 9(1): 1–10.

Handschel J, Simonowska M, Naujoks C, Depprich RA, Ommerborn MA, Meyer U, Kübler NR. A histomorphometric meta-analysis of sinus elevation with various grafting materials. Head Face Med. **2009** Jun 11; 5: 12.

Handschin AE, Trentz OA, Hoerstrup SP, Kock HJ, Wanner GA, Trentz O. Effect of low molecular weight heparin (dalteparin) and fondaparinux (Arixtra) on human osteoblasts in vitro. Br J Surg. **2005** Feb; 92(2): 177–183.

Hanlon JT, Handler S, Maher R, Schmader KE. Geriatric Pharmacotherapy and Polypharmacy. In: Fillit H, Rockwood K, Woodhouse K (eds). Brocklehurst's textbook of geriatric medicine and gerontology. 7th edition. Philadelphia: WB Saunders. **2010**. 880–885.

Hanna LA, Hughes CM. Public's views on making decisions about over-the-counter medication and their attitudes towards evidence of effectiveness: a cross-sectional questionnaire study. Patient Educ Couns. **2011** Jun; 83(3): 345–351.

Hansen J. Common cancers in the elderly. Drugs Aging. **1998** Dec; 13(6): 467–478.

Harding SM, Guzzo MR, Richter JE. The prevalence of gastroesophageal reflux in asthma patients without reflux symptoms. Am J Respir Crit Care Med. **2000** Jul; 162(1): 34–39.

Harpur P. From universal exclusion to universal equality: regulating ableism in a digital age. **2013**; Northern Kentucky Law Review 40(3): 529–565.

Harris MI, Flegal KM, Cowie CC, Eberhardt MS, Goldstein DE, Little RR, Wiedmeyer HM, Byrd-Holt DD. Prevalence of diabetes, impaired fasting glucose, and impaired glucose tolerance in U.S. adults. The Third National Health and Nutrition Examination Survey, 1988–1994. Diabetes Care. **1998** Apr; 21(4): 518–524.

Harrison JS, Stratemann S, Redding SW. Dental implants for patients who have had radiation treatment for head and neck cancer. Spec Care Dentist. **2003** Nov 1; 23(6): 223–229.

Hartmann R, Müller F. Clinical studies on the appearance of natural anterior teeth in young and old adults. Gerodontology. **2004** Aug; 21(1): 10–16.

Hasegawa M, Umekawa Y, Nagai E, Ishigami T. Retentive force and magnetic flux leakage of magnetic attachment in various keeper and magnetic assembly combinations. J Prosthet Dent. **2011** Apr; 105(4): 266–271.

Haugeberg G. Focal and generalized bone loss in rheumatoid arthritis: Separate or similar concepts? Nat Clin Pract Rheumatol. **2008** Aug; 4(8): 402–403.

Haynes RB, McKibbon KA, Kanani R. Systematic review of randomised trials on interventions to assist patients to follow prescriptions for medications. Lancet. **1996** Aug 10; 348(9024): 383–386. [Erratum: Lancet. 1997 Apr 19; 349(9059): 1180.]

Heaney RP, Gallagher JC, Johnston CC, Neer R, Parfitt AM, Whedon GD. Calcium nutrition and bone health in the elderly. Am J Clin Nutr. **1982** Nov; 36(5 Suppl): 986–1013.

Heath MR. The effect of maximum biting force and bone loss upon masticatory function and dietary selection of the elderly. Int Dent J. **1982** Dec; 32(4): 345–356.

Hebling E, Pereira AC. Oral health-related quality of life: a critical appraisal of assessment tools used in elderly people. Gerodontology. **2007** Sep; 24(3): 151–161.

Heckmann SM, Heckmann JG, Weber HP. Clinical outcomes of three Parkinson's disease patients treated with mandibular implant overdentures. Clin Oral Implants Res. **2000** Dec; 11(6): 566–567.

Heckmann SM, Heckmann JG, Linke JJ, Hohenberger W, Mombelli A. Implant therapy following liver transplantation: clinical and microbiological results after 10 years. J Periodontol **2004** Jun; 75 (6): 909–913.

Heino TJ, Kurata K, Higaki H, Väänänen K. Evidence of the role of osteocytes in the initiation of targeted remodeling. Technol Health Care. **2009**; 17(1): 49 – 56.

Heitz-Mayfield LJ. Peri-implant diseases: diagnosis and risk indicators. J Clin Periodontol. **2008** Sep; 35(8 Suppl): 292 – 304.

Hernández G, Lopez-Pintor RM, Arriba L, Torres J, de Vicente J C. Implant treatment in patients with oral lichen planus: a prospective-controlled study. Clin Oral Implants Res. **2012** Jun; 23(6): 726 – 732.

Heschl A, Payer M, Clar V, Stopper M, Wegscheider W, Lorenzoni M. Overdentures in the edentulous mandible supported by implants and retained by a Dolder bar: a 5-year prospective study. Clin Implant Dent Relat Res. **2013** Aug; 15(4): 589 – 599.

Heydecke G, Klemetti E, Awad MA, Lund JP, Feine JS. Relationship between prosthodontic evaluation and patient ratings of mandibular conventional and implant prostheses. Int J Prosthodont. **2003** May – Jun; 16(3): 307 – 312. (**a**)

Heydecke G, Locker D, Awad MA, Lund JP, Feine JS. Oral and general health-related quality of life with conventional and implant dentures. Community Dent Oral Epidemiol. **2003** Jun; 31(3): 161 – 168. (**b**)

Heydecke G, Penrod JR, Takanashi Y, Lund JP, Feine JS, Thomason JM. Cost-effectiveness of mandibular two-implant overdentures and conventional dentures in the edentulous elderly. J Dent Res. **2005** Sep; 84(9): 794 – 799.

Hoeksema AR, Visser A, Raghoebar GM, Vissink A, Meijer HJ. Influence of age on clinical performance of mandibular two-implant overdentures: a 10-year prospective comparative study. Clinical implant dentistry and related research. **2015** Apr 29. [Epub ahead of print.]

Hoff AO, Toth BB, Altundag K, Johnson MM, Warneke CL, Hu M, Nooka A, Sayegh G, Guarneri V, Desrouleaux K, Cui J, Adamus A, Gagel RF, Hortobagyi GN. Frequency and risk factors associated with osteonecrosis of the jaw in cancer patients treated with intravenous bisphosphonates. J Bone Miner Res. **2008** Jun; 23 (5): 826 – 836.

Hofmann M, Pröschel P. Funktionelle Wechselbeziehung zwischen perioraler. Muskulatur und totaler Prothese. [Mandibular dynamics and the mastication pattern of complete denture wearers and of subjects with a full set of teeth]. Dtsch Zahnärztl Z. **1982** Sep; 37(9): 763 – 771.

Hofschneider U, Tepper G, Gahleitner A, Ulm C. Assessment of the blood supply to the mental region for reduction of bleeding complications during implant surgery in the interforaminal region. Int J Oral Maxillofac Implants. **1999** May – Jun; 14(3): 379 – 383.

Holm-Pedersen P, Folke LEA, Gawronski TH. Composition and metabolic activity of dental plaque from healthy young and elderly individuals. J Dent Res. **1980** May; 59 (5): 771 – 776.

Holtzman JM, Akiyama H. Symptoms and the decision to seek professional care. Gerodontics. **1985** Feb; 1(1): 44 – 49.

Hong CH, Napenas JJ, Brennan MT, Furney SL, Lockhart PB. Frequency of bleeding following invasive dental procedures in patients on low-molecular-weight heparin therapy. J Oral Maxillofac Surg. **2010** May; 68(5): 975 – 979.

Horne BD, Anderson JL. Haptoglobin 2-2 genotyping for refining standard cardiovascular risk assessment: a promising proposition in need of validation. J Am Coll Cardiol. **2015** Oct 20; 66(16): 1800 – 1802.

Horner K, Devlin H, Alsop CW, Hodgkinson IM, Adams JE. Mandibular bone mineral density as a predictor of skeletal osteoporosis Br J Radiol. **1996** Nov; 69(827): 1019 – 1025.

Hubbard BM, Squier M. The physical aging of the neuromuscular system. In: Tallis J (ed). The clinical neurology of old age. London: John Wiley and Sons. **1989**: 137 – 142.

Hui SL, Slemenda CW, Johnston CC Jr. Age and bone mass as predictors of fracture in a prospective study. J Clin Invest. **1988** Jun; 81(6): 1804 – 1809.

Huja SS, Fernandez SA, Hill KJ, Li Y: Remodeling dynamics in the alveolar process in skeletally mature dogs. Anat Rec A Discov Mol Cell Evol Biol. **2006** Dec; 288(12): 1243 – 1249.

Hultin M, Svensson KG, Trulsson M. Clinical advantages of computer-guided implant placement: a systematic review. Clin Oral Implants Res. **2012** Oct; 23(Suppl 6): 124 – 135.

Hwang D, Wang HL. Medical contraindications to implant therapy: part I: absolute contraindications. Implant Dent. **2006** Dec; 15(4): 353–360.

Iber FL, Nurohy PA, Connor ES. Age-related changes in the gastrointestinal system. Effects on drug therapy. Drugs Aging. **1994** Jul; 5(1): 34–48.

Iida S, Tanaka N, Kogo M, Matsuya T. Migration of a dental implant into the maxillary sinus. A case report. Int J Oral Maxillofac Surg. **2000** Oct; 29(5): 358–359.

Iinuma T, Arai Y, Abe Y, Takayama M, Fukumoto M, Fukui Y, Iwase T, Takebayashi T, Hirose N, Gionhaku N, Komiyama K. Denture wearing during sleep doubles the risk of pneumonia in the very elderly. J Dent Res. **2015** Mar 94(3 Suppl): 28S-36S.

Ikebe K, Wada M, Kagawa R, Maeda Y. Is old age a risk factor for dental implants? Japanese Dental Science Review. **2009** ; 4(1): 59–64.

Ikebe K, Hazeyama T, Ogawa T, Kagawa R, Matsuda K, Wada M, Gonda T, Maeda Y. Subjective values of different age groups in Japan regarding treatment for missing molars. Gerodontology. **2011** Sep; 28(3): 192–196.

Incel NA, Sezgin M, As I, Cimen OB, Sahin G. The geriatric hand: correlation of hand-muscle function and activity restriction in elderly. Int J Rehabil Res. **2009** Sep; 32(3): 213–218.

International Diabetes Federation. IDF Diabetes Atlas. Sixth edition. **2014**. http://www.idf.org/diabetesatlas. Last accessed December 29, 2014.

Isaacson TJ. Sublingual hematoma formation during immediate placement of mandibular endosseous implants. J Am Dent Assoc. **2004** Feb; 135(2): 168–172.

Isaksson R, Becktor JP, Brown A, Laurizohn C, Isaksson S. Oral health and oral implant status in edentulous patients with implant-supported dental prostheses who are receiving long-term nursing care. Gerodontology. **2009** Dec; 26(4): 245–249.

Isidor F, Brøndum K, Hansen H J, Jensen J, Sindet-Pedersen S. Outcome of treatment with implant-retained dental prostheses in patients with Sjögren syndrome. Int J Oral Maxillofac Implants. **1999** Sep – Okt; 14(5): 736–743.

Israelson H, Plemons JM, Watkins P, Sory C. Barium-coated surgical stents and computer-assisted tomography in the preoperative assessment of dental implant patients. Int J Periodontics Restorative Dent. **1992**; 12(1): 52–61.

Jacobs R, Schotte A, van Steenberghe D, Quirynen M, Naert I. Posterior jaw bone resorption in osseointegrated implant-supported overdentures. Clin Oral Implants Res. **1992** Jun; 3(2): 63–70.

Jacobs R, Ghyselen J, Koninckx P, van Steenberghe D. Long-term bone mass evaluation of mandible and lumbar spine in a group of women receiving hormone replacement therapy. Eur J Oral Sci. **1996** Feb; 104(1): 10–16.

Jacobs JW, Bijlsma JW, van Laar JM. Glucocorticoids in early rheumatoid arthritis: are the benefits of joint-sparing effects offset by the adverse effect of osteoporosis? The effects on bone in the utrecht study and the CAMERA-II study. Neuroimmunomodulation. **2015**; 22(1–2): 66–71.

Jainkittivong A, Aneksuk V, Langlais RP. Oral mucosal conditions in elderly dental patients. Oral Dis. **2002** Jul; 8(4): 218–223.

Javed F, Almas K. Osseointegration of dental implants in patients undergoing bisphosphonate treatment: a literature review. J Periodontol. **2010** Apr; 81(4): 479–484.

Jeffcoat MK. Safety of oral bisphosphonates: controlled studies on alveolar bone. Int J Oral Maxillofac Implants. **2006** May–Jun; 21(53): 349–353.

Jemt T, Chai J, Harnett J, Heath MR, Hutton JE, Johns RB, McKenna S, McNamara DC, van Steenberghe D, Taylor R, Watson RM, Herrmann I. A 5-year prospective multicenter follow-up report on overdentures supported by osseointegrated implants. Int J Oral Maxillofac Implants. **1996** May–Jun; 11(3): 291–298. (**a**)

Jemt T, Book K. Prosthesis misfit and marginal bone loss in edentulous implant patients. Int J Oral Maxillofac Implants. **1996** Sep – Oct; 11(5): 620–625. (**b**)

Jerjes W, Upile T, Nhembe F, Gudka D, Shah P, Abbas S, et al. Experience in third molar surgery: an update. Br Dent J. **2010** Jul 10; 209(1): E1.

Jevon P. Emergency oxygen therapy in the dental practice: administration and management. Br Dent J. **2014** Feb; 216(3): 113–115.

Jisander S, Grenthe B, Alberius P. Dental implant survival in the irradiated jaw: a preliminary report. Int J Oral Maxillofac Implants. **1997** Sep – Oct; 12(5):643 – 648.

Jones R, Jones RO, McCowan C, Montgomery AA, Fahey T. The external validity of published randomized controlled trials in primary care. BMC Fam Pract. **2009** Jan 19; 10: 5.

Joshi A, Douglass CW, Feldman H, Mitchell P, Jette A. Consequences of success: do more teeth translate into more disease and utilization? J Public Health Dent. **1996** Summer; 56(4): 190 – 197.

Jyrkkä J, Enlund H, Lavikainen P, Sulkava R, Hartikainen S. Association of polypharmacy with nutritional status, functional ability and cognitive capacity over a three-year period in an elderly population. Pharmacoepidemiol Drug Saf. **2010** May; 20(5): 514 – 522.

Kale SS, Yende S. Effects of aging on inflammation and hemostasis through the continuum of critical illness. Aging Dis. **2011** Dec; 2(6): 501 – 511.

Kalpidis CD, Setayesh RM. Hemorrhaging associated with endosseous implant placement in the anterior mandible: a review of the literature. J Periodontol. **2004** May; 75(5): 631 – 645.

Kalpidis CD, Setayesh RM. Haemorrhaging associated with endosseous implant placement in the anterior mandible: a review of the literature. J Periodontol. **2004** May; 75(5): 631 – 645.

Kan JY, Rungcharassaeng K, Bohsali K, Goodacre CJ, Lang BR. Clinical methods for evaluating implant framework fit. J Prosthet Dent. **1999** Jan; 81(1), 7 – 13.

Kang B, Cheong S, Chaichanasakul T, Bezouglaia O, Atti E, Dry SM, Pirih FQ, Aghaloo TL, Tetradis S. Periapical disease and bisphosphonates induce osteonecrosis of the jaws in mice. J Bone Miner Res. **2013** Jul 28(7): 1631 – 1640.

Kaplan DM, Attal U, Kraus M. Bilateral benign paroxysmal positional vertigo following a tooth implantation. J Laryngol Otol. **2003** Apr; 117(4): 312 – 313.

Kapur K. Masticatory performance and efficiency in denture wearers. J Prosthet Dent. **1964**; 14: 687 – 694.

Kapur KK, Garrett NR, Hamada MO, Roumanas ED, Freymiller E, Han T, Diener RM, Levin S, Wong WK. Randomized clinical trial comparing the efficacy of mandibular implant-supported overdentures and conventional dentures in diabetic patients. Part III: comparisons of patient satisfaction. J Prosthet Dent. **1999** Oct; 82(4): 416 – 427.

Katon WJ, Lin EH, Von Korff M, Ciechanowski P, Ludman EJ, Young B, Peterson D, Rutter CM, McGregor M, McCulloch D. Collaborative care for patients with depression and chronic illnesses. N Engl J Med. **2010** Dec 10; 363(27): 2611 – 2620.

Katsoulis J, Walchli J, Kobel S, Gholami H, Mericske-Stern R. Complications with computer-aided designed/computer-assisted manufactured titanium and soldered gold bars for mandibular implant-overdentures: short-term observations. Clin Implant Dent Relat Res. **2015** Jan; 17(Suppl 1): e75 – e85.

Kaufman DW, Kelly JP, Rosenberg L, Anderson TE, Mitchell AA. Recent patterns of medication use in the ambulatory adult population of the United States: the Slone survey. JAMA. **2002** Jan 16; 287(3): 337 – 344.

Kay EJ, Nuttall NM, Knill-Jones R. Restorative treatment thresholds and agreement in treatment decision-making. Community Dent Oral Epidemiol. **1992** Oct; 20(5): 265 – 268.

Kay EJ, Nuttall N. Clinical decision making—an art or a science? Part V: Patient preferences and their influence on decision making. Br Dent J. **1995** Mar; 178(6): 229 – 233.

Käyser AF. Shortened dental arches and oral function. J Oral Rehabil. **1981** Sep; 8(5): 457 – 462.

Keefe DM, Schubert MM, Elting LS, Sonis ST, Epstein JB, Raber-Durlacher JE, Migliorati CA, McGuire DB, Hutchins RD, Peterson DE. Updated clinical practice guidelines for the prevention and treatment of mucositis. Cancer. **2007** Mar 1; 109(5): 820 – 831.

Keller EE. Placement of dental implants in the irradiated mandible: A protocol without adjunctive hyperbaric oxygen. J Oral Maxillofac Surg. **1997** Sep; 55(9): 972 – 980.

Kelly E. Changes caused by a mandibular removable partial denture opposing a maxillary complete denture. J Prosthet Dent. **1972** Feb; 27(2): 140 – 150.

Kennedy E. Partial denture construction. Dent Items Interest. **1928**; 1: 3 – 8.

Khadivi V, Anderson J, Zarb GA. Cardiovascular disease and treatment outcomes with osseointegration surgery. J Prosthet Dent. **1999** May; 81(5): 533–536.

Khan AA, et al. International consensus on diagnosis and management of osteonecrosis of the jaw: a systematic review and international consensus. J Bone Miner Res. **2015** Jan; 30(1) 3–23.

Kilmartin CM. Managing the medically compromised geriatric patient. J Prosthet Dent. **1994** Nov; 72(5): 492–499.

Kim YK, Yun PY, Kim SG, Lim SC. Analysis of the healing process in sinus bone grafting using various grafting materials. Oral Surg Oral Med Oral Pathol Oral Radiol Endod. **2009** Feb; 107(2): 204–211.

Kim MS, Lee JK, Chang BS, Um HS. Benign paroxysmal positional vertigo as a complication of sinus floor elevation. J Periodontol Implant Sci. **2010** Apr; 40(2): 86–89.

Kimura T, Wada M, Suganami T, Miwa S, Hagiwara Y, Maeda Y. Dental implant status of patients receiving long-term nursing care in Japan. Clin Implant Dent Relat Res. **2015** Jan; 17(Suppl 1): e163-167.

Klein MO, Schiegnitz E, Al-Nawas B. Systematic review on success of narrow-diameter dental implants. Int J Oral Maxillofac Implants. **2014**; 29(Suppl): 43–54.

Klemetti E. Is there a certain number of implants needed to retain an overdenture? J Oral Rehabil. **2008** Jan; 35(Suppl 1): 80–84.

Ko YJ, Kim JY, Lee J, Song HJ, Kim JY, Choi NK, Park BJ. Levothyroxine dose and fracture risk according to the osteoporosis status in elderly women. J Prev Med Public Health. **2014** Jan 29; 47(1): 36–46.

Kobayashi M, Srinivasan M, Ammann P, Perriard J, Ohkubo C, Müller F, Belser UC, Schimmel M. Effects of in vitro cyclic dislodging on retentive force and removal torque of three overdenture attachment systems. Clin Oral Implants Res. **2014** Apr; 25(4): 426–434.

Koch WM, Patel H, Brennan J, Boyle JO, Sidransky D. Squamous cell carcinoma of the head and neck in the elderly. Arch Otolaryngol Head Neck Surg. **1995** Mar; 121(3): 262–265.

Koller MM. [Geriatric dentistry: medical problems as well as disease- and therapy-induced oral disorders].

Schweiz Rundsch Med Prax. **1994** Mar 8; 83(10): 273–282.

Kotsovilis S, Karoussis IK, Fourmousis I. A comprehensive and critical review of dental implant placement in diabetic animals and patients. Clin Oral Implants Res. **2006** Oct; 17(5): 587–599.

Kovács AF. Clinical analysis of implant losses in oral tumor and defect patients. Clin Oral Implants Res. **2000** Oct; 11(5): 494–504. (**a**)

Kovács L, Török T, Bari F, Kéri Z, Kovács A, Makula E, Pokorny G. Impaired microvascular response to cholinergic stimuli in primary Sjögren's syndrome. Ann Rheum Dis. **2000** Jan; 59(1): 48–53. (**b**)

Kowar J, Eriksson A, Jemt. Fixed implant-supported prostheses in elderly patients: a 5-year retrospective comparison between partially and completely edentulous patients aged 80 years or older at implant surgery. Clin Implant Dent Relat Res. **2013** Feb; 15(1): 37–46.

Kreisler M, Behneke N, Behneke A, d'Hoedt B. Residual ridge resorption in the edentulous maxilla in patients with implant-supported mandibular overdentures: an 8-year retrospective study. Int J Prosthodont. **2003** May–Jun; 16(3): 295–300.

Kremer U, Schindler S, Enkling N, Worni A, Katsoulis J, Mericske-Stern R. Bone resorption in different parts of the mandible in patients restored with an implant overdenture. A retrospective radiographic analysis. Clin Oral Implants Res. **2014** Nov 22. [Epub ahead of print.]

Krennmair G, Seemann R, Piehslinger E. Dental implants in patients with rheumatoid arthritis: clinical outcome and peri-implant findings. J Clin Periodontol. **2010** Oct; 37(19): 928–936.

Kripalani S, LeFevre F, Phillips CO, Williams MV, Basaviah P, Baker DW. Deficits in communication and information transfer between hospital-based and primary care physicians: implications for patient safety and continuity of care. JAMA. **2007** Feb 28; 297(8): 831–841.

Kronstrom M, Davis B, Loney R, Gerrow J, Hollender L. A prospective randomized study on the immediate loading of mandibular overdentures supported by one or two implants; a 3 year follow-up report. Clin Implant Dent Relat Res. **2014** Jun; 16(3): 323–329.

Kshirsagar AV, Craig RG, Moss KL, Beck JD, Offenbacher S, Kotanko P, Klemmer PJ, Yoshino M, Levin NW, Yip JK, Almas K, Lupovici EM, Usvyat LA, Falk RJ. Periodontal disease adversely affects the survival of patients with end-stage renal disease. Kidney Int. **2009** Apr; 75(7): 746 – 751.

Kuehl S, Payer M, Zitzmann NU, Lambrecht JT, Filippi A. Technical accuracy of printed surgical templates for guided implant surgery with the coDiagnostiX™ software. Clin Implant Dent Relat Res. **2015** Jan; 17(Suppl 1): e177 – 182.

Kuluski K, Gill A, Naganathan G, Upshur R, Jaakkimainen RL, Wodchis WP. A qualitative descriptive study on the alignment of care goals between older persons with multi-morbidities, their family physicians and informal caregivers. BMC Fam Pract. **2013** Sep 8; 14: 133.

Kunchur R, Need A, Hughes T, Goss A. Clinical investigation of C-terminal cross-linking telopeptide test in prevention and management of bisphosphonate-associated osteonecrosis of the jaws. J Oral Maxillofac Surg. **2009** Jun 1; 67(6): 1167 – 1173.

Kyrgidis A, Vahtsevanos K, Koloutsos G, Andreadis C, Boukovinas I, Teleioudis Z, Patrikidou A, Triaridis S. Bisphosphonate-related osteonecrosis of the jaws: a case-control study of risk factors in breast cancer patients. J Clin Oncol. **2008** Oct 1; 26(28): 4634 – 4638.

Lam NP, Donoff RB, Kaban LB, Dodson TB. Patient satisfaction after trigeminal nerve repair. Oral Surg Oral Med Oral Pathol Oral Radiol Endod. **2003** May; 95(5): 538 – 543.

Lambert FE, Weber HP, Susarla SM, Belser UC Gallucci GO. Descriptive analysis of implant and prosthodontic survival rates with fixed implant-supported rehabilitations in the edentulous maxilla. J Periodontol. **2009** Aug; 80(8): 1220 – 1230.

Lambrecht JT, Filippi A, Arrigoni J. Cardiovascular monitoring and its consequences in oral surgery. Ann Maxillofac Surg. **2011** Jul; 1(2): 102 – 106.

Landesberg R, Cozin M, Cremers S, Woo V, Kousteni S, Sinha S, Garrett-Sinha L, Raghavan S. Inhibition of oral mucosal cell wound healing by bisphosphonates. J Oral Maxillofac Surg. **2008** May; 66(5): 839 – 847.

Lang PO, Michel JP, Zekry D. Frailty syndrome: a transitional state in a dynamic process. Gerontology. **2009**; 55(5): 539 – 549.

Lang NP, Berglundh T. Periimplant diseases: where are we now?—Consensus of the Seventh European Workshop on Periodontology. J Clin Periodontol. **2011** Mar; 38(Suppl 11): 178 – 181. (**a**)

Lang NP, Bosshardt DD, Lulic M. Do mucositis lesions around implants differ from gingivitis lesions around teeth? J Clin Periodontol. **2011** Mar; 38(Suppl 11): 182 – 187. (**b**)

Lanza FL, Hunt RH, Thomson AB, Provenza JM, Blank MA. Endoscopic comparison of esophageal and gastroduodenal effects of risedronate and alendronate in post- menopausal women. Gastroenterology. **2000** Sep; 119 (3): 631 – 638.

Larrazabal-Morón C, Boronat-López A, Peñarrocha-Diago M, Peñarrocha-Diago M. Oral rehabilitation with bone graft and simultaneous dental implants in a patient with epidermolysis bullosa: a clinical case report. J Oral Maxillofac Surg. **2009** Jul 1; 67(7): 1499 – 1502.

Larsen PE. Placement of dental implants in the irradiated mandible: a protocol involving adjunctive hyperbaric oxygen. J Oral Maxillofac Surg. **1997** Sep; 55(9): 967 – 971.

Laurell KA, Gegauff AG, Rosenstiel SF. Magnetic resonance image degradation from prosthetic magnet keepers; J Prosthet Dent. **1989** Sep; 62(3): 344 – 348.

Law C, Bennani V, Lyons K, Swain M. Mandibular flexure and its significance on implant fixed prostheses: a review. J Prosthodont, **2012** Apr; 21(3): 219 – 224.

Lawton MP, Brody EM. Assessment of older people: self-maintaining and instrumental activities of daily living. Gerontologist. **1969** Autumn; 9(3): 179 – 186.

Leblebicioglu B, Ersanli S, Karabuda C, Tosun T, Gokdeniz H. Radiographic evaluation of dental implants placed using an osteotome technique. J Periodontol. **2005** Mar; 76(3): 385 – 390.

Lecka-Czernik B. Bone loss in diabetes: use of antidiabetic thiazolidinediones and secondary osteoporosis. Curr Osteoporos Rep. **2010** Sep 1; 8(4): 178 – 184.

Ledermann PD, Schenk RK, Buser D. Long-lasting osseointegration of immediately loaded, bar-connected TPS screws after 12 years of function: a histologic case report of a 95-year-old patient. Int J Periodontics Restorative Dent. **1998** Dec; 18(6): 552 – 563.

Lee RH, Lyles KW, Colón-Emeric C. A review of the effect of anticonvulsant medications on bone mineral density and fracture risk. Am J Geriatr Pharmacother. **2010** Feb; 8(1): 34–46.

Leesungbok R. Dr. Lee's Top-Down Implant Dentistry [in Korean]. Myung-Moon Publishing; **2004**.

Leiss W, Méan M, Limacher A, Righini M, Jaeger K, Beer HJ, Osterwalder J, Frauchiger B, Matter CM, Kucher N, Angelillo-Scherrer A, Cornuz J, Banyai M, Lämmle B, Husmann M, Egloff M, Aschwanden M, Rodondi N, Aujesky D. Polypharmacy is associated with an increased risk of bleeding in elderly patients with venous thromboembolism. J Gen Intern Med. **2014** Jan 30; 30(1): 17–24.

Lekholm U, Zarb G. Patient selection and preparation. In: Brånemark PI, Zarb G, Albrektsson T (eds). Tissue-integrated prostheses. Chicago: Quintessence. **1985**: 199–211.

Lim KO, Zipursky RB, Watts MC, Pfefferbaum A. Decreased gray matter in normal aging: an in vivo magnetic resonance study. J Gerontol. **1992** Jan; 47(1): B26–B30.

Lindhardsen J, Ahlehoff O, Gislason GH, Madsen OR, Olesen JB, Torp-Pedersen C, Hansen PR. The risk of myocardial infarction in rheumatoid arthritis and diabetes mellitus: a Danish nationwide cohort study. Ann Rheum Dis. **2011** Jun; 70(6): 929–934.

Lindquist LW, Rockler B, Carlsson GE. Bone resorption around fixtures in edentulous patients treated with mandibular fixed tissue-integrated prostheses. J Prosthet Dent. **1988** Jan; 59(1): 59–63.

Lindquist LW, Carlsson GE, Jemt T. A prospective 15-year follow-up study of mandibular fixed prostheses supported by osseointegrated implants. Clinical results and marginal bone loss. Clin Oral Implants Res. **1996** Dec; 7(4): 329–336.

Linsen SS, Martini M, Stark H. Long-term results of endosteal implants following radical oral cancer surgery with and without adjuvant radiation therapy. Clin Implant Dent Relat Res. **2012** Apr; 14(2): 250–258.

Lipschitz DA, Mitchell CO, Thompson C: The anemia of senescence. Am J Hematol. **1981**; 11(1): 47–57.

Listgarten MA, Lang NP, Schroeder HE, Schroeder A. Periodontal tissues and their counterparts around endosseous implants Clin Oral Implants Res. **1991** Jan–Mar; 2(3): 1–19.

Little JW, Miller CS, Henry RG, McIntosh BA. Antithrombotic agents: implications in dentistry. Oral Surg Oral Med Oral Pathol Oral Radiol Endod. **2002** May; 93(5): 544–551.

Lo JC, O'Ryan FS, Gordon NP, Yang J, Hui RL, Martin D, Hutchinson M, Lathon PV, Sanchez G, Silver P, Chandra M, McCloskey CA, Staffa JA, Willy M, Selby JV, Go AS. Prevalence of osteonecrosis of the jaw in patients with oral bisphosphonate exposure. J Oral Maxillofac Surg. **2010** Feb; 68(2): 243–253.

Locker D, Jokovic A. Using subjective oral health status indicators to screen for dental care needs in older adults. Community Dent Oral Epidemiol. **1996** Dec; 24(6): 398–402.

Locker D. Dental status, xerostomia and the oral health-related quality of life of an elderly institutionalized population. Spec Care Dentist. **2003**; 23(3): 86–93.

Lockhart PB, Gibson J, Pond SH, Leitch J. Dental management considerations for the patient with an acquired coagulopathy. Part 2: Coagulopathies from drugs. Br Dent J. **2003** Nov 8; 195(9): 405–501.

Loftus MJ, Peterson LJ. Delayed healing of mandibular fracture in idiopathic myxedema. Oral Surg Oral Med Oral Pathol. **1979** Mar; 47(3): 233–237.

Logemann JA. Evaluation and treatment of swallowing disorders. Austin: Pro-Ed. **1998**.

Loo WJ, Burrows NP. Management of autoimmune skin disorders in the elderly. Drugs Aging. **2004**; 21(12): 767–777.

López-Jornet P, Camacho-Alonso F, Martínez-Canovas A, Molina-Miñano F, Gómez-García F, Vicente-Ortega V. Perioperative antibiotic regimen in rats treated with pamidronate plus dexamethasone and subjected to dental extraction: A study of the changes in the jaws. J Oral Maxillofac Surg. **2011** Oct; 69(10): 2488–2493.

Lugtenberg M, Burgers JS, Clancy C, Westert GP, Schneider EC. Current guidelines have limited applicability to patients with comorbid conditions: a systematic analysis of evidence-based guidelines. PLoS One. **2011**; 6(10): e25987.

Lulic M, Brägger U, Lang NP, Zwahlen M, Salvi, GE. Ante's (1926) law revisited: a systematic review on survival rates and complications of fixed dental prostheses (FDPs) on severely reduced periodontal tissue support. Clin Oral Implants Res. **2007** Jun; 18(Suppl 3): 63 – 72.

MacEntee MI, Walton JN, Glick N. A clinical trial of patient satisfaction and prosthodontic needs with ball and bar attachments for implant-retained complete overdentures: three-year results. J Prosthet Dent. **2005** Jan; 93(1): 28 – 37.

MacEntee MI, Müller F, Wayatt C (eds). Oral healthcare and the frail elder: a clinical perspective. Wiley-Blackwell. **2010**.

Madland G, Newton-John T, Feinmann C. Chronic idiopathic orofacial pain: I: What is the evidence base? Br Dent J. **2001** Jul 14; 191(1): 22 – 24.

Madrid C, Sanz M. What impact do systemically administrated bisphosphonates have on oral implant therapy? A systematic review. Clin Oral Implants Res. **2009** Sep; 20(Suppl 4): 87 – 95. (**a**)

Madrid C, Sanz M. What influence do anticoagulants have on oral implant therapy? A systematic review. Clin Oral Implants Res. **2009** Sep; 20(Suppl 4): 96 – 106. (**b**)

Maeda Y, Walmsley DA (ed). Implant dentistry with new generation magnetic attachments. Chicago: Quintessence. **2005**. (**a**)

Maeda Y, Sogo M, Tsutsumi S. Efficacy of a posterior implant support for extra shortened dental arches: a biomechanical model analysis. J Oral Rehabil. **2005** Sep; 32(9): 656 – 660. (**b**)

Maher RL, Hanlon J, Hajjar ER. Clinical consequences of polypharmacy in elderly. Expert Opin Drug Saf. **2014** Jan; 13(1): 57 – 65.

Mahoney FI, Barthel DW. Functional evaluation: the Barthel index. Md State Med J. **1965** Feb; 14: 61 – 65.

Malamed SF. Handbook of local anesthesia. 4th ed. St. Louis: Mosby; **1997**.

Malan J, Ettinger K, Naumann E, Beirne OR. The relationship of denosumab pharmacology and osteonecrosis of the jaws. Oral Surg Oral Med Oral Pathol Oral Radiol. **2012** Dec; 114(6): 671 – 676.

Malden N, Lopes V: An epidemiological study of alendronate-related osteonecrosis of the jaws. A case series from the south-east of Scotland with attention given to case definition and prevalence. J Bone Miner Metab. **2012** Mar; 30(2): 171 – 182

Malmstrom K, Daniels S, Kotey P, Seidenberg BC, Desjardins PJ. Comparison of rofecoxib and celecoxib, two cyclooxygenase-2 inhibitors, in postoperative dental pain: a randomized, placebo- and active comparator-controlled clinical trial. Clin Ther. **1999** Oct; 21(10): 1653 – 1663.

Maloney WJ, Weinberg MA. Implementation of the American Society of Anesthesiologists physical status classification system in periodontal practice. J Periodontol. **2008** Jul; 79(7): 1124 – 1126.

Mancha de la Plata M, Gías LN, Díez PM, Muñoz-Guerra M, González-García R, Lee GY, Castrejón-Castrejón S, Rodríguez-Campo FJ. Osseointegrated implant rehabilitation of irradiated oral cancer patients. J Oral Maxillofac Surg. **2012** May; 70(5): 1052 – 1063.

Mangoni AA, Jackson SHD. Age-related changes in pharmacokinetics and pharmacodynamics: basic principles and practical applications. Br J Clin Pharmacol. **2004** Jan; 57(1): 6 – 14.

Mannucci PM, Nobili A; REPOSI Investigators. Multimorbidity and polypharmacy in the elderly: lessons from REPOSI. Intern Emerg Med. **2014** Oct; 9(7): 723 – 734.

Marengoni A, Angleman S, Melis R, Mangialasche F, Karp A, Garmen A, Meinow B, Fratiglioni L. Aging with multimorbidity: a systematic review of the literature. Ageing Res Rev. **2011** Sep 1; 10(4): 430 – 439.

Marques MA, Dib LL: Periodontal changes in patients undergoing radiotherapy. J Periodontol. **2004** Sep; 75(9): 1178 – 1187.

Marx JJ: Normal iron absorption and decreased red cell iron uptake in the aged. Blood. **1979** Feb; 53(2): 204 – 211.

Marx RE, Johnson RP. Studies in the radiobiology of osteoradionecrosis and their clinical significance. Oral Surg Oral Med Oral Pathol. **1987** Oct; 64(4): 379 – 390.

Marx RE. Bisphosphonate-induced osteonecrosis of the jaws: A challenge, a responsibility, and an opportunity. Int J Periodontics Restorative Dent. **2008** Feb; 28(1): 5 – 6.

Masarachia P, Weinreb M, Balena R, Rodan GA: Comparison of the distribution of 3H-alendronate and 3H-etidronate in rat and mouse bones. Bone. **1996** Sep; 19(3): 281 – 290.

Mason ME, Triplett RG, Van Sickels JE, Parel SM. Mandibular fractures through endosseous cylinder implants: report of cases and review. J Oral Maxillofac Surg. **1990**; 48: 311 – 317.

Mattheos N, Caldwell P, Petcu EB, Ivanovski S, Reher P. Dental implant placement with bone augmentation in a patient who received intravenous bisphosphonate treatment for osteoporosis. J Can Dent Assoc. **2013**; 79: d2.

Mauri D, Valachis A, Polyzos IP, Polyzos NP, Kamposioras K, Pesce LL. Osteonecrosis of the jaw and use of bisphosphonates in adjuvant breast cancer treatment: a meta-analysis. Breast Cancer Res Treat. **2008** Aug; 116(3): 433 – 439.

Mavrokokki T, Cheng A, Stein B, Goss A. Nature and frequency of bisphosphonate-associated osteonecrosis of the jaws in Australia. J Oral Maxillofac Surg. **2007** Mar; 65(3): 415 – 423.

McComsey G, Kitch D, Daar E, et al. Bone mineral density and fractures in anti-retroviral-naive persons randomized to receive abacavir-lamivudine or tenofovir disoproxil fumarate-emtricitabine along with efavirenz or atazanavir-ritonavir: AIDS clinical trials group A5224s, a substudy of ACTG A5202. J Infect Dis. **2011** Jun 15; 203(12): 1791 – 1801.

Meijer HJ, Raghoebar GM, Van't Hof MA, Geertman ME, Van Oort RP. Implant-retained mandibular overdentures compared with complete dentures; a 5-years' follow-up study of clinical aspects and patient satisfaction. Clin Oral Implants Res. **1999** Jun; 10(3): 238 – 244.

Meijer HJ, Raghoebar GM, Van 't Hof MA. Comparison of implant-retained mandibular overdentures and conventional complete dentures: a 10-year prospective study of clinical aspects and patient satisfaction. Int J Oral Maxillofac Implants. **2003** Nov – Dec; 18(6): 879 – 885.

Meijer HJ, Raghoebar GM, Van't Hof MA, Visser A. A controlled clinical trial of implant-retained mandibular overdentures: 10 years' results of clinical aspects and aftercare of IMZ implants and Brånemark implants. Clin Oral Implants Res. **2004** Aug; 15(4): 421 – 427.

Meijer HJ, Raghoebar GM, Batenburg RH, Visser A, Vissink A. Mandibular overdentures supported by two or four endosseous implants: a 10-year clinical trial. Clin Oral Implants Res. **2009** Jul; 20(7): 722 – 728.

Meraw SJ, Reeve CM. Dental considerations and treatment of the oncology patient receiving radiation therapy. J Am Dent Assoc. **1998** Feb; 129(2): 201 – 205.

Mericske-Stern R, Oetterli M, Kiener P, Mericske E. A follow-up study of maxillary implants supporting an overdenture: clinical and radiographic results. Int J Oral Maxillofac Implants. **2002** Sep – Oct; 17(5): 678 – 686.

Merriam Webster. Medical Dictionary. **2015.** http://www.merriam-webster.com/dictionary/polypharmacy. Last accessed October 29, 2015.

Mersel A, Babayof I, Rosin A. Oral health needs of elderly short-term patients in a geriatric department of a general hospital. Spec Care Dentist. **2000** Mar – Apr; 20(2): 72 – 74.

Micheelis W, Schiffner U. Vierte Deutsche Mundgesundheitsstudie (DMS IV). Cologne: Deutscher Zahnärzte Verlag. **2006.**

Millwood J, Heath MR. Food choice by older people: the use of semi-structured interviews with open and closed questions. Gerodontology. **2000** Jul; 17(1): 25 – 32.

Minsk L, Polson AM. Dental implant outcomes in postmenopausal women undergoing hormone replacement. Compend Contin Educ Dent. **1998** Sep; 19(9): 859 – 864.

Mioche L, Bourdiol P, Monier S, Martin JF, Cormier D. Changes in jaw muscles activity with age: effects on food bolus properties. Physiol Behav. **2004** Sep 30; 82(4): 621 – 627.

Mitrani R, Brudvik JS, Phillips KM. Posterior implants for distal extension removable prostheses: a retrospective study. Int J Periodontics Restorative Dent. **2003** Aug; 23(4): 353 – 359.

Mojon P, Budtz-Jørgensen E, Michel JP, Limeback H. Oral health and history of respiratory tract infection in frail institutionalised elders. Gerodontology. **1997** Jul; 14(1): 9 – 16.

Mojon P. The world without teeth: demographic trends. In: Feine J, Carlsson GE (eds). Implant overdentures: the standard of care for edentulous patients. Chicago: Quintessence. **2003**: 3 – 14.

Mombelli A, van Oosten MA, Schurch E, Jr., Lang NP. The microbiota associated with successful or failing osseointegrated titanium implants. Oral Microbiol Immunol. **1987** Dec; 2(4): 145 – 151.

Mombelli A, Buser D, Lang NP. Colonization of osseointegrated titanium implants in edentulous patients. Early results. Oral Microbiol Immunol. **1988** Sep; 3(3): 113 – 120.

Mombelli A, Lang NP. Antimicrobial treatment of peri-implant infections. Clin Oral Implants Res. **1992** Dec; 3(4): 162 – 168.

Mombelli A. Aging and the periodontal and peri-implant microbiota. Periodontol 2000. **1998** Feb; 16: 44 – 52.

Mombelli A, Cionca N. Systemic diseases affecting osseointegration therapy. Clin Oral Implants Res. **2006** Oct; 17(Suppl 2), 97 – 103.

Montagnani A, Gonnelli S, Alessandri M, Nuti R. Osteoporosis and risk of fracture in patients with diabetes: an update. Aging Clin Exp Res. **2011** Apr; 23(2): 84 – 90.

Moore JG, Tweedy C, Christian PE, Datz FL. Effect of age on gastric emptying of liquid-solid meals in man. Dig Dis Sci. **1983** Apr; 28(4); 340 – 344.

Moore KL, Boscardin WJ, Steinman MA, Schwartz JB. Age and sex variation in prevalence of chronic medical conditions in older residents of U.S. nursing homes. J Am Geriatr Soc. **2012** Apr; 60(4): 756 – 764.

Moraguez OD, Belser UC. The use of polytetrafluoroethylene tape for the management of screw access channels in implant-supported prostheses. J Prosthet Dent. **2011** Mar; 103(3): 189 – 191.

Morais JA, Heydecke G, Pawliuk J, Lund JP, Feine JS. The effects of mandibular two-implant overdentures on nutrition in elderly edentulous individuals. J Dent Res. **2003** Jan; 82(1): 53 – 58.

Morales MP, Carvallo AP, Espinosa KA, Murillo EE. A young man with myelosuppression caused by clindamycin: a case report. J Med Case Rep. **2014** Jan 5; 8: 7.

Morley JE. Anorexia in older persons: epidemiology and optimal treatment. Drugs Aging. **1996** Feb; 8(2): 134 – 155.

Morneburg TR, Pröschel PA. Success rates of microimplants in edentulous patients with residual ridge resorption. Int J Oral Maxillofac Implants. **2008** Mar – Apr; 23(2): 270 – 276.

Mosca M, Virdis A, Tani C, Ghiadoni L, Versari D, Duranti E, d'Ascanio A, Salvetti A, Taddei S, Bombardieri S. Vascular reactivity in patients with undifferentiated connective tissue diseases. Atherosclerosis. **2009** Mar; 203(1): 185 – 191.

Moussavi S, Chatterji S, Verdes E, Tandon A, Patel V, Ustun B. Depression, chronic diseases, and decrements in health: results from the World Health Surveys. Lancet. **2007**; 370(9590): 851 – 858.

Moy PK, Medina D, Shetty V, Aghaloo TL. Dental implant failure rates and associated risk factors. Int J Oral Maxillofac Implants. **2005** Jul – Aug; 20(4): 569 – 577.

Moynihan PJ. The relationship between nutrition and systemic and oral well-being in older people. J Am Dent Assoc. **2007** Apr; 138(4): 493 – 497.

Mozzati M, Arata V, Gallesio G: Tooth extraction in patients on zoledronic acid therapy. Oral Oncol. **2012** Sep; 48(8): 817 – 821.

Muir JM, Andrew M, Hirsh J, Weitz JI, Young E, Deschamps P, Shaughnessy SG. Histomorphometric analysis of the effects of standard heparin on trabecular bone in vivo. Blood. **1996** Aug 15; 88(4): 1314 – 1320.

Muller JE, Tofler GH, Stone PH. Circadian variation and triggers of acute cardiovascular disease. Circulation. **1989** Apr; 79(4): 733 – 743.

Müller F, Hasse-Sander I. Experimental studies of adaptation to complete dentures related to ageing. Gerodontology. **1993** Jul; 10(1): 23 – 27.

Müller F, Link I, Fuhr K, Utz KH. Studies on adaptation to complete dentures. Part II: Oral stereognosis and tactile sensibility. J Oral Rehabil. **1995** Oct; 22(10): 759 – 767.

Müller F, Heath MR, Ferman AM, Davis GR. Modulation of mastication during experimental loosening of complete dentures. Int J Prosthodont. **2002** Nov – Dec; 15(6): 553 – 558.

Müller F, Naharro M, Carlsson GE. What are the prevalence and incidence of tooth loss in the adult and elderly population in Europe? Clin Oral Impl Res. **2007** Jun; 18(Suppl 3): 2–14.

Müller F. Tooth loss and dental prostheses in the oldest old. Eur Geriatr Med. **2010**; 1(4): 239–243.

Müller F, Bergendal B, Wahlmann U, Wagner W. Implant-supported fixed dental prostheses in an edentulous patient with dystrophic epidermolysis bullosa. Int J Prosthodont. **2010** Jan–Feb; 23(1): 42–48.

Müller F, Salem K, Barbezat C, Herrmann FR, Schimmel M. Knowledge and attitude of elderly persons towards dental implants. Gerodontology. **2012** Jun; 29(2): e914–e923. (**a**)

Müller F, Hernandez M, Grutter L, Aracil-Kessler L, Weingart D, Schimmel M. Masseter muscle thickness, chewing efficiency and bite force in edentulous patients with fixed and removable implant-supported prostheses: a cross-sectional multicenter study. Clin Oral Implants Res. **2012** Feb; 23(2): 144–150. (**b**)

Müller F, Duvernay E, Loup A, Vazquez L, Herrmann FR, Schimmel M. Implant-supported mandibular overdentures in very old adults: a randomized controlled trial. J Dent Res. **2013** Dec; 92(12 Suppl): 154S–160S.

Müller F. Interventions for edentate elders—what is the evidence? Gerodontology. **2014** Feb; 31(Suppl 1): 44–51.

Müller F, Al-Nawas B, Storelli S, Quirynen M, Hicklin S, Castro-Laza J, Bassetti R, Schimmel M; Roxolid Study Group. Small-diameter titanium grade IV and titanium-zirconium implants in edentulous mandibles: five-year results from a double-blind, randomized controlled trial. BMC Oral Health. **2015** Oct; 15(1); 123.

Nabil S, Samman N: Incidence and prevention of osteoradionecrosis after dental extraction in irradiated patients: a systematic review. Int J Oral Maxillofac Surg. **2011** Mar; 40(3): 229–243.

Naert I, Quirynen M, Theuniers G, van Steenberghe D. Prosthetic aspects of osseointegrated fixtures supporting overdentures. A 4-year report. J Prosthet Dent. **1991** May; 65(5): 671–680.

Naert I, Alsaadi G, van Steenberghe D, Quirynen M. A 10-year randomized clinical trial on the influence of splinted and unsplinted oral implants retaining mandibular overdentures: peri-implant outcome. Int J Oral Maxillofac Implants. **2004** Sep–Oct; 19(5): 695–702.

Nagaya M, Sumi Y. Reaction time in the submental muscles of normal older people. J Am Geriatr Soc. **2002** May; 50(5): 975–976.

Naik AA, Xie C, Zuscik MJ, Kingsley P, Schwarz EM, Awad H, Guldberg R, Drissi H, Puzas JE, Boyce B, Zhang X, O'Keefe RJ. Reduced COX-2 expression in aged mice is associated with reduced fracture healing. J Bone Miner Res. **2009** Feb; 24(2): 251–264.

Naitoh M, Hiraiwa Y, Aimiya H, Gotoh K, Ariji E. Accessory mental foramen assessment using cone-beam computed tomography. Oral Surg Oral Med Oral Pathol Oral Radiol Endod. **2009** Feb; 107(2): 289–294.

Nakayama H. Osteoporosis in the patients with rheumatoid arthritis (3): The efficacy and the selection of the osteoporosis therapeutic drug [in Japanese]. Clin Calcium. **2007** Oct; 17(10): 1607–1612.

Napeñas JJ, Hong CH, Brennan MT, Furney SL, Fox PC, Lockhart PB. The frequency of bleeding complications after invasive dental treatment in patients receiving single and dual antiplatelet therapy. J Am Dent Assoc. **2009** Jun; 140(6): 690–695.

Nedelman CI, Bernick S. The significance of age changes in human alveolar mucosa and bone. J Prosthet Dent. **1978** May; 39(5): 495–501.

Nelson K, Heberer S, Glatzer C. Survival analysis and clinical evaluation of implant-retained prostheses in oral cancer resection patients over a mean follow-up period of 10 years. J Prosthet Dent. **2007** Nov; 98(5): 405–410.

Newton JP, Abel EW, Robertson EM, Yemm R. Changes in human masseter and medial pterygoid muscles with age: a study by computed tomography. Gerodontics. **1987** Aug; 3(4): 151–154.

Newton JP, Yemm R, Abel RW, Menhinick S. Changes in human jaw muscles with age and dental state. Gerodontology. **1993** Jul; 10(1): 16–22.

Newton JP, McManus FC, Menhenick S. Jaw muscles in older overdenture patients. Gerodontology. **2004** Mar; 21(1): 37–42.

Ney DM, Weiss JM, Kind AJ, Robbins J. Senescent swallowing: impact, strategies, and interventions. Nutr Clin Pract. **2009** Jun – Jul; 24(3): 395 – 413.

Niamtu J 3rd. Near-fatal airway obstruction after routine implant placement. Oral Surg Oral Med Oral Pathol Oral Radiol Endod. **2001** Dec; 92(6): 597 – 600.

NICE (National Institute for Health and Care Excellence). Clinical Knowledge Summaries. **2014**. http://cks.nice.org.uk/osteoporosis-prevention-of-fragility-fractures#!topicsummary. Last accessed December 27, 2014.

NICE (National Institute for Health and Care Excellence). Ensuring the safe and effective use of medicines. **2015** Mar. https://www.nice.org.uk/news/article/ensuring-the-safe-and-effective-use-of-medicines. Last accessed February 20, 2016.

Nitschke I, Ilgner A, Müller F. Barriers to provision of dental care in long-term care facilities: the confrontation with ageing and death. Gerodontology. **2005** Sep; 22(3): 123 – 129.

Niwa H, Sato Y, Matsuura H. Safety of dental treatment in patients with previously diagnosed acute myocardial infarction or unstable angina pectoris. Oral Surg Oral Med Oral Pathol Oral Radiol Endod. **2000** Jan; 89(1): 35 – 41.

Nobili A, Garattini S, Mannucci PM. Multiple diseases and polypharmacy in the elderly: challenges for the internist of the third millennium. Journal of Comorbidity. **2011**; 1(1): 28 – 44.

Nooh N. Dental implant survival in irradiated oral cancer patients: a systematic review of the literature. Int J Oral Maxillofac Implants. **2013** Sep – Oct; 28(5): 1233 – 1242.

North Carolina State University. The principles of universal design. **1997**: https://www.ncsu.edu/ncsu/design/cud/about_ud/udprinciples.htm+D559

Nyomba BL, Verhaegue J, Tomaste M, Nyomba BL, Verhaeghe J, Thomasset M, Lissens W, Bouillon R. Bone mineral homeostasis in spontaneously diabetic BB rats. I. Abnormal vitamin D metabolism and impaired active intestinal calcium absorption. Endocrinology. **1989** Feb; 124(2): 565 – 572.

O'Halloran M, Boyd N, Smith A. Denosumab and osteonecrosis of the jaws—the pharmacology, pathogenesis and a report of two cases. Aust Dent J. **2014** Dec; 59(4): 516 – 519.

O'Neill PA, Davies I, Fullerton KJ, Bennett D. Stress hormone and blood glucose response following acute stroke in the elderly. Stroke. **1991** Jul; 22(7): 842 – 847.

O'Neill JE, Yeung SC. Do dental implants preserve and maintain alveolar bone? J Investig Clin Dent. **2011** Nov; 2(4): 229 – 235.

Oczakir C, Balmer S, Mericske-Stern R. Implant-prosthodontic treatment for special care patients: a case series study. Int J Prosthodont. **2005** Sep-Oct; 18(5), 383 – 389.

Oertel R, Ebert U, Rahn R, Kirch W. The effect of age on pharmacokinetics of the local anesthetic drug articaine. Reg Anesth Pain Med. **1999** Nov – Dec; 24(6): 524 – 528.

Oettle AC, Fourie J, Human-Baron R, van Zyl AW. The midline mandibular lingual canal: importance in implant surgery. Clin Implant Dent Relat Res. **2015** Feb; 17(1): 93 – 101.

Office for National Statistics. Population trends. PT 118, table 1.4 (population age and sex). London: ONS. **2004**.

Oghalai JS. Aspiration of a dental appliance in a patient with Alzheimer disease. JAMA. **2002** Nov; 288(20): 2543 – 2544.

Ohkubo C, Kurihara D, Shimpo H, Suzuki Y, Kokubo Y, Hosoi T. Effect of implant support on distal extension removable partial dentures: in vitro assessment. J Oral Rehab. **2007** Jan; 34(1): 52 – 56.

Ohkubo C, Kobayashi M, Suzuki Y, Hosoi T. Effect of implant support on distal-extension removable partial dentures: in vivo assessment. Int J Oral Maxillofac Implants. **2008** Nov – Dec; 23(6): 1095 – 1101.

Olerud E, Hagman-Gustafsson ML, Gabre P. Oral status, oral hygiene, and patient satisfaction in the elderly with dental implants dependent on substantial needs of care for daily living. Spec Care Dentist. **2012** Mar; 32(2): 49 – 54.

Olesen C, Harbig P, Barat I, Damsgaard EM. Absence of "over-the-counter" medicinal products in on-line prescription records: a risk factor of overlooking interactions in the elderly. Pharmacoepidemiol Drug Saf. **2013** Feb; 22(2): 145 – 150.

Ong CT, Ivanovski S, Needleman IG, Retzepi M, Moles DR, Tonetti MS, Donos N. Systematic review of implant outcomes in treated periodontitis subjects. J Clin Periodontol. **2008** May; 35(5): 438–462.

Op Heij DG, Opdebeeck H, van Steenberghe D, Quirynen M. Age as compromising factor for implant insertion. Periodontol 2000. **2003**; 33: 172–184.

Oral Cancer Foundation. Oral cancer facts. Rates of occurrence in the United States. **2012**. http://www.oralcancerfoundation.org/facts. Last accessed December 21, 2014.

Osterberg T, Carlsson GE, Sundh V. Trends and prognoses of dental status in the Swedish population: analysis based on interviews in 1975 to 1997 by Statistics Sweden. Acta Odontol Scand. **2000** Aug; 58(4): 177–182.

Osterberg T, Carlsson GE, Sundh V, Steen B. Number of teeth—a predictor of mortality in the elderly? A population study in three Nordic localities. Acta Odontol Scand. **2007** Nov; 65(6): 335–340.

Ostuni E. Stroke and the dental patient. J Am Dent Assoc. **1994** June; 125(6): 721–727.

Ott SM. Bone disease in CKD. Curr Opin Nephrol Hypertens. **2012** Jul; 21(4): 376–381.

Oyebode O. Cardiovascular disease. In: Craig R, Mindell J (eds). Health survey for England—2011. Vol 1: Health, social care and lifestyles. Leeds: Health and Social Care Information Centre. **2012**: 21–62.

Packer M, Nikitin V, Coward T, Davis DM, Fiske J. The potential benefits of dental implants on the oral health quality of life of people with Parkinson's disease. Gerodontology. **2009** Mar; 26(1): 11–18.

Palmqvist S, Carlsson GE, Öwall B. The combination syndrome: a literature review. J Prosthet Dent. **2003** Sep; 90(3): 270–275.

Pandya A, Gaziano TA, Weinstein MC, Cutler D. More Americans living longer with cardiovascular disease will increase costs while lowering quality of life. Health Aff. **2013**; 32(10): 1706–1714.

Papaspyridakos P, Chen CJ, Singh M, Weber HP, Gallucci GO. Success criteria in implant dentistry: a systematic review. J Dent Res. **2012** Mar; 91(3): 242–248.

Papaspyridakos P, Chen CJ, Chuang SK, Weber HP, Gallucci GO. A systematic review of biologic and technical complications with fixed implant rehabilitations for edentulous patients. Int J Oral Maxillofac Implants. **2012** Jan; 27(1): 102–110.

Parlesak A, Klein B, Schecher K, Bode JC, Bode C. Prevalence of small bowel bacterial overgrowth and its association with nutrition intake in nonhospitalized older adults. J Am Geriatr Soc. **2003** Jun; 51(6); 768–773.

Passia N, Wolfart S, Kern M. Six-year clinical outcome of single implant-retained mandibular overdentures—a pilot study. Clin Oral Implants Res. **2015** Oct; 16(19: 1191–1194.

Patel KV. Epidemiology of anemia in older adults. Semin Hematol. **2008** Oct; 45(4): 210–217.

Pauly L, Stehle P, Volkert D. Nutritional situation of elderly nursing home residents. Z Gerontol Geriatr. **2007** Feb; 40(1): 3–12.

Pawelec G, Solana R, Remarque E, Mariani E. Impact of aging on innate immunity. J Leukoc Biol. **1998** Dec; 64(8): 703–712.

Payne AG, Lownie JF, Van Der Linden WJ. Implant-supported prostheses in patients with Sjögren's syndrome: a clinical report on three patients. Int J Oral Maxillofac Implants. **1997** Sep–Oct; 12(5): 679–685.

Payne AGT, Solomons YF. The prosthodontic maintenance requirements of mandibular mucosa- and implant-supported overdentures: a review of the literature. Int J Prosthodont. **2000** May–Jun; 13(3): 238–245.

Payne AG, Tawse-Smith A, De Silva RK, Duncan WJ. Early loading of two implants in the mandible and final restoration with a retentive-anchor-supported RPD. In: Wismeijer D, Buser D, Belser U (eds). ITI Treatment Guide, Vol 2: Loading protocols in implant dentistry. Berlin: Quintessence Publishing Co (Ltd); **2010**.

Peltola P, Vehkalahti MM, Wuolijoki-Saaristo K. Oral health and treatment needs of the long-term hospitalised elderly. Gerodontology. **2004** Jun; 21(2): 93–99.

Peñarrocha-Diago M, Serrano C, Sanchis JM, Silvestre FJ, Bagán JV. Placement of endosseous implants in patients with oral epidermolysis bullosa. Oral Surg Oral Med Oral Pathol Oral Radiol Endod. **2000** Nov; 90(5): 587 – 590.

Peñarrocha M, Rambla J, Balaguer J, Serrano C, Silvestre J, Bagán JV. Complete fixed prostheses over implants in patients with oral epidermolysis bullosa. J Oral Maxillofac Surg. **2007** Jul; 65(7): 103 – 106. [Erratum: J Oral Maxillofac Surg. 2008 Oct; 66(10): 2195 – 2196.] (**a**)

Peñarrocha M, Larrazábal C, Balaguer J, Serrano C, Silvestre J, Bagán JV. Restoration with implants in patients with recessive dystrophic epidermolysis bullosa and patient satisfaction with the implant-supported superstructure. Int J Oral Maxillofac Implants. **2007** Jul – Aug; 22(4): 651 – 655. (**b**)

Peñarrocha-Diago M, Rambla-Ferrer J, Perez V, Pérez-Garrigues H. Benign paroxysmal vertigo secondary to placement of maxillary implants using the alveolar expansion technique with osteotomes: a study of 4 cases. Int J Oral Maxillofac Implants. **2008** Jan – Feb; 23(1): 129 – 132.

Percival RS, Challacombe SJ, Marsh PD. Flow rates of resting whole and stimulated parotid saliva in relation to age and gender. J Dent Res. **1994** Aug; 73(8): 1416 – 1420.

Petersen PE. The World Oral Health Report 2003: continuous improvement of oral health in the 21st century—the approach of the WHO Global Oral Health Programme. Community Dent Oral Epidemiol. **2003** Dec; 31(Suppl 1):3 – 23.

Peyron MA, Blanc O, Lund JP, Woda A. Influence of age on adaptability of human mastication. J Neurophysiol. **2004** Aug; 92(2): 773 – 779.

Pierrisnard L, Renouard F, Renault P, Barquins M. Influence of implant length and bicortical anchorage on implant stress distribution. Clin Implant Dent Relat Res. **2003**; 5(4): 254 – 262.

Pinto A, Glick M. Management of patients with thyroid disease: oral health considerations. J Am Dent Assoc. **2002** Jul; 133(7): 849 – 858.

Pirih FQ, Zablotsky M, Cordell K, McCauley LK. Case report of implant placement in a patient with Paget's disease on bisphosphonate therapy. J Mich Dent Assoc. **2009** May; 91(5): 38 – 43.

Pjetursson BE, Brägger U, Lang NP, Zwahlen M. Comparison of survival and complication rates of tooth-supported fixed dental prostheses (FDPs) and implant-supported FDPs and single crowns (SCs). Clin Oral Implants Res. **2007**; 18 (Suppl. 3): 97 – 113.

Pjetursson BE, Thoma D, Jung R, Zwahlen M, Zembic A. A systematic review of the survival and complication rates of implant-supported fixed dental prostheses (FDPs) after a mean observation period of at least 5 years. Clin Oral Implants Res. **2012** Oct; 23(Suppl 6): 22 – 38.

Pjetursson BE, Asgeirsson AG, Zwahlen M, Sailer I. Improvements in implant dentistry over the last decade: comparison of survival and complication rates in older and newer publications. Int J Oral Maxillofac Implants. **2014**; 29(Suppl): 308 – 324.

Plun-Favreau H, Lewis PA, Hardy J, Martins LM, Wood NW. Cancer and neurodegeneration: between the devil and the deep blue sea. PLoS Genet. **2010** Dec 23; 6(12): e1001257.

Porter SR, Scully C. Adverse drug reactions in the mouth. Clin Dermatol. **2000** Sep – Oct; 18(5): 525 – 532.

Prasad M, Hussain MZ, Shetty SK, Kumar TA, Khaur M, George SA, Dalwai S. Median mandibular flexure at different mouth opening and its relation to different facial types: A prospective clinical study. J Nat Sci Biol Med. **2013** Jul; 4(2): 426 – 430.

Pretty IA, Ellwood RP, Lo EC, MacEntee MI, Müller F, Rooney E, Murray Thomson W, Van der Putten GJ, Ghezzi EM, Walls A, Wolff MS. The Seattle Care Pathway for securing oral health in older patients. Gerodontology. **2014** Feb; 31(Suppl 1): 77 – 87.

Price EA. Aging and erythropoiesis: Current state of knowledge. Blood Cells Mol Dis. **2008** Sep – Oct; 41(2): 158 – 165.

Proctor R, Kumar N, Stein A, Moles D, Porter S. Oral and dental aspects of chronic renal failure. J Dent Res. **2005** Mar; 84(3): 199 – 208.

Qato DM, Alexander GC, Conti RM, Johnson M, Schumm P, Lindau ST. Use of prescription and over-the-counter medications and dietary supplements among older adults in the United States. JAMA. **2008** Dec 24; 300(24): 2867 – 2878.

Qi WX, Tang LN, He AN, Yao Y, Shen Z. Risk of osteo-necrosis of the jaw in cancer patients receiving denosumab: a meta-analysis of seven randomized controlled trials. Int J Clin Oncol. **2014** Apr; 19(2): 403 – 410.

Quagliarello V, Ginter S, Han L, Van Ness P, Allore H, Ti-netti M. Modifiable risk factors for nursing home-ac-quired pneumonia. Clin Infec Dis. **2005** Jan; 40(1): 1 – 6.

Quirynen M, Mraiwa N, van Steenberghe D, Jacobs R. Morphology and dimensions of the mandibular jaw bone in the interforaminal region in patients requir-ing implants in the distal areas. Clin Oral Implants Res. **2003** Jun; 14(3): 280 – 285.

Quirynen M, Al-Nawas B, Meijer HJ, Razavi A, Reichert TE, Schimmel M, Storelli S, Romeo E; Roxolid Study Group. Small-diameter titanium Grade IV and tita-nium-zirconium implants in edentulous mandibles: three-year results from a double-blind, randomized controlled trial. Clin Oral Implants Res. **2015** Jul; 26(7): 831 – 840.

Rabkin JM, Hunt TK. Infection and oxygen. In: Davis JC, Hunt TK (eds). Problem wounds: the role of oxygen. New York: Elsevier. **1988**: 1 – 16.

Raghoebar GM, Stellingsma K, Batenburg RH, Vissink A. Etiology and management of mandibular fractures associated with endosteal implants in the atrophic mandible. Oral Surg Oral Med Oral Pathol Oral Radi-ol Endod. **2000** May; 89(5): 553-559.

Raj DV, Abuzar M, Borromeo GL. Bisphosphonates, healthcare professionals and oral health. Gerodon-tology. **2014** Jul 15. [Epub ahead of print.]

Rajgopal R, Bear M, Butcher MK, Shaughnessy SG. The effects of heparin and low molecular weight hepa-rins on bone. Thrombosis Research. **2008**; 122(3): 293 – 298.

Rankin K, Jones DL (eds). Oral health in cancer therapy. A guide for health care professionals. Austin: Texas Cancer Council; **1999**: 1 – 48.

Rashid F, Awad MA, Thomason JM, Piovano A, Spielberg GP, Scilingo E, Mojon P, Müller F, Spielberg M, Hey-decke G, Stoker G, Wismeijer D, Allen F, Feine JS. The effectiveness of 2-implant overdentures—a prag-matic international multicentre study. J Oral Rehabil. **2011** Mar; 38(3): 176 – 184.

Rasmussen JM, Hopfensperger ML. Placement and res-toration of dental implants in a patient with Paget's disease in remission: literature review and clinical report. J Prosthodont. **2008** Jan; 17(1): 35 – 40.

Regan RF, Rogers B. Delayed treatment of haemoglo-bin neurotoxicity. J Neurotrauma. **2003** Jan; 20(1): 111 – 120.

Reid IR, Bolland MJ, Grey AB: Is bisphosphonate-associ-ated osteonecrosis of the jaw caused by soft tissue toxicity? Bone. **2007** Sep; 41(3): 318 – 320.

Rémond D, Machebeuf M, Yven C, Buffière C, Mioche L, Mosoni L, Patureau Mirand P. Postprandial whole-body protein metabolism after a meat meal is influ-enced by chewing efficiency in elderly subjects. Am J Clin Nutr. **2007** May; 85(5): 1286 – 1292.

Renouard F, Nisand D. Impact of implant length and diameter on survival rates. Clin Oral Implants Res. **2006** Oct; 17(Suppl 2): 35-51.

Renton T, Woolcombe S, Taylor T, Hills CM. Oral surgery: part 1. Introduction and the management of the medically compromised patient. Br Dent J. **2013** Sep; 215(5): 213 – 223.

Renton T, Yilmaz Z. Managing iatrogenic trigeminal nerve injury: a case series and review of the liter-ature. Int J Oral Maxillofac Surg. **2012** May; 41(5): 629 – 637.

Ribera-Casado JM. Ageing and the cardiovascular sys-tem. Z Gerontol Geriatr. **1999** Dec; 32(6): 412 – 419.

Riesen M, Chung JP, Pazos E, Budtz-Jorgensen E. Inter-ventions bucco-dentaires chez les personnes âgées. Rev Med Suisse. **2002**; 2414: 2178 – 2188.

Riley MA, Walmsley AD, Harris IR. Magnets in pros-thetic dentistry. J Prosthet Dent. **2001** Aug; 86(2): 137 – 142.

Ripamonti CI, Maniezzo M, Campa T, Fagnoni E, Brunelli C, Saibene G, Bareggi C, Ascani L, Cislaghi E. Decreased occurrence of osteonecrosis of the jaw after implementation of dental preventive measures in solid tumour patients with bone metastases treated with bisphosphonates. The experience of the National Cancer Institute of Milan. Ann Oncol. **2009** Jan; 20(1): 137 – 145.

Ristow O, Gerngroß C, Schwaiger M, Hohlweg-Majert B, Kehl V, Jansen H, Hahnefeld L, Koerdt S, Otto S,

Pautke C. Effect of antiresorptive drugs on bony turnover in the jaw: denosumab compared with bisphosphonates. Br J Oral Maxillofac Surg. **2014** Apr; 52(4): 308 – 313.

Robert Wood Johnson Foundation. **2010**; http://www. rwjf.org/pr/product.jsp?id=50968.

Roberts HW, Mitnitsky EF. Cardiac risk stratification for postmyocardial infarction dental patients. Oral Surg Oral Med Oral Pathol Oral Radiol Endod. **2001** Jun; 91(6): 676 – 681.

Rocchietta I, Fontana F, Simion M. Clinical outcomes of vertical bone augmentation to enable dental implant placement: a systematic review. J Clin Periodontol. **2008** Sep; 35(Suppl): 203 – 215.

Roccuzzo M, Bonino F, Gaudioso L, Zwahlen M, Meijer HJ. What is the optimal number of implants for removable reconstructions? A systematic review on implant-supported overdentures. Clin Oral Implants Res. **2012** Oct; 23(Suppl 6): 229 – 237.

Rofes L, Arreola V, Romea M, Palomera E, Almirall J, Cabré M, Serra-Prat M, Clavé P. Pathophysiology of oropharyngeal dysphagia in the frail elderly. Neurogastroenterol Motil. **2010** Aug; 22(8): 851 – 858.

Rohlin M, Mileman PA. Decision analysis in dentistry—the last 30 years. J Dent. **2000** Sep; 28(7): 453 – 468.

Romano MM, Soares MS, Pastore CA, Tornelli MJ, de Oliveira Guaré R, Adde CA. A study of effectiveness of midazolam sedation for prevention of myocardial arrhythmias in endosseous implant placement. Clin Oral Implants Res. **2012** Apr; 23(4): 489 – 495.

Rosenberg ES, Torosian JP, Slots J. Microbial differences in 2 clinically distinct types of failures of osseointegrated implants. Clin Oral Implants Res. **1991** Jul – Sep; 2(3): 135 – 144.

Rossi MI, Young A, Maher R, Rodriguez KL, Appelt CJ, Perera S, Hajjar ER, Hanlon JT. Polypharmacy and health beliefs in older outpatients. Am J Geriatr Pharmacother. **2007** Dec; 5(4): 317 – 323.

Rothman SLG, Schwarz MS, Chafetz NI. High-resolution computerized tomography and nuclear bone scanning in the diagnosis of postoperative stress fractures of the mandible: a clinical report. Int J Oral Maxillofac Implants. **1995** Nov – Dec; 10(6): 765 – 768.

Roubenoff R. The pathophysiology of wasting in the elderly. J Nutr. **1999** Jan; 121(1S Suppl): 256S – 259S.

Ruggiero SL, Dodson TB, Assael LA, Landesberg R, Marx RE, Mehrotra B. American Association of Oral and Maxillofacial Surgeons position paper on bisphosphonate-related osteonecrosis of the jaws—2009 update. J Oral Maxillofac Surg. **2009** May; 67(5 Suppl): 2 – 12.

Ruggiero SL, Dodson TB, Fantasia J, Goodday R, Aghaloo T, Mehrotra B, O'Ryan F. American Association of Oral and Maxillofacial Surgeons position paper on medication-related osteonecrosis of the jaw—2014 update. J Oral Maxillofac Surg. **2014** Oct; 72(10): 1938 – 1956.

Ruospo M, Palmer SC, Craig JC, Gentile G, Johnson DW, Ford PJ, Tonelli M, Petruzzi M, De Benedittis M, Strippoli GF. Prevalence and severity of oral disease in adults with chronic kidney disease: a systematic review of observational studies. Nephrology Dialysis Transplantation. **2014** Feb; 29(2): 364 – 375.

Russell RG, Croucher PI, Rogers MJ. Bisphosphonates: pharmacology, mechanisms of action and clinical uses. Osteoporos Int. **1999**; 9(Suppl 2): S66 – S80.

Ryan Camilon P, Stokes WA, Nguyen SA, Lentsch EJ. The prognostic significance of age in oropharyngeal squamous cell carcinoma. Oral oncol. **2014** May; 50(5): 431 – 436.

Saad F, Brown JE, Van Poznak C, Ibrahim T, Stemmer SM, Stopeck AT, Diel IJ, Takahashi S, Shore N, Henry DH, Barrios CH, Facon T, Senecal F, Fizazi K, Zhou L, Daniels A, Carrière P, Dansey R. Incidence, risk factors, and outcomes of osteonecrosis of the jaw: integrated analysis from three blinded active-controlled phase III trials in cancer patients with bone metastases. Ann Oncol. **2012** May; 23(5): 1341 – 1347.

Saarela RK, Lindroos E, Soini H, Hiltunen K, Muurinen S, Suominen MH, Pitkälä KH. Dentition, nutritional status and adequacy of dietary intake among older residents in assisted living facilities. Gerodontology. **2014** Aug 28.

Sakakura CE, Marcantonio Jr E, Wenzel A, Scaf G. Influence of cyclosporin A on quality of bone around integrated dental implants: a radiographic study in rabbits. Clin Oral Implants Res. **2007** Feb; 18(1): 34 – 39.

Salvi GE, Aglietta M, Eick S, Sculean A, Lang NP, Ramseier CA. Reversibility of experimental peri-implant mucositis compared with experimental gingivitis in humans. Clin Oral Implants Res. **2012** Feb; 23(2): 182–190.

Santana RB, Xu L, Chase HB, Amar S, Graves DT, Trackman PC. A role for advanced glycation end products in diminished bone healing in type 1 diabetes. Diabetes. **2003** Jun; 52(6): 1502–1510.

Santini D, Vincenzi B, Dicuonzo G, Avvisati G, Massacesi C, Battistoni F, Gavasci M, Rocci L, Tirindelli MC, Altomare V, Tocchini M, Bonsignori M, Tonini G. Zoledronic acid induces significant and long-lasting modifications of circulating angiogenic factors in cancer patients. Clin Cancer Res. **2003** Aug 1; 9(8): 2893–2897.

Sarajlic N, Topic B, Brkic H, Alajbeg IZ. Aging quantification on alveolar bone loss. Coll Antropol. **2009** Dec; 33(4): 1165–1170.

Scannapieco FA, Stewart EM, Mylotte J. Colonization of dental plaque by respiratory pathogens in medical intensive care patients. Crit Care Med. **1992** Jun; 20(6): 740–745.

Schein OD, Hochberg MC, Muñoz B, Tielsch JM, Bandeen-Roche K, Provost T, Anhalt GJ, West S. Dry eye and dry mouth in the elderly: a population- based assessment. Arch Intern Med. **1999** Jun 28; 159(12): 1359–1363.

Schembri A, Fiske J. The implications of visual impairment in an elderly population in recognizing oral disease and maintaining oral health. Spec Care Dentist. **2001** Nov–Dec; 21(6): 222–226.

Schilcher J, Koeppen V, Aspenberg P, Michaëlsson K. Risk of atypical femoral fracture during and after bisphosphonate use. N Engl J Med. 2014 Sep; 371(10): 974–976.

Schimmel M, Schoeni P, Zulian GB, Müller F. Utilisation of dental services in a university hospital palliative and long-term care unit in Geneva. Gerodontology. **2008** Jun; 25(2): 107–112.

Schimmel M, Loup A, Duvernay E, Gaydarov N, Müller F. The effect of lower denture abstention on masseter muscle thickness in a 97 year-old patient: a case report. Int J Prosthodont. **2010** Sep–Oct; 23(5): 418–420.

Schimmel M, Srinivasan M, Herrmann FR, Müller F. Loading protocols for implant-supported overdentures in the edentulous jaw: a systematic review and meta-analysis. Int J Oral Maxillofac Implants. **2014**; 29(Suppl): 271–286.

Schneider D, Witt L, Hämmerle CH. Influence of the crown-to-implant length ratio on the clinical performance of implants supporting single crown restorations: a cross-sectional retrospective 5-year investigation. Clin Oral Implants Res. **2012** Feb; 23(2): 169–174

Schneider D, Schober F, Grohmann P, Hämmerle CH, Jung RE. In-vitro evaluation of the tolerance of surgical instruments in templates for computer-assisted guided implantology produced by 3-D printing. Clin Oral Implant Res. **2015** Mar; 26(3): 320–325.

Schoen F. The heart. In: Kumar V (ed). Robbins and Cotran pathologic basis of disease. 7th ed. St. Louis: Saunders. **2005**: 584–586.

Schropp L, Isidor F. Timing of implant placement relative to tooth extraction. J Oral Rehabil. **2008** Jan; 35(Suppl. 1): 33–43.

Schuldt Filho G, Dalago HR, Oliveira de Souza JG, Stanley K, Jovanovic S, Bianchini MA. Prevalence of peri-implantitis in patients with implant-supported fixed prostheses. Quintessence Int. **2014** Nov; 45(10): 861–868.

Schulte J, Flores AM, Weed M. Crown-to-implant ratios of single tooth implant-supported restorations. J Prosthet Dent. **2007** Jul; 98(1): 1–5.

Scott J, Valentine JA, St Hill CA, Balasooriya BA. A quantitative histological analysis of the effects of age and sex on human lingual epithelium. J Biol Buccale. **1983** Dec; 11(4): 303–315.

Scully C, Boyle P. Reliability of a self-administered questionnaire for screening for medical problems in dentistry. Community Dent Oral Epidemiol. **1983** Apr; 11(2): 105–108.

Scully C: Scully's medical problems in dentistry. 7th ed. Elsevier Health Sciences. **2014**: 167–168.

Seddon HJ. A classification of nerve injuries. Br Med J. **1942** Aug 29; 2(4260): 237–239.

Sedghizadeh PP, Kumar SK, Gorur A, Schaudinn C, Shuler CF, Costerton JW. Identification of microbial biofilms in osteonecrosis of the jaws secondary to bisphosphonate therapy. J Oral Maxillofac Surg. **2008** Apr; 66(4): 767 – 775.

Sedghizadeh PP, Kumar SK, Gorur A, Schaudinn C, Shuler CF, Costerton JW. Microbial biofilms in osteomyelitis of the jaw and osteonecrosis of the jaw secondary to bisphosphonate therapy. J Am Dent Assoc. **2009** Oct; 140(10): 1259 – 1265.

Seitz HK, Stickel F. Alcoholic liver disease in the elderly. Clin Geriatr Med. **2007** Nov; 23(4): 905 – 921.

Seymour DG, Vaz FG. A prospective-study of elderly general surgical patients: II. Post-operative complications. Age Ageing. **1989** Sep; 18(5): 316 – 326.

Sharkey S, Kelly A, Houston F, O'Sullivan M, Quinn F, O'Connell B. A radiographic analysis of implant component misfit. Int J Oral Maxillofac Implants. **2011** Jul – Aug; 26(4): 807 – 815.

Sharma L. Epidemiology of osteoarthritis. In: Moskovitz RW, Howell OS, Altman RD, Buckwater JA, Goldberg VM (eds). Osteoarthritis: Diagnosis and medical surgical management. 3rd edition. Philadelphia: Saunders; **2001**: 3 – 17.

Shaw JE, Sicree RA, Zimmet PZ. Global estimates of the prevalence of diabetes for 2010 and 2030. Diabetes Res Clin Pract. **2010** Jan; 87(1): 4 – 14.

Shay K. Identifying the needs of the elderly dental patient. The geriatric dental assessment. Dent Clin North Am. **1994** Jul; 38(3): 499 – 523.

Sheehy C, Gaffney K, Mukhtyar C. Standardized grip strength as an outcome measure in early rheumatoid arthritis. Scand J Rheumatol. **2013**; 42(4): 289 – 293.

Sheiham A, Steele JG, Marcenes W, Lowe C, Finch S, Bates CJ, Prentice A, Walls AW. The relationship among dental status, nutrient intake, and nutritional status in older people. J Dent Res. **2001** Feb; 80(2): 408 – 413.

Sheikh JI, Yesavange JA. Geriatric Depression Scale (GDS). Recent evidence and development of a shorter version. In: Bring T (ed). Clinical gerontology: a guide to assessment and interventions. New York: Haworth Press. **1986**: 165 – 173.

Shepherd AM, Hewick DS, Moreland TA, Stevenson IH. Age as a determinant of sensitivity to warfarin. Br J Clin Pharmacol. **1977** Jun; 4(3): 315 – 320.

Shet UK, Oh HK, Kim HJ, Chung HJ, Kim YJ, Kim OS, Choi HR, Kim OJ, Lim HJ, Lee SW. Quantitative analysis of periodontal pathogens present in the saliva of geriatric subjects. J Periodontal Implant Sci. **2013** Aug; 43(4): 183 – 190.

Ship JA, Pillemer SR, Baum BJ. Xerostomia in the geriatric patient. J Am Geriatr Soc. **2002** Mar; 50(3): 535 – 543.

Shulman KI. Clock-drawing: is it the ideal cognitive screening test? Int J Geriatr Psychiatry. **2000** Jun; 15(6): 548 – 561.

Shuman SK, Bebeau MJ. Ethical issues in nursing home care: practice guidelines for difficult situations. Special Care Dentist. **1996** Jul – Aug; 16(4): 170 – 176.

Sihvo S, Klaukka T, Martikainen J, Hemminki E. Frequency of daily over-the-counter drug use and potential clinically significant over-the-counter prescription drug interactions in the Finnish adult population. Eur J Clin Pharmacol. **2000** Sep; 56(6 – 7): 495 – 499.

Sjögren P, Nilsson E, Forsell M, Johansson O, Hoogstraate J. A systematic review of the preventive effect of oral hygiene on pneumonia and respiratory tract infection in elderly people in hospitals and nursing homes: effect estimates and methodological quality of randomized controlled trials. J Am Geriatr Soc. **2008** Nov; 56(11): 2124 – 2130.

Slade GD, Spencer AJ. Development and evaluation of the Oral Health Impact Profile. Community Dent Health. **1994** Mar; 11(1): 3 – 11.

Slade GD. Assessment of oral health related quality of life. In: Inglehart MR, Bagramian RA (eds). Oral health related quality of life. Chicago: Quintessence. **2002**.

Slagter KW, Raghoebar GM, Vissink A. Osteoporosis and edentulous jaws. Int J Prosthodont. **2008** Jan – Feb; 21(1): 19 – 26.

Slotte C, Grønningsæter A, Halmøy AM, Öhrnell LO, Stroh G, Isaksson S, Johansson LÅ, Mordenfeld A, Eklund J, Embring J. Four-millimeter implants supporting fixed partial dental prostheses in the severely resorbed posterior mandible: two-year results.

Clin Implant Dent Relat Res. **2012** May;14(Suppl 1): e46 – e58.

Soehardi A, Meijer GJ, Manders R, Stoelnga PJ. An inventory of mandibular fractures associated with implants in atrophic edentulous mandibles: a survey of Dutch oral and maxillofacial surgeons. Int J Oral Maxillofac Implants. **2010** Sep – Oct; 26(5): 1087 – 1093.

Soteriades ES, Evans JC, Larson MG, Chen MH, Chen L, Benjamin EJ, Levy D. Incidence and prognosis of syncope. N Engl J Med. **2002** Sep 19; 347(12): 878 – 885.

Sreebny LM, Schwartz SS. A reference guide to drugs and dry mouth—2nd edition. Gerodontology. **1997** Jul; 14(1): 33 – 47.

Srinivasan M, Vazquez L, Rieder P, Moraguez O, Bernard JP, Belser UC. Survival rates of short (6 mm) micro-rough surface implants: a review of literature and meta-analysis. Clin Oral Implants Res. **2014** May; 25(5): 539 – 545. (**a**)

Srinivasan M, Schimmel M, Riesen M, Ilgner A, Wicht MJ, Warncke M, Ellwood RP, Nitschke I, Müller F, Noack MJ. High-fluoride toothpaste: a multicenter randomized controlled trial in adults. Community Dent Oral Epidemiol. **2014** Aug; 42(4): 333 – 340. (**b**)

Srinivasan M, Makarov NA, Herrmann FR, Müller F. Implant survival in 1- versus 2-implant mandibular overdentures: a systematic review and meta-analysis. Clin Oral Implants Res. **2016** Jan; 27(1): 63 – 72.

Stamberger H. Functional endoscopic sinus surgery. Philadelphia: Mosby Year Book/BC Decker. **1991**.

Stanford CM. Dental implants. A role in geriatric dentistry for the general practice? J Am Dent Assoc. **2007** Sep; 138(Suppl): 34S – 40S.

Stanford CM. Surface modification of biomedical and dental implants and the processes of inflammation, wound healing and bone formation. Int J Mol Sci. **2010** Jan 25; 11(1): 354 – 369.

Starr ME, Saito H. Sepsis in old age: review of human and animal studies. Aging Dis. **2014** Apr 1; 5(2): 126 – 136.

Stoehr GP, Ganguli M, Seaberg EC, Echement DA, Belle S. Over-the-counter medication use in an older rural community: the MoVIES Project. J Am GeriatrSoc. **1997** Feb; 45(2): 158 – 165.

Stone AA, Schwartz JE, Broderick JE, Deaton A. A snapshot of the age distribution of psychological well-being in the United States. Proc Natl Acad Sci U.S.A. **2010** Jun; 107(22): 9985 – 9990.

Strippoli GF, Palmer SC, Ruospo M, Natale P, Saglimbene V, Craig JC, Pellegrini F, Petruzzi M, De Benedittis M, Ford P, Johnson DW, Celia E, Gelfman R, Leal MR, Torok M, Stroumza P, Bednarek-Skublewska A, Dulawa J, Frantzen L, Ferrari JN, del Castillo D, Hegbrant J, Wollheim C, Gargano L. Oral disease in adults treated with hemodialysis: prevalence, predictors, and association with mortality and adverse cardiovascular events: the rationale and design of the ORAL Diseases in hemodialysis (ORAL-D) study, a prospective, multinational, longitudinal, observational, cohort study. BMC Nephrology. **2013** Apr 19; 14: 90.

Stuck AE, Beers MH, Steiner A, Aronow HU, Rubenstein LZ, Beck JC. Inappropriate medication use in community-residing older persons. Arch Intern Med. **1994** Oct 10; 154(19), 2195 – 2200.

Summers RB. Sinus floor elevation with osteotomes. J Esthet Dent. **1998**; 10(3): 164-171.

Sweeney MP, Williams C, Kennedy C, Macpherson LM, Turner S, Bagg J. Oral health care and status of elderly care home residents in Glasgow. Community Dent Health. **2007** Mar; 24(1): 37 – 42.

Swelem AA, Gurevich KG, Fabrikant EG, Hassan MH, Aqou S. Oral health-related quality of life in partially edentulous patients treated with removable, fixed, fixed-removable, and implant-supported prostheses. Int J Prosthodont. **2014** Jul – Aug; 27(4): 338 – 347.

Swift ME, Burns AL, Gray KL, DiPietro LA. Age-related alterations in the inflammatory response to dermal injury. J Invest Dermatol. **2001** Nov; 117(5): 1027 – 1035.

Syrjälä AM, Ylöstalo P, Ruoppi P, Komulainen K, Hartikainen S, Sulkava R, Knuuttila M.Dementia and oral health among subjects aged 75 years or older. Gerodontology. **2012** Mar; 29(1): 36 – 42.

Taguchi T, Fukuda K, Sekine H, Kakizawa T. Intravenous sedation and hemodynamic changes during dental implant surgery. Int J Oral Maxillofac Implants. **2011** Nov – Dec; 26(6): 1303 – 1308.

Tahmaseb A, Wismeijer D, Coucke W, Derksen W. Computer technology applications in surgical implant dentistry: a systematic review. Int J Oral Maxillofac Implants. **2014**; 29(Suppl): 25 – 42.

Taji T, Yoshida M, Hiasa K, Abe Y, Tsuga K, Akagawa Y. Influence of mental status on removable prosthesis compliance in institutionalized elderly persons. Int J Prosthodont. **2005** Mar – Apr; 18(2): 146 – 149.

Tallgren A. The continuing reduction of the residual alveolar ridges in complete denture wearers: a mixed-longitudinal study covering 25 years. J Prosthet Dent. **1972** Feb; 27(2): 120 – 132.

Tan K, Pjetursson BE, Lang NP, Chan ES. A systematic review of the survival and complication rates of fixed partial dentures (FPDs) after an observation period of at least 5 years. Clin Oral Implants Res. **2004** Dec; 15(6): 654 – 666.

Tan WC, Lang NP, Zwahlen M, Pjetursson BE. A systematic review of the success of sinus floor elevation and survival of implants inserted in combination with sinus floor elevation. Part II: transalveolar technique. J Clin Periodontol. **2008** Sep; 35(8 Suppl): 241 – 254.

Tepper G, Haas R, Zechner W, Krach W, Watzek G. Three-dimensional finite element analysis of implant stability in the atrophic posterior maxilla: a mathematical study of the sinus floor augmentation. Clin Oral Implants Res. **2002** Dec; 13(6): 657 – 665.

Tepper G, Haas R, Mailath G, Teller C, Bernhart T, Monov G, Watzek G. Representative marketing-oriented study on implants in the Austrian population. II. Implant acceptance, patient-perceived cost and patient satisfaction. Clin Oral Implants Res. **2003** Oct; 14(5): 634 – 642.

Terpenning MS, Taylor GW, Lopatin DE, Kerr CK, Dominguez BL, Loesche WJ. Aspiration pneumonia: dental and oral risk factors in an older veteran population. J Am Geriatr Soc. **2001** May; 49(5): 557 – 563.

Thiel CP, Evans DB, Burnett RR. Combination syndrome associated with a mandibular implant-supported overdenture: a clinical report. J Prosthet Dent. **1996** Feb; 75(2): 107 – 113.

Thomas DR. Age-related changes in wound healing. Drugs Aging. **2001**; 18(8): 607 – 620.

Thomason JM, Feine J, Exley C, Moynihan P, Müller F, Naert I, Ellis JS, Barclay C, Butterworth C, Scott B,

Lynch C, Stewardson D, Smith P, Welfare R, Hyde P, McAndrew R, Fenlon M, Barclay S, Barker D. Mandibular two implant-supported overdentures as the first choice standard of care for edentulous patients—the York Consensus Statement. Br Dent J. **2009** Aug; 207(4): 185 – 186.

Thompson R, Phillips J, McCauley S, Elliott JR, Moran CG. Atypical femoral fractures and bisphosphonate treatment. Journal of Bone and Joint Surgery. **2012** Mar; 94(3): 385 – 390.

Tinetti ME, Bogardus ST, Agostini JV. Potential pitfalls of disease-specific guidelines for patients with multiple conditions. N Engl J Med. **2004** Dec 30; 351(27): 2870 – 2874.

Tjia J, Velten SJ, Parsons C, Valluri S, Briesacher BA.. Studies to reduce unnecessary medication use in frail older adults: a systematic review. Drugs Aging. **2013** May; 30(5): 285 – 307.

Toffler M. Osteotome-mediated sinus floor elevation: a clinical report. Int J Oral Maxillofac Implants. **2004** Mar – Apr; 19(2): 266 – 273.

Tokmakidis SP, Kalapotharakos VI, Smilios I, Parlavantzas A. Effects of detraining on muscle strength and mass after high or moderate intensity of resistance training in older adults. Clin Physiol Funct Imaging. **2009** Jul 29(4): 316 – 319.

Tomkinson A, Reeve J, Shaw RW, Noble BS. The death of osteocytes via apoptosis accompanies estrogen withdrawal in human bone. J Clin Endocrinol Metab. **1997** Sep; 82(9): 3128 – 3135.

Torres J, Tamimi F, Garcia I, Herrero A, Rivera B, Sobrino JA, Hernández G. Dental implants in a patient with Paget disease under bisphosphonate treatment: a case report. Oral Surg Oral Med Oral Pathol Oral Radiol Endod. **2009** Mar; 107(3): 387 – 392.

Trisi P, Rao W. Bone classification: clinical histomorphometric comparison. Clin Oral Implants Res. **1999** Feb; 10(1): 1 – 7.

Tsao C, Darby I, Ebeling PR, Walsh K, O'Brien-Simpson N, Reynolds E, Borromeo G. Oral health risk factors for bisphosphonate-associated jaw osteonecrosis. J Oral Maxillofac Surg. **2013** Aug; 71(8): 1360 – 1366.

Turkyilmaz I, Company AM, McGlumphy EA. Should edentulous patients be constrained to removable complete dentures? The use of dental implants to improve the quality of life for edentulous patients. Gerodontology. **2010** Mar; 27(1): 3 – 10.

Turner MD, Ship JA. Dry mouth and its effects on the oral health of elderly people. J Am Dent Assoc. **2007** Sep; 138(Suppl): 15S – 20S. [Erratum: J Am Dent Assoc. 2008 Mar; 139(3): 252 – 253.]

Tymstra N, Raghoebar GM, Vissink A, Meijer HJ. Maxillary anterior and mandibular posterior residual ridge resorption in patients wearing a mandibular implant-retained overdenture. J Oral Rehabil. **2011** Jul; 38(7): 509 – 516.

Tzakis MG, Osterberg T, Carlsson GE. A study of some masticatory functions in 90-year old subjects. Gerodontology. **1994** Jul; 11(1): 25 – 29.

Ueda M, Kaneda T. Maxillary sinusitis caused by dental implants: report of two cases. J Oral Maxillofa Surg. **1992** Mar; 50(3): 285 – 287.

Ungar A, Morrione A, Rafanelli M, Ruffolo E, Brunetti MA, Chisciotti VM, Masotti G, Del Rosso A, Marchionni N. The management of syncope in older adults. Minerva Med. **2009** Aug; 100(4): 247 – 258.

United Nations, Department of Economic and Social Affairs, Population Division. World Population Ageing 2013. **2013**. United Nations publication ST/ESA/SER.A/348.

Vahtsevanos K, Kyrgidis A, Verrou E, Katodritou E, Triaridis S, Andreadis CG, Boukovinas I, Koloutsos GE, Teleioudis Z, Kitikidou K, Paraskevopoulos P, Zervas K, Antoniades K. Longitudinal cohort study of risk factors in cancer patients of bisphosphonate-related osteonecrosis of the jaw. Journal of Clinical Oncology. **2009** Nov 10; 27(32): 5356 – 5362.

Valenti G, Ferrucci L, Lauretani F, Ceresini G, Bandinelli S, Luci M, Ceda G, Maggio M, Schwartz RS. Dehydroepiandrosterone sulfate and cognitive function in the elderly: The InCHIANTI Study. J Endocrinol Invest. **2009** Oct; 32(9): 766 – 772.

van den Akker M, Buntinx F, Roos S, Knottnerus JA. Problems in determining occurrence rates of multimorbidity. J Clin Epidemiol. **2001** Jul; 54(7): 675 – 679.

van den Bergh JP, Bruggenkate ten CM, Disch FJ, Tuinzing DB. Anatomical aspects of sinus floor elevations. Clin Oral Implants Res. **2000** Jun; 11(3): 256-265.

van der Bilt A, van Kampen FM, Cune MS. Masticatory function with mandibular implant-supported overdentures fitted with different attachment types. Eur J Oral Sci. **2006** Jun; 114(3): 191 – 196.

van der Bilt A, Burgers M, van Kampen FM, Cune MS. Mandibular implant-supported overdentures and oral function. Clin Oral Implants Res. **2010** Nov; 21(11): 1209 – 1213.

van der Maarel-Wierink CD, Vanobbergen JN, Bronkhorst EM, Schols JM, de Baat C. Meta-analysis of dysphagia and aspiration pneumonia in frail elders. J Dent Res. **2011** Dec; 90(12): 1398 – 1404.

Van der Sleen MI, Slot DE, Van Trijffel E, Winkel EG, Van der Weijden GA. Effectiveness of mechanical tongue cleaning on breath odour and tongue coating: a systematic review. Int J Dent Hyg. **2010** Nov; 8(4): 258 – 268.

van Kampen FM, van der Bilt A, Cune MS, Fontijn-Tekamp FA, Bosman F. Masticatory function with implant-supported overdentures. J Dent Res. **2004** Sep; 83(9): 708 – 711.

van Steenberghe D, Vanherle GV, Fossion E, Roelens J. Crohn's disease of the mouth, report of case. J Oral Surg. **1976** Jul; 34(7): 635 – 638.

van Steenberghe D, Jacobs R, Desnyder M, Maffei G, Quirynen M. The relative impact of local and endogenous patient-related factors on implant failure up to the abutment stage. Clin Oral Implants Res. **2002** Dec; 13(6): 617 – 622.

van Steenberghe D, Quirynen M, Molly L, Jacobs R. Impact of systemic diseases and medication on osseointegration. Periodontol 2000. **2003**; 33: 163 – 171.

Vandone AM, Donadio M, Mozzati M, Ardine M, Polimeni MA, Beatrice S, Ciuffreda L, Scoletta M. Impact of dental care in the prevention of bisphosphonate-associated osteonecrosis of the jaw: A single-center clinical experience. Ann Oncol. **2012** Jan; 23 (1): 193 – 200.

Vercruyssen M, Marcelis K, Coucke W, Naert I, Quirynen M. Long-term, retrospective evaluation (implant and patient-centred outcome) of the two-implants-supported overdenture in the mandible. Part 1: survival rate. Clin Oral Implants Res. **2010** Apr; 21(4): 357 – 365. (**a**)

Vercruyssen M, Quirynen M. Long-term, retrospective evaluation (implant and patient-centred outcome) of the two-implant-supported overdenture in the mandible. Part 2: marginal bone loss. Clin Oral Implants Res. **2010** May; 21(5): 466 – 472. (**b**)

Vernamonte S, Mauro V, Vernamonte S, Messina AM. An unusual complication of osteotome sinus floor evaluation: benign paroxysmal positional vertigo. Int J Oral Maxillofac Surg. **2011** Feb; 40(2): 216 – 218.

Vernooij-Dassen M, Leatherman S, Rikkert MO. Quality of care in frail older people: the balance between receiving and giving. BMJ. **2011** Mar 25; 342: 1062 – 1063.

Vigild M. Benefit related assessment of treatment need among institutionalised elderly people. Gerodontology. **1993** Jul; 10(1): 10 – 15.

Visentin GP, Liu CY. Drug-induced thrombocytopenia. Hematol Oncol Clin North Am. **2007** Aug; 21(4): 685 – 696, vi.

Visser A, Raghoebar GM, Meijer HJ, Vissink A. Implant-retained maxillary overdentures on milled bar suprastructures: a 10-year follow-up of surgical and prosthetic care and aftercare. Int J Prosthodont. **2009** Mar – Apr; 22(2): 181 – 192.

Visser A, de Baat C, Hoeksema AR, Vissink A. Oral implants in dependent elderly persons: blessing or burden? Gerodontology. **2011** Mar; 28(1): 76 – 80.

Vitlic A, Khanfer R, Lord JM, Carroll D, Phillips AC. Bereavement reduces neutrophil oxidative burst only in older adults: role of the HPA axis and immunesenescence. Immun Ageing. **2014** Aug 29; 11: 13.

Vogeli C, Shields AE, Lee TA, Gibson TB, Marder WD, Weiss KB, Blumenthal D. Multiple chronic conditions: prevalence, health consequences, and implications for quality, care management, and costs. J Gen Intern Med. **2007** Dec; 22(Suppl. 3): 391 – 395.

von Wowern N, Melsen F. Comparative bone morphometric analysis of mandibles and iliac crests. Scand J Dent Res. **1979** Oct; 87(5): 351 – 357.

von Wowern N, Storm TL, Olgaard K. Bone mineral content by photon absorptiometry of the mandible compared with that of the forearm and the lumbar spine. Calcif Tissue Int. **1988** Mar; 42(3): 157 – 161.

von Wowern N, Gotfredsen K. Implant-supported overdentures, a prevention of bone loss in edentulous mandibles? A 5-year follow-up study. Clin Oral Implants Res. **2001** Feb; 12(1): 19 – 25.

Vos T et al. Years lived with disability (YLDs) for 1160 sequelae of 289 diseases and injuries 1990 – 2010: a systematic analysis for the Global Burden of Disease Study 2010. Lancet. **2012** Dec 15; 380(9859): 2163 – 2196. [Erratum: Lancet. 2013 Feb 23; 381(9867): 628.]

Wagner W, Esser E, Ostkamp K. Osseointegration of dental implants in patients with and without radiotherapy. Acta Oncol. **1998**; 37(7 – 8): 693 – 696.

Walton JN, MacEntee MI, Glick N. One-year prosthetic outcomes with implant overdentures: a randomized clinical trial. Int J Oral Maxillofac Implants. **2002** May – Jun; 17(3): 391 – 398.

Walton JN, MacEntee MI. Choosing or refusing oral implants: a prospective study of edentulous volunteers for a clinical trial. Int J Prosthodont. **2005** Nov – Dec; 18(6): 483 – 488.

Walton JN, Glick N, Macentee MI. A randomized clinical trial comparing patient satisfaction and prosthetic outcomes with mandibular overdentures retained by one or two implants. Int J Prosthodont. **2009** Jul – Aug; 22(4): 331 – 339.

Wang HL, Weber D, McCauley LK. Effect of long-term oral bisphosphonates on implant wound healing: literature review and a case report. J Periodontol. **2007** Mar; 78(3): 584 – 594.

Warrer K, Buser D, Lang NP, Karring T. Plaque-induced peri-implantitis in the presence or absence of keratinized mucosa. An experimental study in monkeys. Clin Oral Implants Res. **1995** Sep; 6(3): 131 – 138.

Watson RM, Jemt T, Chai J, Harnett J, Heath MR, Hutton JE, Johns RB, Lithner B, McKenna S, McNamara DC, Naert I, Taylor R. Prosthodontic treatment, patient response, and the need for maintenance of complete implant-supported overdentures: an appraisal of 5 years of prospective study. Int J Prosthodont. **1997** Jul – Aug; 10(4): 345 – 354.

Wawruch M, Kuzelova M, Foltanova T, Ondriasova E, Luha J, Dukat A, Murin J, Shah R. Characteristics of elderly patients who consider over-the-counter medications as safe. Int J Clin Pharm. **2013** Feb; 35(1): 121 – 128.

Weinlander M, Krennmair G, Piehslinger E. Implant prosthodontic rehabilitation of patients with rheumatic disorders: a case series report. Int J Prosthodont. **2010** Jan – Feb; 23(1): 22 – 28.

Weischer T, Mohr C. Ten-year experience in oral implant rehabilitation of cancer patients: treatment concept and proposed criteria for success. Int J Oral Maxillofac Implants. **1999** Jul – Aug; 14(4): 521 – 528.

Weiss RE, Gorn AH, Nimni ME. Abnormalities in the biosynthesis of cartilage and bone proteoglycans in experimental diabetes. Diabetes. **1981** Aug; 30(8): 670 – 677.

Weiss A, Beloosesky Y, Boaz M, Yalov A, Kornowski R, Grossman E. Body mass index is inversely related to mortality in elderly subjects. J Gen Intern Med. **2008** Jan; 23(1): 19 – 24.

Welsh G, Grey N, Potts S. The use of liaison psychiatry service in restorative dentistry. CPD Dent. **2000**; 1(1): 32 – 34.

Welte T, Torres A, Nathwani D. Clinical and economic burden of community-acquired pneumonia among adults in Europe. Thorax. **2012** Jan; 67(1): 71 – 79.

Wennström JL, Derks J. Is there a need for keratinized mucosa around implants to maintain health and tissue stability? Clin Oral Implants Res. **2012** Oct; 23(Suppl 6): 136 – 146.

Werbitt MJ, Goldberg PV. The immediate implant: bone preservation and bone regeneration. Int J Periodontics Restorative Dent. **1992**; 12(3): 206 – 217.

Weyant RJ, Pandav RS, Plowman JL, Ganguli M. Medical and cognitive correlates of denture wearing in older community-dwelling adults. J Am Geriatr Soc. **2004** Apr; 52(4): 596 – 600.

White H. Weight change in Alzheimer's disease. J Nurt Health Aging. **1998**; 2(2): 110 – 112.

Whitfield LR, Schentag JJ, Levy G. Relationship between concentration and anticoagulant effect of heparin in plasma of hospitalized patients: magnitude of predictability of interindividual differences. Clin Pharmacol Ther. **1982** Oct; 32(4): 503 – 516.

WHO Definition of palliative care. **1990**. http://www.who.int/cancer/palliative/definition/en/. Last accessed November 23, 2015.

Williams S, Malatesta K, Norris K. Vitamin D and chronic kidney disease. Ethn Dis. **2009** Autumn; 19(4 Suppl 5): S5 – 8 – 11.

Wiltfang J, Schultze-Mosgau S, Merten HA, Kessler P, Ludwig A, Engelke W. Endoscopic and ultrasonographic evaluation of the maxillary sinus after combined sinus floor augmentation and implant insertion. Oral Surg Oral Med Oral Pathol Oral Radiol Endod. **2000** Mar; 89(3): 288 – 291.

Winkler S, Garg AK, Mekayarajjananonth T, Bakaeen LG, Khan E. Depressed taste and smell in geriatric patients. J Am Dent Assoc. **1999** Dec; 130(12): 1759 – 1765.

Winwood K, Zioupos P, Currey JD, Cotton JR, Taylor M. The importance of the elastic and plastic components of strain in tensile and compressive fatigue of human cortical bone in relation to orthopaedic biomechanics. J Musculoskelet Neuronal Interact. **2006** Apr – Jun; 6(1): 134 – 141.

Wiseman M. The treatment of oral problems in the palliative patient. J Can Dent Assoc. **2006** Jun; 72(5): 453 – 458.

Wismeijer D, VanWaas MAJ, Vermeeren J, Mulder J, Kalk W. Patient satisfaction with implant-supported mandibular overdentures. A comparison of three treatment strategies with ITI-dental implants. Int J Oral Maxillofac Surg. **1997** Aug 26(4): 263 – 267.

Wismeijer D, Tawse-Smith A, Payne AG. Multicentre prospective evaluation of implant-assisted mandibular bilateral distal extension removable partial dentures: patient satisfaction. Clin Oral Implants Res. **2013** Jan; 24(1): 20 – 27.

Wolfe M, Lichtenstein D, Singh G. Gastrointestinal toxicity of nonsteroidal antiinflammatory drugs. N Engl J Med. **1999** Jun 17; 340(24): 1888 – 1889.

Wolff B, Berger T, Frese C, Max R, Blank N, Lorenz HM, Wolff D. Oral status in patients with early rheumatoid arthritis: a prospective, case-control study. Rheumatology (Oxford). **2014** Mar; 53(3): 526 – 431.

Wood J, Bonjean K, Ruetz S, Bellahcène A, Devy L, Foidart JM, Castronovo V, Green JR. Novel antiangiogenic effects of the bisphosphonate compound zoledronic acid. J Pharmacol Exp Ther. **2002** Sep; 302(3): 1055 – 1061.

Wood MR, Vermilyea SG; Committee on Research in Fixed Prosthodontics of the Academy of Fixed Prosthodontics. A review of selected dental literature on evidence-based treatment planning for dental implants: report of the Committee on Research in Fixed Prosthodontics of the Academy of Fixed Prosthodontics. J Prosthet Dent. **2004** Nov; 92(5): 447 – 462.

World Health Organization. Statistical Dataset. **2000**. http://www.who.int/respiratory/copd/burden/en/index.html. Last accessed Jan 1, 2015.

World Health Organization. Global status report on noncommunicable diseases 2010. **2011**. http://www.who.int/nmh/publications/ncd_report_full_en.pdf.

Wurtman JJ, Lieberman H, Tsay R, Nader T, Chew B. Caloric and nutrient intake of elderly and young subjects measured under identical conditions. J Gerontol. **1988** Nov; 43(6): B174 – B180.

Xiao W, Li Z, Shen S, Chen S, Wang Y, Wang J. Theoretical role of adjunctive implant positional support in stress distribution of distal-extension mandibular removable partial dentures. Int J Prosthodont. **2014** Nov – Dec; 27(6): 579 – 581.

Yacoub N, Ismail YH, Mao JJ. Transmission of bone strain in the craniofacial bones of edentulous human skulls upon dental implant loading. J Prosthet Dent. **2002** Aug; 88(2): 192 – 199.

Yoneyama T, Yoshida M, Matsui T, Sasaki H. Oral care and pneumonia. Oral Care Working Group. Lancet. **1999** Aug; 354(9177): 515.

Yoon V, Maalouf NM, Sakhaee K. The effects of smoking on bone metabolism. Osteoporos Int. **2012** Aug; 23(8): 2081 – 2092.

Zarb GA, Schmitt A. Implant therapy alternatives for geriatric edentulous patients. Gerodontology. **1993** Jul 1; 10(1): 28 – 32.

Zembic A, Kim S, Zwahlen M, Kelly JR. Systematic review of the survival rate and incidence of biologic, technical, and esthetic complications of single implant abutments supporting fixed prostheses. Int J Oral Maxillofac Implants. **2014**; 29(Suppl): 99 – 116. (**a**)

Zembic A, Wismeijer D. Patient-reported outcomes of maxillary implant-supported overdentures compared with conventional dentures. Clin Oral Implants Res. **2014** Apr; 25(4): 441 – 450.

Zermansky AG, Alldred DP, Petty DR, Raynor DK, Freemantle N, Eastaugh J, Bowie P. Clinical medication review by a pharmacist of elderly people living in care homes—randomised controlled trial. Age Ageing. **2006** Nov; 35(6): 586 – 591.

Zimmer CM, Zimmer WM, Williams J, Liesener J. Public awareness and acceptance of dental implants. Int J Oral Maxillofac Implants. **1992** Summer; 7(2): 228 – 232.

Zitzmann NU, Sendi P, Marinello CP. An economic evaluation of implant treatment in edentulous patients: preliminary results. Int J Prosthodont. **2005** Jan – Feb; 18(1): 20 – 27.

Zitzmann NU, Hagmann E, Weiger R. What is the prevalence of various types of prosthetic dental restorations in Europe? Clin Oral Implants Res. **2007** Jun; 18(Suppl 3): 20 – 33.

Zitzmann NU, Staehelin K, Walls AW, Menghini G, Weiger R, Zemp Stutz E. Changes in oral health over a 10-yr period in Switzerland. Eur J Oral Sci. **2008** Feb; 116(1): 52 – 59. (**a**)

Zitzmann NU, Berglundh T (2008). Definition and prevalence of peri-implant diseases. J Clin Periodontol. **2008** Sep; 35(8 Suppl): 286 – 291. (**b**)

Zou H, Zhao X, Sun N, Zhang S, Sato T, Yu H, Chen Q, Weber HP, Dard M, Yuan Q, Lanske B. Effect of chronic kidney disease on the healing of titanium implants. Bone. **2013** Oct; 56(2): 410 – 415.